I0099929

American AGONY

The Opioid War Against Patients in Pain

Helen Borel, RN, PhD

American AGONY

The Opioid War Against Patients in Pain

Helen Borel, RN, PhD

Fresh Ink Group
Guntersville

American AGONY:
The Opioid War Against Patients in Pain

Fresh Ink Group
An Imprint of:
The Fresh Ink Group, LLC
1021 Blount Avenue, #931
Guntersville, AL 35976
Email: info@FreshInkGroup.com
FreshInkGroup.com

Edition 1.0 2019

Book design by Amit Dey / FIG
Cover design by Stephen Geez / FIG
Associate publisher Lauren A. Smith / FIG

Cataloging-in-Publication Recommendations:
MED023000 MEDICAL / Drug Guide
PSY038000 PSYCHOLOGY / Psychopathology / Addiction
PSY000000 PSYCHOLOGY / General

ISBN-13: 978-1-947867-68-0 Papercover
ISBN-13: 978-1-947867-69-7 Hardcover
ISBN-13: 978-1-947867-70-3 Ebooks

FROM AGONY TO OPIOID FREEDOM FROM PAIN

Opiohysterics: The Bad, the Ugly, the Deadly

- **VA opiophobes** cause Veteran suicides
- **DEA raids**, asset seizures curtail MD paincare
- **DOJ targets**, imprisons innocent MDs
- **State Medical Boards abandon** paincare MDs
- **Exposé** Critique of *CDC Guideline*
- **All over America, Pain Patients speak out**
- **PROPagenda** and Suboxone Hoax decried
- **State Attorneys-General and DOJ GREED**
  vs. Pharm manufacturers of medically-safe Opioids

Memorial and Dirge for Pain Patient Suicides

Restoring Prescription Opioid Rights

DEMAND Congress nullify VA, DOJ, and DEA anti-Rx-Opioid objectives

SUE doctors, clinics, hospitals that cancel paincare, deny Rx Opioids

BRING lawsuits,Class Actions: Negligence Medical malpractice,Wrongful Death

SUE Federal and State government agencies

VOTE all opiophobes out of office

Plus:

Your PETITION, Advocacy Contacts

Resources and 237 References

Pain Patients' Battle Cry

S.O.S. SAVE OPIOID SCRIPTS

TABLE OF CONTENTS

PRECIS

Restoring Opioids for Pain is a National Emergency

The facts, detailed in ***American AGONY: The Opioid War Against Patients in Pain***, challenge and disprove the egregious lies – publicized as truths throughout our country by federal, state and other officials – that drug addicts are dying because physicians are prescribing opioid medications for patients in pain. Clearly, patients suffering various diseases, genetic conditions, injuries or surgeries – leaving them in chronic, intractable pain that requires prescription opioids – have zero to do with drug addicts who choose illicit substances to get "high". (Patients on opioids for analgesia, don't experience a "high," simply pain relief.)

Neither do physicians or other prescribing clinicians, who treat pain patients with opioid analgesics at dosages their medical conditions warrant, have anything to do with drug addicts choosing to use illicit street drugs.

Nor do pharmaceutical manufacturers – who pioneer research and development of the pharmacologic treatment, cure and pain relief of a myriad of human physical and psychiatric ailments – have a scintilla of responsibility for the drug addict who (even these days, with life-saving naloxone readily available) dies using adulterated fentanyl, fentanylized heroin, or the latter in combination with ethanol and/or anxiolytics. All the latter tainted narcotics plus alcohol and benzodiazepines ought to be interdicted by the lax Drug Enforcement Administration (DEA) as they arrive in America from China, Mexico and the Internet. But the DEA is too busy haunting and raiding doctors' offices, seizing assets, dictating opioid dosages, curtailing various classes of opioids and other prescription medications so that there are shortages – turning quality medical practice into chaos. In collusion with these injustices, is the DEA's parent agency, the Department of Justice (DOJ).

Also, starting many years ago with the Veterans Administration (VA) crackdown against VA physicians prescribing opioids for pain, it didn't take long for DOJ prosecutors to zero in on physicians all over America who dare to treat various kinds and levels of pain appropriately with opioid medications. The proof is that over a thousand physicians, other clinicians and pharmacists are imprisoned, some for 25 years, others for a lifetime, while others died in this witch-hunt process, in prison or awaiting trial. (See Chapter 16, "Plight of the Paincare Physicians".)

Thus, with the DOJ's implicit carte blanche, the DEA has managed to divert (speaking of "diversion") the nation's attention from its real drug deterrence responsibility to the key medications for pain– opioids. And so, both the DEA and DOJ have created an opiophobia that has so infected our country, due to their operatives unconscionable assertions of baseless connections between legal opioid prescriptions for pain and unsafe street-bought illicits. Due, also, to their DOJ lawyers and DEA agents irresponsible television announcements and press releases that whipped up an opiohysteria the likes of which rivals the fever pitch of the 13th Century Torquemada era.

These federal agents would have Americans believe that opioid medication tablets walk themselves out of medicine cabinets around the nation and, somehow, find their ways into the bodies of dead drug addicts. By now, the majority of Americans believe this hogwash because this DOJ, DEA and VA propaganda is ongoing. And government functionaries at these three agencies continue these falsehoods – because of a silent Congress that lacks oversight, it appears – continuing to conflate tainted chemicals killing addicts with safe, consistently manufactured, scientifically-accurate, pure and reliable medicinal opioids marketed by pharmaceutical manufacturers.

Adding to this nationwide pandemonium, another two agencies decided to chime in, hurt pain patients even more, and further interfere with the Hippocratic practice of medicine. Enter the Department of Health and Human Services (HHS) giving the go-ahead to its Centers for Disease Control and Prevention (CDC) to develop a primer for physicians about how to manage their patients' various pain-sufferings. As though physicians are kindergartners requiring instruction from bureaucrats mainly concerned about arriving at those pensions of theirs. Whereupon, with nary a pain specialist consulted, the government published its 2016 *CDC Guideline for Prescribing Opioids for Chronic Pain.* Despite mea culpas subsequently reminding State medical boards and doctors everywhere that these were only "recommendations," it morphed swiftly into mandate, depriving millions of their usual and effective opioids, crippling the qualities of their lives, losing them their jobs, causing many daily, including ailing veterans, to commit suicide. Thereby, the Guideline has become an instrument of suffering and death. (See my Critique of the Guideline in Chapter 7.)

As you read the facts in this book, you will come to see how, perhaps usually enlightened health professionals working in government, can become blinded to the everyday clinical challenges medical professionals encounter, and to the severities of human suffering they no longer have access to, nor are treating, in their bureaucratic roles. That the pressures of government protocols and exigencies of budgets and politics outweigh, and are far removed from, daily medical practice.

In other words, they've forgotten what it is a doctor really does clinically and what a doctor stands for ethically. And they are far removed from patients' illnesses and symptoms. Ensconced in their bubble of government rules and regulations, what can be more appropriate than developing an insidious document chock full of more rules and regulations?

But, this time, they stretched credulity implementing "recommendations" they were fully aware would have dire consequences: (1) Because they know that overdose deaths from illicits have zero to do with Intractable Pain Patients (IPPs) long stabilized on their prescription opioids. (2) And they absolutely know that less than 1% of drug abuse is via prescription narcotics. (3) Thus, they know too, that they've conflated drug addicts on street illicits with well-functioning IPPs on legally prescribed opioids for pain. Nonetheless, justifying to themselves the scare tactics and hysteria now invoked by even the word "opioids".

Predicated on bad science and skewed "statistics," the 2016 *CDC Guideline* diverted national focus from the real problems, the failures of federal policing, interdiction and prosecution to curb easy access to harmful chemicals by addicts.

Also, the CDC's "experts" should rethink their reliance on Suboxone® (buprenorphine/naloxone), now known as "The Legal Morphine," supposedly treating opioid withdrawal. Suboxone® detox protocols are being questioned as to their efficacy. And what can't be ignored is the nationwide Suboxone® windfall for its many prescribers, and addiction facilities. All the while, paradoxically touted by a small but vocal group of anti-opioid zealots.

Evidence-based treatment requires that Suboxone® prescribers honestly ask themselves these questions:

1. Does it really help addicts to detox and become drug-free?
2. Does it really work for alcoholics? (It's being given to them, too.)
3. Do we need to add IPPs to the list of Suboxone® detox failures?

Note: Millions of pain patients suddenly cold-turkeyed off their opioids have been labeled "drug seekers." forced to detox facilities, forced to take Suboxone. (See Chapter 20, "The Suboxone Hoax".)

As a Registered Nurse, Medical and Pharmaceutical Writer and Psychotherapist, I am sorely wounded by the unconscionable actions of our government agencies, many headed by nonmedical bureaucrats with zero knowledge of anatomy, physiology, neurology, nociceptors, pain-causing diseases, injuries, and zilch about pharmacology. Nor do they grasp the intricacies of pain management for a wide variety of complex conditions. For example, Alex Azar, who heads HHS, is a lawyer and former Eli Lilly executive. Chances are he's familiar with internal corporate concerns in the pharmaceutical industry. But he's not knowledgeable about what concerns medical clinicians and pain specialists in particular.

In my years in nursing, I cared for hundreds of patients with various acute and chronic illnesses subjecting them to all kinds and degrees of pain. I've administered oral as well as injectable narcotics. I've witnessed the benefits of taking care of pain. Known definitely (1) When pain is controlled, acute illnesses and surgical wounds heal faster. (2) When chronic pain is quelled, patients' qualities of life improve dramatically. They can work and partake in life with family and friends to degrees impossible without their prescribed opioids.

Counterpoint to the blaming of prescription opioids for drug addicts' deaths is one journalist's revelation, putting this street drug crisis in tragic focus. David Browne's Rolling Stone article (July, 2018) demonstrates the deadliness of illegal, impure chemical substances addicts permit themselves to risk taking into their bodies. He pointed out, in addition to heroin, American streets are now flooded with adulterated forms of fentanyl, an opioid 30 to 50 times more potent than heroin. It's dangerous. On the other hand, medicinal fentanyl prescribed by a physician, is ordered for short time periods such as a week, and is only available in slow-absorption formulations – a dermal patch or a lollipop.

Importantly, therefore, street fentanyl pills are perilous. Browne lists various musicians who died taking illicit street drugs including adulterated fentanyl. He points out, because of its strength and rapid action within a minute or so of swallowing, it is illegal to produce fentanyl in pill form. Which hasn't stopped criminal chemists from formulating the pill form, nor criminal dealers, who feel no guilt, from selling death via fentanyl pills to their fellow humans. Further, Browne reports, street fentanyl is cheap, only $10, is 50 to 100 times stronger than legally-made prescription fentanyl, and is deadly.

Throughout this exposê, expert pain management physicians speak out, in quotes. However, many other doctors, out of fear of DEA police raids on medical practices, have requested anonymity which I've honored when reporting something they've said. Other physician empaths speak out, too. Suffering IPPs speak out. And, the American Medical Association has spoken, rebutting and rebuking the 2016 *CDC Guideline* for its harm to patients. Many physicians do remember PRIMUM NON NOCERE. Dr. Hippocrates would be proud.

This book gets into the most minute details of the issues causing incalculable suffering to 50,000,000 American patients in pain and severely restricting the medical professionals who prescribe opioids for them. Any paincare doctor not yet jailed by the DOJ after being targeted by its DEA is living in fear of such gestapo tactics. Thus, currently hogtied by federal and state government strangulatory intrusions into autonomous opioid prescribing, both pain patients and their doctors are suffering. This needs to stop!

To grasp what pain patients are now enduring without their opioids due to nonconsentual tapering and sudden cold-turkeying, *American AGONY* delves, in depth, into all the egregious government actions shackling physicians' rights to prescribe opioids. First, you'll read about pain itself, some serious painful conditions, and the narcotics which treat pain. Throughout the book, you'll read quotes from various pain patients and the anguish caused when their opioid medications are wrongly withdrawn.

You'll also read about the hundreds of clinicians from various parts of the United States who are in prison due to nefarious and bogus DOJ prosecutorial license. Some of these doctors died – long before any adjudications. Some suicided. To be remembered is that, though many cases had not yet been brought to court, our government has conferred *carte blanche* on DOJ prosecutors to empower their DEA police to seize all professional and personal assets of their targeted doctors. Another catch-22 by these DOJ weasels: How do you defend yourself against government lies when you haven't a penny to your name to defend yourself with? You'll read more about the witch hunts and unjust prosecutions of physicians and other healthcare professionals by DOJ prosecutors and their treacherous "conspiracy" charge (carrying 25 years in prison) if a doctor defendant doesn't agree to plead to lesser, though also bogus, charges.

There is also a Memorial Section (see Chapter 18, "In Memoriam: Suicides Due to Untreated Pain".) Related to which is Chapter 17, "Veterans in Pain, Suiciding at Alarming Rates". No, those suicides of veterans you read about in newspapers are not due to posttraumatic stress syndrome. They're due to unbearable, untreated pain – a vicious policy of deliberate torture by the VA, which is supposed to ease the lives of our hurting soldiers.

Finally, you'll arrive at Section VII about solutions, which also honors "pain warriors" both patients and physicians, suggested actions to turn the tide, to vote out all legislators who are allowing these injustices to continue, legal recourse, class actions, what Congress must do, and the need to dissolve the DEA in its current gestapo form.

And, in that same section, there's a petition you have permission to use or alter to your heart's content to suit the goals you have when you approach the local, state and federal legislators you are appealing to. Which is followed by a Resources section and, finally, a lengthy bibliography. I dedicate this book to you, the pain-concerned reader.

Section I

PAIN:
DESCRIBED, PRESCRIBED, UNTREATED

Chapter One

PAIN DESCRIBED – WHAT IS PAIN?

Despite what we all endure when parts of our bodies hurt, we recognize that pain is positive because 1) it warns us to stop doing what we're doing, right now, that's causing the noxious sensation or 2) it notifies us that something is inexplicably wrong and we need to go get it diagnosed and treated.

A Pain-free Woman Thrives. Her Genes May Hold the Analgesic Key.

Anecdotally, a condition which many longtime pain sufferers might envy was reported by Heather Murphy on March 29, 2019 in the *New York Times* article, "A Woman, 71, Doesn't Feel Pain. Now, Scientists Know Why: A Mutation". Not only is she pain-free, she also heals more quickly than normal people. Why discovery of and studying this woman's genetic painlessness is important is that her genetic glitch could lead scientists to developing more precise, more on-target treatments for the vast majority of us who can't escape pain. And, an excellent side effect from FAAH-OUT (this gene's scientific name) is that it can promote swifter healing. Furthermore, another added benefit of this genetic anomaly is that any injuries she didn't feel, over the decades of her life, tended to leave no scars. Pain-Free, Faster Healing. Zero Scars. Now that's an advertising campaign slogan any product manager at any commercial healthcare company could gleefully embrace. Wholeheartedly. Meantime, the rest of us can't escape pain.

Thus, everyone – except that rare genetically charmed woman, and the few others who may be out there, never experiencing varied physical pain – has suffered acute, sudden pain, many have endured postsurgical pain, all have experienced dental pain. Varied kinds and intensities of pain are unmistakable. They hurt. They pinch. They burn. They shock. They sometimes instigate nausea, vomiting, vertigo. And inability to do daily chores, participate in social activities, keep their jobs.

However, you see how ordinary pain – that warns us to take care of something because something's physically wrong with us right now – differs from everlasting pain that, sometimes, can be easily explained because it's pathognomonic for the condition causing it. But, excruciatingly, a large number of patients, who endure pain that never goes away, are diagnosed with pain-producing sufferings that can't always be precisely implicated. Because there are some things about the Central Nervous System (CNS = Brain and Spinal Cord) and the peripheral nerves that do their own thing – sending and receiving sensations, sometimes noxious – without any easy explanation.

Tissue and Organ Healing Don't Always Assure Pain Relief

And, as one orthopedic surgeon discovered, to his dismay, after years and years of performing delicate spinal surgeries and fusions for vertebrae-related pathologies, a majority of his patients did not become pain-free, and were never so, long past the post-surgical healing. Such sad outcomes despite complete repair of the pain-producing problem. Finally, this orthopedist realized that it had to be the brain continuing to inform the distant body part to continue to perceive pain, due to some physically-entrenched neurologic mechanism, that apparently couldn't shut itself off, even after the physical problem was cured. Thereafter, he quit doing back surgeries and began to focus on other possibilities for helping patients manage pain.

With those two surprising examples about the evanescence of the pain experience – and the potential origins and unrelentingness of chronic pain, let's now focus on chronic pain itself and the sources of it.

The Chronic Pain Perspective

Pain lasting three months or longer is deemed chronic. Pain prevalence in America, as far back as 1999 to 2001, was tabulated as ranging from 10 million to 60 million sufferers. These included millions of patients without cancer but, nevertheless, with severe, intractable pain conditions.

Two Kinds of Pain: Nociceptive and Neuropathic

Any pain specialist will tell you that the origins of pain vary widely, thus pain's sources are difficult to pinpoint. Damage to tissues that stimulate pain receptors produce what is known as nociceptive pain. And damage to the Brain and Spinal Cord, or to the peripheral nerves, cause neuropathic pain. I elaborate on these concepts further along in the segment **Pain Sufferings Beyond Ordinary**. Additionally, to complicate the diagnosis and adequate treatment of either of these pain conditions, peripheral and CNS actions affect each other, either modulating or magnifying pain.

Cytokines, Immune System Substances, have Dramatic Effects on Cells, Organs and Pain Production

Among its many other chemicals, the immune system produces cytokines, which can be either inflammatory or anti-inflammatory. Scientists have shown that certain cytokines can instigate pain and, also, can maintain the persistence of pathologic pain due to their ability to activate nociceptive sensory neurons. Central sensitization due to nerve injury can result from some inflammatory cytokines. Many pathologic pain conditions can be attributed to inflammatory Brain, Spinal Cord and Peripheral responses to some of these cytokines in everyone's immune system which include monocytes, lymphocytes, chemokines, interferon, interleukin, lymphokines and tumor necrosis factor. And there are more immune system chemicals like those which can excite, maybe incite, the body's mechanisms for experiencing pain.

While arthritis is an example of immune system cytokines (like interferon, interleukin and growth factors, secreted by the immune system and affecting other cells in the body) inflaming nociceptors, peripheral (outer, more surface aspects of the body distant from the Central Nervous System) injuries are also subject to pain production by excitation of cytokines.

Pain is Considered a Disease Condition Itself

Despite the naysayers and federal troublemakers, now beleaguering pain patients and their physicians – patients forced back into pain (left without their prescription narcotic analgesics), physicians going to prison – in the assessment and treatment of pain, the pain management specialist physician, as do nonspecialists, recognizes that pain itself should be considered a disease condition. And that it should be sought for as "the fifth vital sign" among the traditional other four: Pulse, Temperature, Respirations, Blood Pressure.

Pain care experts agree that years-long, even lifelong, opioid therapy substantially helps a majority of Intractable Pain Patients live better lives and maintain employment. Patients so medicated also require reduced healthcare visits and incur lower related costs. The experts' focus, too, is on carefully selecting out those (less than 1% of pain patients) who are not candidates for narcotics because they might be addiction-vulnerable. These would be pain patients with a prior history of substance abuse, including alcoholism.

Pain Sufferings Beyond Ordinary

Normally, babies, children, adults feel pain when they are hurt by an injury or an illness. Such as a scraped knee, a fall, a bronchitic chest cold, an accidental burn at the kitchen stove. Also, of course, pain is felt when one has appendicitis, has a neck injury from an automobile accident, has swimmer's cramp, carpal tunnel syndrome, a tension headache, or a fracture. Each of these can be treated with pain-relief (analgesic) medications among which a physician has several choices. Some of these are temporary conditions with pain that lasts for a short period. Some are intermediary in suffering time, so to speak, in expectation of pain, such as post-surgical pain from the removal of an organ, from plastic surgery, from a colostomy, from reduction of a fracture, from dental surgery. And many of these are relieved by an opiate (narcotic derived from opium) or opioid (synthetic or semi-synthetic opiate, laboratory-manufactured) and prescribed for the limited time the particular pain lingers.

But, there are many other diseases, post-surgical residual states and even hereditary conditions like migraine headaches and diabetes mellitus (which can lead to both blindness and leg amputations) that are inherently chronic, from which patients never again are free of pain. Another dire example is Sickle Cell Disease, a type of severe anemia with its risks of Sickle Cell Crises that cause excruciating pain, often from bleeding into a joint like the knee. In addition to those latter three chronic diseases, there are many other conditions that are so unrelentingly painful that, but for regular prescription narcotic medications, their sufferers would be permanently wheelchair-bound, often bedridden, always housebound. It is about this latter group of patients, who've come to be known as Intractable Pain Patients (IPPs), upon whom this book is strongly focused, and for whom this book is meant to be a tool to change the government-caused painful status quo. As well, this book also discusses many other kinds and durations of pain requiring prescription opioids which government fiat has intimidated professionals from prescribing.

Everyone knows the reason life has evolved to experience pain is to warn us to take care of what is wrong with that body part that is hurting, or to get out of danger if, for example, we've just touched hot boiling water, to pull our hand away. Evolution probably didn't mean to leave the human being in permanent extremis. Therefore, pain has no function when the cause of it is eliminated. Ergo, it's supposed to stop when the disease or injury or condition is corrected. Unfortunately, that's not the way the Central Nervous System works. (And, also, some diseases are progressive, worsening as time passes.) Its pain receptors or irritators too often send interminable pain signals to patients, subjecting them to constant pain.

Intractable pain is persistent. Algesia, from the Greek, is the medical word for pain. And another name for painkillers is analgesics. Aspirin is an analgesic, as is morphine. They each counteract pain in different ways. As everyone knows, aspirin is meant for milder forms of pain like ordinary headaches, sprains, strains – in other words, where some anti-inflammatory action is also required.

Unrelenting Pain is Often Either Neuropathic or is Nociceptor-Related

Your nociceptors are nerve endings responsible for pain perception. Neuropathic pain results from damaged CNS nerves or damaged peripheral nerves. Perception of pain is the responsibility of these sensate systems which can produce never-ending pain. Any number of a variety of conditions can afflict a patient with permanent, unrelenting pain that will render the patient hopeless and even suicidal if not treated empathically with the best narcotic at the optimal dosage and frequency, or a narcotic in combination with another ancillary drug carefully dosed, to quell at least a major portion of the suffering these patients will otherwise endure.

More in-depth: When there's tissue damage that generates one's pain, it's called Nociceptive Pain. When its your brain and spinal cord messaging you with pain, this is called Neuropathic Pain. Carpal Tunnel Syndrome and Plantar Fasciitis are nociciptive. Sciatica and Lumbar Radiculopathy are neuropathic.

In contrast with the short-duration conditions and injuries, whose pain diminishes and subsides in a relatively short period of time, in the suffering of unrelenting, intractable pain, pain receptors keep firing, even after the patient's condition appears to have healed physically. This can continue for years and decades, a lifetime of suffering. Whatever triggered this permanent life-sentence of pain, a bone condition, an injury, cancer, certain hereditary bodily conditions, these patients are *in extremis* unless adequately treated, most often with prescription narcotics.

Aging is a Fragile Time, Pain Ever-Looming

And one's susceptibility to persistent pain is heightened during the aging process because that's the time when osteoporosis with fracture is a risk, when muscle loss is common (unless one is a fit athlete), when synovial fluid (which lubricates the joints) begins to disappear limiting ambulation and balance (setting elders on the road to that "I've fallen and I can't get up" emergency phone call), adding protracted pain to a system winding down with progressively limited reserves.

Many Intractable Pain Conditions Occur Frequently in Our Population

Low Back Pain is a major culprit. Pain from a **cancer** condition is another. Patients with **Parkinson's Disease** and **Multiple Sclerosis** experience progressive worsening of their diseases with persistent pain from damage to brain and spinal cord nerves. And, in the case of MS, due to demyelination (loss of unpredictable areas of the fatty substance insulating the spinal cord).

Many other conditions produce unbearable pain that never goes away without prescription narcotic help. There is Chronic Primary Pain which encompasses such sufferings as the diffuse musculoskeletal Chronic Widespread Pain (where 3 or more body quadrants, as in Fibromyalgia and Complex Regional Pain Syndrome (CRPS) are affected. Some people suffer Chronic Headaches, Chronic Orofacial Pain as in TMJ (temporomandibular joint pain), and there's Trigeminal Autonomic Cephalagia, Chronic Tension Headache, Chronic Primary Visceral Pain, Chronic Burning Mouth Pain, Chronic Primary Chest Pain, Irritable Bowel Syndrome, and many more chronic specific conditions too numerous to mention, except for a few more examples, I'll discuss as this chapter proceeds.

Unempathic, Nonexperts Attribute Physical Pain to Emotional Instability

Despite all the scientific evidence of the microscopic and visibly evident origins of pain, some sources and too many government bureaucrats far removed from clinical medicine, are determined to attribute physical pain to psychological causations. A ready way to exit from the necessity of providing a prescription opioid (which I will discuss in greater depth later on in this chapter). However, rarely do lifelong pain patients benefit – except tangentially – from physical modalities, from meditation, Oriental practices, psychotherapy, intra-spinal injections, etc. *ad nauseam*. All of these latter, and other analogous "therapies" do not show the results that straightforward relief with a narcotic analgesic demonstrates. And even if they did control pain, which they haven't been proven to do, insurers will not reimburse for these "treatments". And now, of course, insurers are interlopers against normal opioid analgesics, emboldened by the federal government's prescription opioid wars. For they are also refusing to cover prescription narcotics, the proven pain relievers.

The Toll of Intractable Lifetime Pain

According to experts in pain assessment and pain management, intractable pain unrelentingly won't cease unless an effective treatment intervenes. Although such pain can be due to a disease or an injury, there are many pain sufferers for whom an etiology (cause) is never discovered. If pain continues beyond six months, it falls into this category and deserves appropriate treatment, bearing in mind that the current suffering the patient is experiencing may no longer relate to the trauma or illness that initiated it. Nevertheless, such a patient is still suffering because the brain, spinal cord and/or peripheral nerves still appear to be sending and receiving pain signals.

Some chronic and severe pain may be carcinoma-related or due to chemotherapy or radiotherapy. Also implicated are chronic pain conditions like arthritis, lumbar and sacral pain, Sickle Cell Anemia pain, various headache syndromes, neuralgias, TMJ disorder, fibromyalgia and others.

Doctors recognize two pain happenings–"baseline pain" and "breakthrough pain". Physicians caring for these complex cases also see the multi-dimensional aspects of such pain sufferers' lives that are affected by their disabling, noxious sensations. These include restrictions in mobility leading to becoming wheelchair-bound or bedridden with loss of employment inescapable. Too, loss of social interactions with isolation and such a curtailed quality of life that such patients – in addition to not wanting to feel their pain any longer – also want to stop living due to a shriveled existence as well as pain-suffering. They are all at risk of suicide due to hopelessness about their unrelenting pain.

Opioids: The Therapeutic Cornerstone

Opioids for the treatment of such pain levels is considered fundamental to the treatment of both cancer and other lifelong pain conditions. The phrase "therapeutic cornerstone" has been applied to this mainstay for such patients. The aim is to reduce enough of the pain so that as much as possible of the pain patient's prior, more normal existence can be restored, so the patient can participate in normal daily activities, can keep a job, can feel hopeful.

The patient's self-report of the nature, location and quality of his/her pain is fundamental to the doctor's treatment plan. Pain intensity reports are vital information for selection of the particularly appropriate narcotic and its scheduled dosages and timings.

Underdosing is a danger because it assures that all the restrictions on such patients' lives – ambulation, socialization, work, family life – will loom large, cause depression, stress the patient's body to the point of shortening the life span due to new physical ailments, and also to suicide due to pain and despair.

According to all available expert sources, prescription opioids for severe intractable pain and breakthrough pain are the preferred medications for optimal efficacy. With careful patient assessment by an expert, empathic clinician, optimal analgesia can be achieved. Experts also caution that limiting opioid use in these patients, or under-dosing so that pain is never subdued – because of misreported statistics related to illicit drug users – will mean mistreatment of pain patients, terrible suffering, and escalating suicides.

MANY PAINFUL CONDITIONS LAST A LIFETIME

To grasp the dire essence of the very many dangerous, sometimes lethal diseases and conditions that produce severe and, often, unrelenting pain, it is unnecessary to enumerate all known pathologies that produce acute, short-term, intermediate, ongoing, or intractable pain. Thus, I'll simply list a small number of those awful afflictions, specifically those that cause lifelong miseries. And, I'll briefly describe a few of them to give you a sense of the varied sufferings that are sorely impacting the lives of millions of pain-filled Americans.

A Sampling of the Scope and Types of Chronic Pain-Producing Conditions Unremittingly Attacking Patients from All Physical Locations:

Brain and Brain Circulation	- Migraine, Cluster, and Post-trauma Headaches
Joints and Bones	- Arthritis, Fractures, Congenital deformities
Vertebrae (Spinal Bones)	- Vertebral and Discogenic pain
Diabetic (Pancreas)	- Blindness, Neuropathy, Foot Amputations
Nerves, Viral, Herpes zoster	- Acute stage, Shingles, a year or more of pain
Nerves, Herpes zoster	- Post-herpetic Neuralgia lasting a lifetime
Kidneys	- Nephrolithiasis (kidney stones)
Skin, Mucous Membranes	- Pemphigus, Autoimmune disease - mortality 5-15%
Tick Bite - Lyme Disease	- Borrelia burgdorferi, a spirochete bacterium
Blood	- Sickle Cell Disease (genetic)
Connective Tissue Disease	- Ehlers Danlos Syndrome (genetic)
Bladder	- Interstitial Cystitis
Nonspecific	- Fibromyalgia
Immune System	- Lupus erythematosus
Neurofacial & Orofacial	- Trigeminal Neuralgia, Temporomandibular Joint pain

Acute Conditions Warranting Narcotic Treatment

Most likely, acute illnesses, injuries and other sudden conditions would be treated in the Emergency Department of one's nearby hospital. A small sampling, by no means a comprehensive list of such painful afflictions, includes Snake Bites, Shoulder Dislocations, Stab Wounds, Second Degree Burns, Gunshot Wounds, Angina (cardiac pain), Sprained Ankles, and Various types of Headaches. Not all of these require a narcotic analgesic. For example, once the patient's dislocated shoulder is reduced by the physician - the upper humerus plus scapula (shoulder blade) restored to normal, by the doctor swiftly tugging the arm to pop the humerus ball back into its scapular socket, the pain disappears. No narcotic needed. Probably not even an aspirin. However, sutured stab wounds, deep burns, certain headaches, and other conditions ER doctors encounter, will benefit from a stronger-than-aspirin analgesic; and these warrant an opioid.

Two Very Painful Disease Examples of What All Intractable Pain Patients Endure

Interstitial Cystitis (IC) and Chronic Pelvic Pain

Researchers report that IC (aka Painful Bladder Syndrome [PBS]) manifests somewhat differently in different patients with different levels of symptoms. Which means there's a wide latitude of how various patients with the same diagnosis respond to treatments, perhaps why some may need higher doses of painkillers than others with the same diagnosis.

To further focus on the varied presentations of patients' IC signs and symptoms, these subtypes differentiate them:

1. There is Ulcerative IC which occurs in 5% to 10% of patients who often suffer, too, from Hunner's ulcers which cause urinary bladder wall bleeding.
2. Non-ulcerative IC occurs in 90% of patients which produce cystic (urinary bladder) glomerulations, which are tiny bladder hemorrhages.

3. End-Stage IC, an even more severe and terminal condition, occurs in 5% of these patients, who suffer hard bladders with low capacity leading to frequent voiding and excruciating pain.

Sickle Cell Disease, a blood condition, in fact the most prevalent heritable hematologic condition, afflicts millions around the world and about 100,000 Americans. It was an evolutionary solution to Malaria, protecting against that infection; however, distorting red blood cells has other dire consequences.

To protect against that mosquito-borne (an Anopheles mosquito bite transmits the plasmodium parasitic illness), a diabolical Darwinian transformation evolved in Malaria-infested geographic regions like the Mediterranean. Thus, wonderful disc-shaped hemoglobin cells were malformed into sickle-shaped blood elements, crippling their ability to effectively carry oxygen, often so severely that they can't do this vital job at all, causing severe health problems and unfathomable pain.

During Sickle Cell Crises, a periodic excruciating pain emergency as well as a hematologic treatment imperative, the sickled red blood cells' curved arcs cause them to periodically stack up and occlude blood vessels. This pathologic occurrence prevents normal blood flow, obstructing tissue oxygenation (red hemoglobin cells in your arteries normally carry oxygen, delivering it to all parts of your body), preventing excretion of impurities, a function of the venous (vein) system that rids the blood of these. Sickle Cell patients are subject to such attacks suddenly. And must endure their periodic occurrences.

When a **Sickle Cell Crisis** occurs, so severely painful and disabling as it is in these acute phases, the disease itself progressively worsens as it continually impacts these sufferers' lives. (Not unlike the toll other lifelong conditions inflict on their victims.) At various times and unexpectedly, the crisis occurs. And thus ensues an emergency in hematologic medical practice and in pain management medical care. It is a crisis of unimaginable pain when these sickle-shaped blood cells, prevent smooth blood flow, robbing tissues and organs of oxygen, inducing excruciating pain that requires STAT (immediate!) pain relief, often in the form of intravenous morphine.

Ominous Denials of Narcotics to Critically Afflicted Sickle Cell Crisis Patients due to Federal Interference

Shamefully, some unschooled or heartless health professionals have, sometimes, malpracticed by denying these patients STAT opioid analgesic medication, and accusing them of "drug-seeking" behavior, a new cruel frame of mind stemming from, and promoted by, the ill-informed "experts" who devised the infamous 2016 *CDC Guideline (*discussed next, in Section II).

Aggressive Opiate or Opioid Treatment for Sickle Cell Crisis is Fundamental

As but one example of the complexities pain specialists (and, in this case, also hematologists) must consider when managing periodic and intractable pain, note what physicians must adhere to when treating the excruciating acute pain of a Sickle Cell Crisis: Pain relief is the fundamental objective. Opioid treatment must be aggressive. Due to their speed of action, the opiate morphine and the opioid Dilaudid® (hydromorphone) are preferred in these instances. Breakthrough pain requires "rescue" dosing of a fourth to a half of the main dose. Additionally, those Sickle Cell patients who've been on longstanding narcotics for their chronic pain should be continued on these as well.

Importantly, due to the 7-to-10 range of Sickle Cell Crisis pain, only pure opioid medications, not combination drugs, should be given. Due to drug tolerance and longstanding illness, these patients often require higher opioid doses. And, because of the hypoxemic (low blood oxygen levels), despite introduction of an intravenous narcotic, some Sickle Cell patients may need to swallow their narcotic or get it subcutaneously (a shot in and under the skin).

After the Acute Pain Crisis

As pain experts know, when an acute pain event has been managed successfully, it's time to reassess the patient's narcotic needs. Gradual tapering off the acute narcotic dosage, timed to minimize negative side reactions and withdrawal symptoms, should begin. Side effects of chronic opioid treatment such as constipation and somnolence are to be noted and addressed by both physician and patient. Rarely, respiratory depression, breaths lower than 12 to 14 per minute, may occur. This is a danger because breathing can, then, all-of-a-sudden, stop. This is what Narcan® (naloxone) rescue injections and intranasal naloxone are for. All patients on narcotics long term should have rescue naloxone (it comes in generic forms, too) on hand, as should their family members and friends when spending time with the patient on a long-term narcotic.

Emboldened Feds are Poised to Destroy Normal Narcotic Pain Care

The above vignette, about the terrible sufferings of Sickle Cell patients, mirrors sharply the various sufferings many other kinds of pain patients endure and some of the tortuous (and torturous) hoops most pain patients go through merely due to their specific illnesses or conditions. Distressingly, some Cold Turkeys in Washington, DC and in state governments throughout our country, have unilaterally decided to invade the professional expert medical care of Intractable Pain Patients, intimidating their narcotic-prescribing physicians, creating shortages of life-sustaining pain-relieving narcotics, barging into doctors' offices, arresting clinicians, stealing patients' confidential medical records, imprisoning physicians and forcing the *cold-turkeying* of so many pain-filled Americans that suicides of untreated chronic pain patients are running into the thousands. This upon, and still rampant today, the debut and heavy pall cast over our country by the noxious 2016 *CDC Guideline*. (See Section II for an overview of this ominous document.

Chapter Two

Prescription Opioids: The Best Treatment for Most Chronic Pain

How **Opioid Narcotics Behave in the Body** Opiates are opium-like substances derived from opium. Related chemicals that also attach to opiate receptors in the brain and elsewhere in the body, are called opioids because, being semi-synthetic or wholly synthetic, the "oid" = "akin," ergo opium-like. **Receptors** are aspects of the Central Nervous System (CNS = Brain and Spinal Cord) and of the peripheral nerves which are sensory segments beyond the CNS. They receive and transmit signals, including pain sensations.

Our natural opioid receptors, to which an opioid drug binds, have VGreek names such as delta, kappa and mu. It is the mu opioid receptor to which an opioid drug binds creating pain relief. Morphine, methadone and oxycodone are called full mu agonists. On the other hand, opioids that occupy, without activating, these receptors are named opioid antagonists which counteract the effects of the mu opioid agonists. Examples are Vivitrol® (naltrexone) and Narcan® (naloxone).

Alkaloids are examples of chemicals from opium poppies that attach to these receptors. They include such well-known narcotics as morphine and codeine. These prescription drugs have been used normally for more than half a century for acute and long-lasting pain. I administered many thousands of doses of these during my years practicing hospital nursing. None of these medical, neurological or surgical patients became addicts due to having been prescribed morphine or codeine or analogous narcotics. Completely synthetic opioids include Darvon® (propoxyphene), fentanyl and methadone.

Some of the Various Medicinal Opioids

Prescription opioids are manufactured in forms for use intravenously (into the vein), orally, and by skin patch. The latter is known as a "dermal patch". Some prescription narcotic formulations combine an opioid with another drug. For example, Vicodin® (hydrocodone + acetaminophen). Other formulations with other opiates or opioids contain aspirin.

Locations of Opioid Actions

As already stated, opioids bind to opioid receptors throughout the CNS and peripherally. And here's where something interesting happens: these same receptors bind to your own endorphins (your brain's own morphines) which normally modulate pain, balance emotions and ease stress. So, narcotics work by sending triggering messages from your brain and nerves to your hurting receptors telling them to stop hurting. Doctors reserve narcotics for moderate to severe pain, which is not expected to respond to milder analgesics.

Commonly Prescribed Semi-Synthetic and Synthetic Opioids Include:

BRANDS	THEIR GENERICS
Dilaudid®	hydromorphone
Exalgo®	hydromorphone
Demerol®	meperidine
Methadone®	methadone
Dolophine®	methadone
Kadian®	morphine
MS Contin®	morphine
Morphabond®	morphine
Oxycontin®	oxycodone

Oxaydo®	oxycodone
Percocet®	oxycodone with acetaminophen
Roxicet®	oxycodone with acetaminophen
(generic only)	oxycodone with naloxone
(generic only)	codeine
Actiq®	fentanyl
Duragesic®	fentanyl
Fentora®	fentanyl
Abstral®	fentanyl
Onsolis®	fentanyl
Hysingla®	hydrocodone
Zyhydro ER®	hydrocodone

Unlike all the other narcotic analgesics mentioned, which are often taken by mouth, fentanyl is applied in a skin patch for consistently slow absorption because oral ingestion would produce too swift an action which would be dangerous. Fentanyl can also be prescribed in lollipop form, also for slow systemic absorption.

Doctors prescribe dosage amounts and how frequently - such as “every 6 hours” or “twice a day” or “every 8 hours as needed”. They may also instruct you when you could take an additional dose for “break-through pain,” that which is uncontrolled by your regularly-scheduled dose.

Pain patients are medically monitored for efficacy of their narcotic’s effect on their specific pain condition. As well as to be sure there aren’t any worrisome side effects. (One could be constipation. Another, somnolence. At times, nausea and vomiting.) So, it’s important to regularly check in with your physician for optimum management of your pain to assure the best quality of life for you as you struggle to live with your incurable pain-producing condition.

It’s also important to never abruptly stop taking your narcotic once you’ve been on it for a time for your chronic condition. To stop, very gradual (and I mean "very, very") tapering-down of your dosage is managed and monitored by your physician, who needs to know all the other prescription and OTC (over-the-counter/nonprescription drugs) medications you are taking as well.

It's imperative to not combine opioids with certain antidepressants, soporifics (sleeping medicines), and specific antibiotics which your doctor will instruct you about.

Importantly, unlike the compulsion for illicit drugs that addicts exhibit, pain patients on long-term narcotic analgesics can develop a tolerance to their prescription narcotic which could require adjustment to a higher dose to maintain pain control. It's very important, too, that government and other nonmedical persons grasp the difference between "dependence" - where the body needs the opioid only to deaden the pain - and "addiction" - where the addict craves illicit drugs to experience a "high".

General Information about Some Prescription Opioids...and Illicits

Hydrocodone is the most frequently-prescribed opioid medication. It is classified as a Schedule II controlled substance. A most effective analgesic, hydrocodone is also useful as an antitussive (cough suppressant), which is why it can be found in certain prescription cough medicines. It's available in tablet form and oral liquid. (Watch out! Government functionaries may be poised to rid the nation of antitussives with a touch of this opioid.)

Morphine, a natural opiate alkaloid from the opium poppy, is used medicinally for both acute and chronic pain management, and also to provide sedation before surgical procedures. It is still one of the most widely used analgesics in hospitals, where it was once available only as an injectable drug. These days, morphine is made in regular and extended-release tablets, in oral solutions, and in suppositories. Morphine remains active for four-to-six hours in the blood. Many synthetic and semi-synthetic narcotics are derived from morphine.

Hydromorphone (Dilaudid®, Exalgo®), a semi-synthetic opioid, is another Schedule II narcotic. It is available as an injectable solution, an oral solution, and as both immediate and controlled-release tablets. It is indispensable in hospitals and clinics because it provides powerful analgesic control.

Codeine, made from the opium poppy, one source of this prescription pharmaceutical. Additionally, most medicinal codeine is synthetically manufactured, relying on morphine as a chemical foundation. Codeine is only available, in America, generically and is a component of other analgesics when combined with acetaminophen, etc. Compared to morphine, codeine is a milder pain reliever and it also has antitussive (cough-controlling) properties.

Methadone. well-known as part of medical detox protocols for addicts, is a synthetic opioid which is also useful as an analgesic.

Fentanyl treats intractable pain and other severe pain. It is 50 to 100 times more potent than morphine and is prescribed to patients who are tolerant to (unable to benefit from)other opioid narcotics. Because of its small molecular nature, it's absorbable on contact with the skin and can be deadly in very small doses. This is why fentanyl is only available from legitimate pharmaceutical manufacturers as a dermal (skin) patch or in lolly-pop form for very slow absorption by the pain patient's system.

Carfentanil, a fentanyl analog, is a veterinary tranquilizer, a powerful opioid narcotic used for anesthetizing large animals. It is one hundred times stronger than fentanyl, five thousand times stronger than heroin, and ten thousand times stronger than morphine. Unfortunately, it has caused fatal outcomes in people buying street illicits which may be "cut" with it unbeknownst to the user.

Buprenorphine is a partial opioid agonist purportedly indicated for analgesia as well as for the treatment of opioid addiction. It is available in different brands as Buprenex®, Butrans®, and Probuphine®. And, in combination with the opioid antagonist drug naloxone, buprenorphine is available as Suboxone®, Zubsolv®, and Bunavail®. In America, over 9 million buprenorphine prescriptions were filled in 2012. Widely used to manage opioid dependence, it's important to note that buprenorphine is also a morphine drug, that it is being abused when some patients, supposedly in detox, illicitly sell it to addicts.

Suboxone® (buprenorphine/naloxone) is a combination of the morphine, buprenorphine, plus its opioid antagonist. Which combination is meant to treat substance addiction while eliminating the addictive and dangerous (e.g., respiratory depression) effects of the synthetic morphine. However, Suboxone® itself is known to be misused by some in whom it is meant to deter abuse.

(Learn more about "The Suboxone Hoax" in Chapter Twenty.)

Finally, medicinal narcotics prescribed to pregnant women have been wrongfully blamed for the later development of ADHD in the child. This unproven "link" belies the fact that most such mothers receive a combination analgesic like Percocet® (oxycodone + acetaminophen) or Vicodin® (hydrocodone + acetaminophen) which contain the widely-ingested over-the-counter analgesic, brand name Tylenol® (acetaminophen) that is known to be hepatotoxic (poisonous to the liver). It must be remembered, in this regard, that acetaminophen is not meant for long-term use - a headache, a sore ankle, a superficial wound that heals quickly, an achy muscle, all temporary events. Unfortunately, the advertising and promotion of this product gives the erroneous impression that this liver toxic chemical can be used frequently and for extended periods. Thus, simple narcotic formulations, for example, oxycodone and hydrocodone are preferred. Caution: when seeking an iatrogenic cause for a childhood illness, blaming the use of pure narcotic pain relievers during pregnancy is specious.

OPIATE AND OPIOID TREATMENT FOR INTRACTABLE PAIN

Opioids Relieve Pain Safely for Decades, Even Lifelong, Without Addiction in Over 98% of IPPs

Despite the hysteria whipped up by CDC and DEA myopic operatives, decades-long and lifelong prescription opiate or opioid medications do not result in pain patient addictions in over 98% of these patients. Dependence on the analgesic (pain relief) component is the rule. Which does not equate with the "high" chased by the illicit street-drug abuser who is addicted. Importantly, too, that missing 1% or so were found to have had a substance abuse problem prior to their painful disease diagnosis. A simple problem that expert pain clinicians can discover when they take a careful medical history at each pain patient's initial examination. Such patients, of course, need alternate treatment modalities because of their propensity for addiction.

Chronic non-cancer pain of moderate to severe intensity is known to respond exceptionally well to prescription opioid treatment. Various scientific studies, conducted by diverse medical institutions which focused on the optimal treatment of pain, consistently report measurable pain reductions with concomitant acceleration of improved mobility, capacity to hold a job, all-around improved quality of life, family and social contacts maintained, and absent risks of addictive behaviors. Nevertheless, due to the hysterical conflation by Federal bureaucrats–who are not participating in direct patient care, who are not neurologists, nor pharmacologists, nor anesthesiologists; who are neither pain specialists nor physicians at all – of drug addicts' illicits with innocent chronic pain patients' prescription opioid medications, millions of human lives, American pain patients, are at risk of being underdosed, tapered without consent, and most horrible of all, *cold-turkeyed.* All without legal or medical protections to rescue them from the horrors of sudden withdrawal symptoms and cardiovascular and other complications leading to death arising out of this sudden disruption in their physiologic equilibrium.

Further muddying the opioid hysteria waters are outright confabulations by the feds (HHS, CDC, DEA) who gossip about a nonexistent drug abuse by patients on medically, ethically and legally prescribed opioid analgesics. And these same autocrats should feel guilty about the multitude of suicides their thoughtless actions have caused and are still causing. For shame!

As long as the powers that be – read "the alphabet soup of arrogant, uninformed, unknowledgeable bureaucrats, encrusted in lifetime, pension-assured jobs at Federal and, now, State agencies" criminally conflate illicit drug addicts and their cravings with intractable pain patients whose prescribed opioid narcotics relieve pain so they can live some kind of a lowered pain existence (because they're never free of pain altogether), that is how long this autocratic oligarchical roughshod ride over the rights of pain patients and their clinicians will endure.

It's been three years, now, since the fatuous 2016 *CDC Guideline* was belched forth from the haughty federal horde of questionable contributors, many of whom gave a tad from each of their multitudes of "specialties," unaware their specific information would be used to distort a whole generation of pain medicine practice, sending thousands of untreated pain patients to their graves by suicide, arming the DEA to invade doctors' offices and steal patients' confidential medical records;prosecuting highly ethical clinicians, sending hundreds of physicians around our nation to prison. All that without proofs of any crimes. Merely American Nazis in full DEA regalia victimizing patients and doctors, lying to the press and the public.

And, not to be overlooked, grieving is an imperative process, essential to enable the IPP to adapt to a life with unremitting pain.

Until the government gets out of medical care, and out of proscribing severe limits on opioid therapy, grief will be a daily presence in pain patients lives. Others who can't wait for common sense to infuse itself into mini-brained government officials will continue to end their lives in suicides. Now, there's an epidemic the CDC should be working to eliminate!

Often Suggested, Non-Opioid Treatments Don't Help

In America, **undertreatment of pain** is considered a major public health problem. And, even before the 2016 *CDC Guideline* was published, scientists reported evidence that many people in pain in our country (remember, pain patients number in the millions) are undertreated (too low dosages of narcotics) or are inadequately treated (don't get the correct medication) for their conditions. Some clinicians prescribe or suggest treatments other than opioids for such patients; however, none of these approaches parallels the pain relief levels these long-suffering people experience when taking their tried-and-true prescription opioids which they've been using appropriately for years, often decades.

In addition to prescription narcotic medications, there are many suggested alternate, and nonpharmaceutical treatments available. I only mention these here to be complete on this subject. However, none of these proposed treatments, simply because they are "available," rule out the salubrious analgesic effects of prescription narcotics safely used long-term by most Intractable Pain Patients (IPPs). Upsetting their equanimity and, often, their decades-long successful subduing of intractable pain by prescription narcotics is senseless and unusually cruel. That's because at least most IPPs have shown they've been able to hold down jobs and live a relatively okay quality of life, and who on long-term opioids never become addicted to them.

In general, what's offered, by various entities eager to benefit from referrals of new patients, are: acupuncture, homeopathy, laser treatments, magnets, prolotherapy, injections of various kinds, pumps, stimulators, even surgery. And more. All more expensive and difficult to access than a simple narcotic pill.

Here, though, I discuss a few of such treatment approaches some people not expert in pain management might prescribe. By no means is this list meant to be comprehensive. Just a smattering of what chronic pain patients are up against when all they need and want is the painkiller that works for them without toxicity and improves their quality of life.

Interventional Procedures For example, the FDA just approved the Accurian Nerve Ablation Platform, a Medtronic company device, that produces a predictable lesion every time to assure ablation of specifically-targeted nerve tissue to reduce chronic pain. Problem with this and any other invasive procedures is that pain patients usually want to avoid any body-invasive procedures, no matter how limited in duration, that will produce yet more pain and potential inflammation or infection, further complicating their already precarious hold on some normalcy. Then, there's **regional anesthesia**, a local infusion of an anesthetic through a catheter into the affected area.

Behavioral Health, otherwise known as psychotherapy, has been suggested as an alternative to prescription narcotic pain treatment. It's meant to change your mind, so to speak. No, your pain isn't as bad as you think it is. Even though you know it's not about what you think, it's about the pain messages your brain, spinal cord and peripheral nervous system are sending you. Listen! Talking to someone empathic to you can always help; however, talking about other things or about the pain itself does not bring relief of the physical hurting. Ouch! A chronic pain patient might get some temporary, during the session, "diversionary relief" from therapy; however, even if insurers paid for it, which they don't in such cases, that relief is merely temporary. The patient's pain still has to receive its quelling narcotic. How do I know this? I'm a psychotherapist. Psychotherapy works for emotional, social, creativity, and psychiatric issues. Severe physical pain due to a lifelong condition can't be talked out of existence. That idea is just plain nonsense.

Non-Narcotic Drugs, which include acetaminophen and the NSAIDs, are generally too mild for the kinds of severe and chronic pain discussed in AMERICAN AGONY. NSAIDs is the acronym for Nonsteroidal Anti-inflammatory Drugs, in contrast to the corticoids, such as cortisone and prednisone which reduce inflammation at a cost to the patient's hormonal and other systemic targets. NSAIDs include the great pain reliever of all time, but not usually for the most severe pain, which is acetylsalicylic acid (Aspirin). Then there's another analgesic, Tylenol ® (acetaminophen) which is meant only for short-term use because it is hepatotoxic (poisonous to the liver). Unfortunately, most people are unaware of this danger, and too often unwisely take this drug for more than a few weeks at a time. This is counter to what a person with a lifelong pain condition requires. And it's another reason why a narcotic that relieves a good portion of one's pain (no medication removes pain completely) reliably, safely, without hepatotoxicity dangers, is preferable.

Other **nonopioid drugs** can be tried. Some can be antidepressants, in very, very low doses, known as tricyclics, like amitriptyline, desipramine, and nortriptyline, which have analgesic properties in certain select conditions. For example, they've been used as partial treatment for the acute stage, which can last many months, of Herpes zoster infections (shingles). However, it's not clear if they actually touch the pain or what they accomplish. Perhaps, there's a bit of a "twilight zone" effect that distances the patient, so to speak, from this pain's severity. Gabapentin, normally used to treat epilepsy, is also useful in diabetic neuropathy and in shingles.

Multidisciplinary Approaches, Often Tried, Not Often Helpful

Suggested are "preoperative psychology," whatever that is, for perioperative (before and after surgery) pain control and really(?) to "manage moderate to severe pain". I can imagine a psychologist coming to the bedside of a patient with acute appendicitis pain, who'd just been prepped for appendectomy and has already had her preoperative anxiolytic (anxiety-reducer) to calm her down due to patient distress about being made unconscious and getting cut with a scalpel, "So, MaryJane, tell me about your childhood; any nightmares?"

And **alternative, nonmedication approaches** have been suggested. These include Acupuncture, Art Therapy, Yoga, Massage, Tai Chi, Mindfulness, Other Meditation methods, and Physiotherapy. As if someone with a most severe level of pain could meditate away that suffering, could exercise it away to oblivion, could psychologize it into disappearing.

It's not that I believe any of these are not well-meant. Nor that some of them couldn't help somewhat, as a diversion perhaps; physiotherapy, with the professional present, could strengthen muscles, provide some flexibility, improve some mobility. However, once the allotted time has passed, the chronic pain intervenes nonetheless.

And, it's not that I believe psychotherapy isn't good in various life and illness circumstances. However, when it comes to physiologic pain, the best that psychotherapy can achieve is some momentary (during sessions and at times on one's own) is distraction. The pain is still present, but when the patient is focused on painting a portrait or playing the piano or intensely talking about prior eras in one's life when physical pain didn't intrude, this diverts the brain. However, it doesn't remove the physical pain. Suggested would be that the patient who does well on their opioid analgesic would still benefit from **supplementary psychotherapy** which would help because of all the life adjustments and givings-up of normal existence, activities and employment that severe, lifelong pain subjects these patients to.

Nevertheless, the infamous 2016 *CDC Guideline* has impelled DEA-frightened and intimidated physicians into cutting off IPPs' normal narcotic prescriptions, destabilizing their lives, reinvigorating their long-time modulated pain to heightened intolerable levels, pushing many off the cliff of ineradicable suffering to suicide. This is an American tragedy which is piling innocent, now dead IPPs on top of one another in the nether world. Why? Who is benefiting from this crusade against patients needing ongoing narcotic pain relief?

All because myopic "advisors" at the CDC and their cohorts at the DEA are ignorantly conflating street fentanyl and heroin (often mixed with alcohol and/or benzodiazepines) overdose deaths with normal chronic pain patients who are not addicted, just pain-relieved.

Anyone who is determined to deprive such patients of their prescription narcotic regimens that are working for years and/or have been stabilizing their lives for decades, must be a closet Torquemada. Because of the cruel torture being inflicted. Because of the mounting numbers of suicides due to this 21st Century Inquisition.

Chapter Three

PAIN ASSESSMENT PROTOCOL and PAIN PATIENTS SPEAK UP

Before presenting the formal overview of how professional pain-managing physicians assess, treat, reassess and adjust treatment for each individual Intractable pain patient, for clarity it's important to review the enormous impact 50,000,000 pain-filled Americans have on society in general, on our economy and on our healthcare system.

Chronic Pain is a Burden, Even Beyond Pain Patients Themselves
Intransigent pain weighs heavily, not only on sufferers, but on their families and on society at large. It is burdensome by shrinking the patient's quality of life, obviating the afflicted's ability to work and earn, impacting the economy at large. Remembering, in that regard, that many millions of Americans fall into this high-level-of pain category. Not only, then, is it an urgent health problem requiring nuanced treatment for the in-pain individual, it encumbers businesses, diminishing profits. For, untreated pain leaves stricken patients incapable of employment, unable to support their families. The latter forcing many to use public assistance funds when they'd rather be productive and employed.

Pain is the top cause of disability in adults, reports the American Pain Association, with one in six Americans struggling with unremitting pain. The cost to businesses of lost workdays due to pain symptoms exceeded $61 billion in 2003. Given the loss of prescription narcotics for most intractable pain sufferers, since the advent of the infamous 2016 *CDC Guideline*, that economic toll must surely have risen considerably higher by now.

Because repetitions of the kinds of intense suffering millions are now being abandoned to is emphatically unnecessary, it's imperative to hold in one's empathic mind and heart, these days, patients with serious afflictions of back pain, neck pain, joint pain (arthritic conditions), headaches like migraine and temporomandibular joint disease, various carcinomas, post-surgical mishaps, Sickle Cell Disease and its periodic crises, Herpes zoster (aka Shingles), a severe viral affliction of nerves on some parts of the upper body, and a multitude of other pain-producing conditions. Far too many such sufferers, due to an egregious absence of federal wisdom or common sense, have been victimized by forced rapid tapering or *cold-turkeying* of their, heretofore, well-stabilized pain control, their once reliable prescription narcotics.

Unremitting pain further injures pain patients' health. For example, if your hip joint hurts and you limit your walking, or can only use a wheelchair, you lose the sturdiness of your nerves, muscles, tendons and ligaments. They atrophy (shrink from lack of use). Circulatory and cardiac problems are risks due to this kind of disabling immobility. And all because some thoughtless bureaucrats in Washington, D.C., can't sense what it would be like to live with such debilitating, dehumanizing painful sensations all day, all night, all month, for years.

Pain is Subjective. Others Can't Feel Yours. You Can't Feel Theirs. However, physicians who specialize in treating difficult painful conditions, normally a subspecialty of anesthesiology, would remind you to think of your pain as an illness that others can't fathom. However, because of this, pain patients are often rejected, regarded suspiciously, ostracized, their suffering disbelieved. The latter negativities fostered on purpose by a dense, clueless DOJ/DEA cabal bearing down on innocent patients requiring simple opioid pain relief.

Never Confuse Dependence for Pain Relief with Addictive Craving Pain patients, dependent for pain relief on their prescription narcotic medication, will experience withdrawal symptoms and signs when rapidly tapered off them or suddenly *cold-turkeyed* (which, morally, should never be done). Thus, the progress made, in modern medicine, in managing various kinds and levels of pain has been suddenly ripped out of the medical sphere, out of the healing hands of pain patients' private physicians, co-opted by the bureaucratic authoritarianism of federal players intent on diverting attention from their negligence on the front line of illicit drug interdiction, dealer prosecution, dilatory distribution of naloxone to the populace to save some unfortunate lives, and negligence in remanding drug addicts to detox facilities.

Pain Management Specialists and Other Clinicians Treating Intractable Pain Patients are keenly aware that prescription narcotic benefits extend beyond pain relief itself. These medical practitioners recognize that the narcotics they are prescribing allow their patients to remain employed, to ambulate rather than be bedridden, to interact with other humans, family and friends, rather than wasting away homebound. Alone. Asocial. Moreover, the monetary and mental health costs of untreated or sparsely treated pain, not to mention the social costs to the pain patient and his or her family, are insurmountable. Intractable Pain Patients, therefore, deserve to receive their usual stabilizing prescriptions for the narcotics that diminish their pain, often never to zero, but enough so they can function with some level of accomplishment in a reasonable life-quality existence.

Pain Assessment and Treatment Protocol

Opiophobia Reigns since the 2016 *CDC Guideline* invaded normal pain management medicine. Recent opiophobic reports by ill-informed journalists, and by irresponsible Federal and State ideologues, have instigated disastrous directions away from normal medical care all the way to unethical, low-dosing of narcotic analgesics for patients in pain. Beyond that, tragically, to underdosing, tapering without patient consent, and to outright *cold-turkeying.*

Under-Assessment of Pain Leads to Under-Treatment and Painful Outcomes

And, according to experts in multiple medical specialty fields, who are focused on the optimal management of simple, varied and complex pain conditions, it is imperative that clinicians carefully assess the signs, symptoms, histories and patient self-reports when deciding upon a specifically targeted treatment approach. It is essential, all professionals agree, to tailor pain care treatment to individually-assessed clinical issues, the source of the pain (whether identifiable or obscure), the patient's living circumstances, ambulating or bedbound, continuous pain or intermittent pain? Plus, how has the patient been coping before this assessment? And so forth.

The Under-dosing Disaster: 90MME (morphine milligram equivalents)

Since pain is a subjective experience, and since, so far, there is no way to measure each patient's pain perceptions objectively, the clinician must rely on both the patient's pain history and must also be astute, from multiple perspectives, when attempting to assess what's generating the suffering, its intensity, its duration and how best to treat it. One admonition from multiple professionals stands out, however: There is no validity to any one-size-fits-all treatment for patients in pain. Therefore, particularly when we are talking about narcotic analgesics, the unfortunate under-dosing "recommendation" generated by a CDC protocol – the infamous 90MME – as a fixed dosage goal for many, even all, patients on prescription opioids along a broad spectrum of ages, life circumstances, disabilities, employment status, pain levels, and pain etiologies is just plain insane.

Pain, subjective as noted, is not quantifiable like a bacterial infection in a petri dish that a physician can wipe out with seven days of 250 mg. q.i.d. of a tetracycline or a penicillin. Pain is evanescent, so to speak.

It does what it wants. It shows up when and how intensely it wants. It sometimes subsides without so much as letting the patient know how that happened. It's a conundrum. It can't be precisely measured. Ergo, it follows that it can't be precisely treated. The best a clinician can do is provide the pain patient with some semblance of relief, for some hours, for half a day, to permit some hours of sleep. And enough to enable a job to be kept. The patient hurts badly. The doctor must treat the pain ethically, adequately, fully aware that only a minute number of pain-experiencing patients ever go on to become addicted to their particular prescribed narcotic.

A Diagnostic Biomarker for Severe, Unrelenting Pain

A consequence of untreated severe chronic pain is overstimulation of the hypothalamic-pituitary-adrenal axis, a system in the brain that maintains physiologic and therefore emotional equilibrium. Under duress, like pain that never lets up, this neurosystem produces excess cortisol (a stress indicator) levels in the blood. Therefore, the presence of excess serum cortisol is one objective measure of a patient's suffering with severe, chronic pain. Which may be used as some future test to pinpoint the height (or depth) of a patient's pain.

PAIN EVALUATION AND TREATMENT APPROACHES

Elemental Pain Assessment

Quality pain assessment, as pain specialists know, includes a history of the patient's health, illnesses, pain experiences, how the patient's family is affected by this pain invasion in their lives, a physical examination and diagnostic studies. The latter can be radiologic (X-ray, Magnetic Resonance Imaging, Computerized Axial Tomography), blood tests to identify something uniquely genetic (e.g., Sickle Cell Disease), infectious (e.g., Lyme Disease) or other possible hematologic clues to the origin(s) of pain in each patient. Additionally, a pain patient may be subjected to biopsies, thoracentesis (an invasive pulmonary procedure), lumbar puncture (a needle inserted into the spinal column to extract cerebrospinal fluid for testing). Furthermore, there are electrodiagnostic tests for both peripheral sensory and peripheral motor nerves.

Finally, it's imperative to reassess physical function and disability... walking, talking, swallowing, reaching, bending, balancing, and so forth. And, of course, respirations. Breathing. Inefficient oxygenation can affect pain and function. Pain itself may hinder breathing. Pain medications, at times, can slow the patient's respiratory rate.

Elements of the Pain Experience

Where is the pain coming from? What is hurting? Is it a skin sensation? Or does it originate internally, as in angina from a cardiac problem or pain from pancreatic inflammation? Are the joints involved, as in arthritis?

Is it pain that is neurally transmitted, as in trigeminal neuralgia? Or as in acute Herpes zoster invasion pain (aka "shingles"), and later, post-herpetic neuralgia that lasts for years, usually forever pain.

Also, certain descriptions of duration and sensation can help the clinician assess and better treat the chronic pain patient. These include sudden bursts of pain, rhythmic occurrences as in throbbing dental or migraine pain. While other conditions may not be so facile to pin down, such as Complex Regional Pain Syndrome (CRPS) with no identifiable specifics of sensate expression. Sometimes, inexplicable nausea and vomiting accompanies certain pain experiences.

Finally, pain expert clinicians, in addition to the patient's subjective reports of his/her pain experiences, have multidimensional assessment tests evaluating varied elements of pain, to help further pinpoint each particular patient's sufferings and how best to treat them. Such parameters include the patient's report of how and where pain occurs – in the body, and where and when in the life setting. How goes the patient's ambulation? Nourishment? Sleep? Socialization? How is the patient emotionally affected by the physical suffering?

Next, there's the **BPI (Brief Pain Inventory)** which helps elicit the severity of the pain and the levels of disability it causes. And the BPI also provides important insight into pain's effect on a patient's daily life and how the prescribed pain treatment is working, or if it's not helping much, if at all.

Then there's the **MPQ (McGill Pain Questionnaire)** which examines multidimensional aspects of the pain experience for diagnostic evaluation and more pin-pointed assessment of the patient's pain experiences. And, always, it's imperative that pain management clinicians bear in mind the quality-of-life level the patient is existing at, now, living with chronic pain; especially when compared with how patients reported their life quality prior to their pain affliction.

Medical Health – Anatomic, Physiologic

Examinations of the pain patient include, also, the usual ones done on any patient such as health history, general health outside of the pain issue, and so forth. After which, evaluation of pain levels along with pain site assessment, with special attention to the neurologic and musculoskeletal systems.

Note too, neuropathic pain should additionally be assessed from its subjective experiential quality for the patient. From his/her perspective. What is the temperature at the site? Cold? Hot? Is it a dull pain or sharp? Is it way internal or is it surface, peripheral? Scales for patients to rate these parameters are graphed from one to ten.

Periodically, each patient's pain experience should be reassessed. Any changes in pain frequency and/or intensity deserves reevaluation. As do any progressive limitations on the chronic pain patient's mobility, social engagement, family participation, and employment. Becoming homebound damages patients' human connections. Becoming wheelchair-bound limits patients' opportunities and ambitions and damages self-esteem. Becoming bedbound leads to further muscle and nerve wasting, thus to other physical limitations and ailments. Then, often, to depression. Finally to suicide.

Thus far, after the unfortunate 2016 *CDC Guideline* was implemented, an enormous toll of suicides by Intractable Pain Patients has occurred. And these are continuing as such patients, striving to adapt to a life of under-dosed (90MME parameter) narcotics without real analgesia and (inexcusably due to DEA agents threatening and DOJ lawyers prosecuting of hundreds of pain care physicians around the country) abrupt *cold-turkeying* of pain-relief-dependent patients. Not to mention the national paranoia all this federal interference in medical practice has caused.

In order to help the physician more accurately determine what the patient is experiencing and how best to treat the pain, a good idea is for pain patients to keep a journal (or a small pad with a pen, in pocket or purse) and note date, time of day, what you were experiencing pain-wise, how you handled or treated it, how you felt once dealt with. Such an ongoing memoir, typed up, will clarify for the physician, the patient's in-the-moment pain experiences, providing an invaluable overview of a-day-in-the-life-of the sufferer. Now the doctor truly gets it. It remains for federal agency policy makers to grasp these essentials, too. And to rescind what the CDC has inflicted on Americans in pain.*

*It also needs to be noted that a great upheaval in normal, healthy, ethical medical care of pain has been abandoned, too, for acute Emergency Department patients, for Postoperative Patients and for Dental Patients. All this latter from the opiophobia falsely injected into the American psyche, infecting every level of clinical medical care with fear of intimidation, arrest, search-and-seizure of confidential patients' records, persecution by DEA operatives via phone calls warning physicians to curb their legitimate prescribing of narcotics, prosecuting honorable physicians, imprisoning faultless physicians for a nebulous invented "crime": "conspiracy". What hath the HHS's CDC wrought? When will the DOJ and its DEA relent?

Following are Some Intractable Pain Patients Describing their Sufferings Since the Feds Began Practicing Medicine:

Intractable Pain Patients are Trapped between Federal Autocrats and Frightened Physicians

Despite highly qualified medical pain specialists' exhortations, to the assortment of federal and state interlopers who breach the intricate workings of pain management, autocratic bureaucrats remain deaf to this expertise and heartless to long-suffering patients in pain.

Due to the onslaught of government powers aligned against their best health and safety interests, and mindful of their rights under the Americans with Disabilities Act (ADA), many IPPs are no longer cowering in silence. They are angry at the injustices. They are determined to get their patients' rights restored. To protect their privacies, I've given people, who've contacted me, initials which don't reflect their real names. They are hurting. And they're not backing down.

In that mind-frame, **G.B.** says, "It's time to sue the abandoners," referring to the doctors who won't treat them any longer and the pain clinics who refuse to set up appointments for them. **L.M.** adds, "What about the ER at my local hospital? They refused to even look at my MRI to see the cause of my pain?" "And what about my drugstore, asks **R.T.**, "where they won't fill my doctor's prescription for my codeine? Can I sue them? I don't know what to do."

On the burdensome extra and expensive doctor visits, **E.B.** laments," Urine tests, extra appointments, rules, long forms to fill out, my health records open to the government, forced to go to addict clinic. Shamed." And **K.V.** reminds other pain "warriors," that the CDC's oppression of pain doctors' narcotic prescribing is based on the nonscientific reliance on baby-dose MMEs (morphine milligram equivalents) which are forced as low as 90MME and even lower – non-analgesic levels for severe chronic pain.

Catastrophic Procedures that Sometimes Lead to Infections, Hemorrhage, Death

All to avoid normal narcotic prescribing, sadly reports **A.J.**, who mourns the death of his friend: "After several back operations, the surgeon wouldn't prescribe him a narcotic to swallow. They put in a morphine pump but it caused an infection in his intestine. The extra pain sent him to the Emergency Room. He died two days later." And **S.M.** adds, "I wouldn't have surgery my orthopedic doctor wanted to do because my cousin went in for back surgery and hemorrhaged to death because they cut into his aorta by mistake."

Decrying the "retiring" of physicians in the wake of the DEA raiders, **K.P.**, says, "It's tragic, Doctors are just stopping practicing medicine, closing their offices, because of harassment by DEA police. I heard many innocent doctors are in prison, prosecuted by the Department of Justice, even though they did nothing wrong, were just taking care of their pain patients." Adds **P.T.**, "All this trouble so my pain doctor suddenly retired. The referred doctor refused to prescribe the pain medicine I've used since 2004, and no sleep meds. I'm angry, sad. In so much pain. Help."

"Really hurt bad," says **A.R.**, "My TMJ pain, for ten years is now not being treated at all. Advil and Aleve don't work. Pain too severe. But that's all they allow now. Severe pain every day, can't work. Can't go out of the house. Can't even brush my teeth. Will anyone help us?" And **D.C.** with a degenerative disease, formerly moderately pain-relieved on adequate hydrocodone dosing for 23 years, has now been cut to an ineffectively low dose of it: "I'm housebound, soon to be bedbound. Pain is so bad. Lost my job. My veterinarian wouldn't treat my dog, Justice, like this."

"Not relieving excruciating pain that never lets up," says **F.T.**, "is outright sadistic". And **R.M.** in pain, says, "Each day I'm forced to stay home because of agonizing pain, I pray for death to take me." Then, **H.A.** adds, "A shame we pain patients are being tortured because our doctors are afraid of the DEA. When will this stop?"

"My doc cut my dose," says **B.K.**, "and now most of my pain has come back. Before it was under good control. I could scream, but I can't cry in front of my children." Adds **G.S.**, "When my doctor dropped me from his care, I didn't know where to turn. I had to relocate to another state to be near a doctor who would prescribe the right medicine for my pain." Finally, **P.G.** reports, I've been told I should learn to live with this pain but it hurts so bad I'd rather be dead."

Chapter Four

PAIN PATIENTS AND EMPATHIC OTHERS SPEAK OUT

Sufferings and Suicide Plans of Pain Patients since the Invidious 2016 *CDC Guideline*

The more I learned that Intractable Pain Patients were having their prescription narcotics, and some ancillary medications, tapered to sub-therapeutic doses or suddenly stopped altogether – because, nationwide, our federal government has empowered itself to invade the confidential physician-patient relationship using the excuse that users of illicit street drugs were overdosing and dying in droves – the more I wanted to scream out, "How dare they? "What do these fools know about the origins of pain? Or about all that is studied in medical school to graduate skilled physicians, and later to specialize in Pain Management, who go on to treat all manner of pain-producing conditions? Who are these Cold Turkeys, anyway?

Thus began my journey into this muddled terrain of meddling federal and, now too, state bureaucrats overriding sound medical judgments about the alleviation of pain. I am still flabbergasted by what I've found and continue to find in my research, both in my readings of scientific papers and on the internet. Websites abound letting America and the world know what the CDC and the DEA are doing to pain patients, and to their physicians and other caring clinicians who have been writing normal narcotic prescriptions for years and decades without negative patient outcomes.

The more I explored the broad spectrum of Intractable Pain Patients' sufferings, the tortuous/adverse conditions imposed on them by federal government bureaucrats, and the diverse diseases/conditions (genetic, developmental, traumatic, and wear-and-tear on tissues, bones, nerves) they've been grappling with all their lives, the more I cried. The more I cried out. For, where is it written, in scientific and empathic medicine, "Let them suffer. Too bad!"?

Isn't it enough for them to live their daily lives crippled by their dire conditions? These kinds of hitlerian rigidities and cruelties do not belong in 21st Century America. Certainly not in today's super-advanced medical world. Even an Artificially Intelligent robot knows that!

Dumbstruck, I discovered website after website, up and running for years, fighting for the God-given and Constitutional rights of persons, even when they are patients, to their basic healthcare, to their right to pain relief prescribed by their physicians. At each reasonable plea, at each endeavor to undo what the clueless powers-that-be wrought (via the infamous *CDC Guideline),* zero moved Health and Human Services, nor its subsidiary, the CDC, nor the Department of Justice, nor its subsidiary, the DEA to alter their onslaughts. Their public attacks that have victimized, instead of allowing opioid treatment of pain patients. That have killed pain physicians' practices, imprisoned hundreds of innocent clinicians nationwide, since this government's holocaust against American pain sufferers had its catastrophic inception in the federal halls of HHS's CDC in 2016.

Cold Turkeys at the CDC and DEA are Condemning Pain Patients to Suicide

The websites I found have, for years now, been broadcasting the horrors and injustices inflicted by Keystone Kop mentalities, filtering down from the CDC to the DEA, making our nation a police state dead set (and I mean DEAD) on killing off patients because they've been on legal prescription narcotics. This haughty behavior exists in the DEA in order to justify their impotence against illicit drug importations, their negligence in vigorous prosecution of drug dealers and criminal chemists manufacturing fatal impure street-bought substances, and their laxness in remanding illicit drug users to medical and psychiatric treatment. The three latter should be their purview. Nothing else. CDC and DEA, by way of HHS, I demand you "Get out of patient care. Get out of physicians' decision-making on behalf of the patients' medical conditions they intimately know!"

Also, what in the world is the DEA doing in yours and my prescription medicine databases nationwide? Known as PDMPs (Prescription Drug Monitoring Programs), these "programs" are actually a way for government goons to access ALL of every American patient's medication history. Is this America? Why are patients allowed to be spied upon? And what are Americans willing to do to handcuff the DEA Nazis and oust the DOJ miscreants who are cutting off quality medical care to pain patients and who are imprisoning physicians nationwide?

There are many websites on this pain patient holocaust that made me cry. Then, immediately, I became furious. Our federal government, by way of its entrenched narrow-thinking bureaucrats, has decided to invade, disrupt and cut off everyone's appropriate medical care and, too bad, you can't do anything about this.

Furthermore, adding more anger to my fire-breathing-dragon against government invading our private healthcare prescriptions, I found yet another website run by a physician which keeps track of the hundreds of physicians and other clinicians (NPs and PAs) from various American states (I feel ashamed to say "America" in this context) who've been persecuted, prosecuted and imprisoned on a legally obscure notion called "conspiracy" even though they're guilty of nothing. Still, our deficient government has them wasting away in jail, unable to provide their medical knowledge to patients who need it, their assets "legally" stolen by the DOJ's DEA, preventing them from acquiring top legal help, completely ruining theirs and their families' lives.

And, Isn't it enough for pain patients to live daily crippled by lifelong pain? Where is it written in scientific and empathic medical practice, "Let them suffer. Too bad."?

These Federal Bureaucrats are COLD TURKEYS

Along comes an imperious blob of insensate federal nincompoops, pretending pain specialty expertise, depth knowledge of morphine metabolism, intricate pharmacologic experience, addiction expertise, while American addicts are dying in droves on DEA-neglected streets. Plus, the unmitigated gall to confound all their tenuous exhortative beliefs by attributing street drug addict deaths to Pain Patients' narcotic prescriptions. Nothing could be further from the truth.

These kinds of Hitlerian rigidities and cruelties do not belong in 21st Century America. Dumbstruck, I discovered website after website, up and running for years since the 2016 *CDC Guideline* debacle debuted, already broadcasting the problems and injustices.

Thus, as I said before, in my travels on the internet to various websites supporting Pain Patients and others supporting Narcotic Prescribing Physicians, I was astounded by the volume of victims (both pain patients and medical personnel), the courage of the voluble ones, and the silence of the government cold turkeys, who are cowardly ignoring all the resulting suicides. This stirred me to search for ways to rectify this gross assault on medical practice, on patients' privacy, and on patients' rights to not suffer. Even Human Rights Watch is getting involved, on the patients' side, of course.

Having read, in depth, about so much of this American horror story, I developed a questionnaire and emailed it to a massive list of my subscribers to my other medical and literary writings. I received a 70% feedback, demonstrating how vital this subject is to so many. They had an opportunity to email me, text me, or telephone me. All three routes of contact were used by my respondents. Now, as I've read, and taken to heart the sufferings of these patients in pain and their alliance-in-spirit with DEA-beleaguered pain specialists, I've been drawn, tearfully, to many of their stories. Most are pain patients. Some are physicians. Others are relatives of pain patients. Some, even, are physicians who are also pain patients. Some are relatives of pain patients who've suicided due to untreated pain. Their recountings are often so moving, they could tear a reader's heart out. You want to hug the person. Send them a prayer. Ask them to hold on. That this government insanity won't last. You want to tear your hair out as you shed tears from the personal sufferings you are reading about or listening to on the phone.

In my case, as a Registered Nurse, the best I can do is write about what I know of the many facets of pain and its varied analgesic treatments. And I write, too, from the perspective of witnessing the salubrious effects of narcotic analgesia, used appropriately by all physicians I've ever worked with, in all kinds of medical, surgical, emergency, obstetric, even pediatric situations. Burns, other injuries, suture removals, migraine episodes, temporomandibular jaw pain, Sickle Cell crises, I could enumerate endlessly...but you get it. Pain has to be treated. And none of these pain conditions equates with addiction disease in illicit drug users. Nor do prescription narcotic patients exceed 1% of overdose occurrences, despite the contorted "statistics" the CDC's hysteria has inflicted on the public's fearful imagination.

Thus, the more months I spent researching the many and varied websites trying to do something to right these terrible wrongs inflicted on pain patients and their clinicians, and the more I received pain-patient feedback from my e-questionnaire, the more I felt compelled to compile their heartrending sentiments, disease descriptions and desperations for proper pain management, the more I knew I must get these expressions out to the public at large. Thus, the poignant stories shared in response to my informal survey of current issues about pain patient abandonment and suffering, are shared here to broadcast the plight of untreated patients in pain.

Always heartbreaking, comments on the horrendous burdens, sufferings and suicides government autocrats have visited on innocent patients in pain are often lengthy. Therefore, I will be quoting some in brief, while others, I will paraphrase at length so as not to omit salient descriptive features that convey all the pain and sorrow and death the DOJ and its DEA are inflicting on these millions. Naturally, I will protect the anonymity of pain patient commentators. Where doctors have spoken up, I've indicated this while, also, keeping them anonymous with initials. (In this climate of gestapo-tactics-engendered fear, this is essential.) It's important these physicians chose not to be secretive about how they feel about these dire times for pain patients and their ethical, empathic medical care.

War Veteran Pain Patients and Other Chronic Pain Patients Speak Out

This is a scary era of Gestapo-like activity by DEA agents phoning MDs, warning them about their prescribing dosages, raiding their offices, and the DOJ prosecuting and imprisoning them. Along with its victimization of pain patients, deprived of appropriate narcotic analgesia, or forced on such low doses that never touch the pain, there's also the sudden *cold-turkeying* of seriously ill patients. Of those who've responded to my e-survey, I am protecting them by using fictitious initials when quoting small samples of their difficult experiences since the 2016 *CDC Guideline* morphed into law, since the DEA turned medical practice for patients in pain into a police state.

Fear of Job loss from Untreated Pain

B.T., a retired teacher, in addition to her pain-causing spinal disease, has to "pee in a cup, count every pill, take a 2-hour trip to the pharmacy to count pills....The pain clinic doctor cut me off my oxycodone. I'm scared I'll lose my job. Too many sick days."

Genocide by Suicide and Physicians Speak Out

As a doctor, sidelined by fibromyalgia, **P.N.** warns, "These guidelines have killed so many by suicide. No government official seems to care about this genocide." **T.M.** accuses "...the CDC and FDA and others for not stopping these suicides by patients abruptly cut off of their opioids. Where is the human empathy? It's genocide by omission. Another doctor, **H.L.**, points out, "What's happening to chronic pain patients is tragic due to medical negligence which is due to the fear the guideline and DEA put into physicians' guts.

T.Y. says, "I'm afraid for my MD license. They're intimidating doctors. As a pain patient myself, I too have experienced pain clinic employees trying to shame pain patients out of describing their true pain levels, out of asking for pain relief. I'm better off dead."

M.N., a businessman, pleads, "Would anyone with a conscience keep doing what the CDC is promoting when the result is more pain and more suicides?" "I keep hurting," **R.V.** says. "But the government keeps making 'recommendations' that are taken as law. We in pain are the victims. Who will save us? One more day in bed all day and suicide feels like a good escape."

A 69-year-old baker, **O.R.** suffers from amputation-related pain. He's contemplating suicide because, he says, "My opioid worked marvelously for 15 years. Then my doctor stopped writing those prescriptions all of a sudden. I can't go on." Desperate, **Y.C.** pleads, "Without my oxycodone, the excruciating pain of my arachnoiditis means it's time to die."

Suicides of Veterans with Untreated Pain Veterans of foreign wars, home after their unimaginable sacrifices, are forced to sacrifice even more—their lives, due to forced tapering of their pain medications, and also many are abruptly *cold-turkeyed* off their narcotic analgesic. **W.W.** is angry because, "Nobody should serve this country to be thrown away like trash. It's damn time we crawl, if we must, to D.C. government offices. Wonderful, free syringes for addicts and Murder Wounded Veterans. Millions of us pain patients need to fight to get government off our backs and give us back our pain medicines." And **G.M.** laments, "Gone is compassionate healthcare for the disabled and for wounded veterans. We are being tortured to death. Living every day with escalating pain. What's the point of living?"

J.P., an Afghanistan veteran given the runaround by his hospital doctor, but zero treatment for his amputation-related pain, reports: "After I made a formal complaint, his office manager, not a doctor mind you, calls me and says I should go see a psychologist. The nerve. So I traveled out of state and found a doctor who cares. She's brave, not afraid of those DEA guys. And I got my pain prescription. She saved my life because I was seriously going to leave this earth." Suicide is imminent for **V.T.**, a war veteran, who says, "I've told my doctor I'm always thinking of killing myself, my only out unless I go to street drugs. I told him I've been writing my suicide letter...planning ways to do it. My pain is excruciating. Don't wish to die, but I have no choice."

The DEA Targets Pain Patients instead of Drug Dealers

B.G.P., focusing on the DEA's tactics, states, "No one will help us pain patients. Because the Justice Department can't handle the cartels and don't prosecute enough drug dealers, they pick on pain patients." And **K.W.** adds, "Our doctors are running scared, pain patients are suffering and dying, the DEA is spying and raiding, the CDC is smiling and uncaring."

Patients' Rights to Quality Medical Care from Doctors, Not Government

S.E., a bedbound mother of two youngsters, whose husband cooks and takes care of their children, reminds Intractable Pain Patients, "We way outnumber CDC officials. We need to fight for our rights as sick patients." And **C.M.** sadly asserts, "The patient-doctor relationship died when the CDC thing came out. They made it so a pain patient is mistreated, talked to like as if I was an addict." **H.E.** demands, "Government get out of the doctor-patient confidential relationship." And a writer from Oregon, a state infamous for its stringent, anti-patient legislation, **T.S.** asks politicians outright: "Are you trying to kill us off? It's alarming how many pain patients are going by suicide since the government took our pain medicines away. Americans **should be ashamed of these killings."**

C.T. is raising her three-year-old grandson because her daughter has a birth defect plus Late Stage Lyme Disease. Now in her late 20s, the young mother would like a job and to socialize. But "her doctor has cut off her hydrocodone because he says DEA agents call and give him warnings." Faulting the CDC and the DEA for their misdirected prohibitions, **F.E.** tells them, "You have made the lives of chronic pain patients a living hell. Stupid, too, you sue manufacturers of opioids which are legal painkillers and, used medically, they make life bearable for us in pain." And **V.B.** says, "The CDC doesn't care about pain patients....The government wants us dead. Less people on Social Security...." A scientist and sufferer of a spinal disease, **M.G.** cries out, "What did we pain patients do to become victims of these vile government agencies? They are empty-headed sadists."

Pain Patient **B.J.** decries all the government groups, panels, reports and so forth, that preach endlessly about opioid use worries and how important it is to rescue illicit drug users, all the while overlooking the dire need for prescription narcotic medications for pain patients. He recalls, "My doctor told me I have to learn to live with the pain."

One group of anonymous pain patients, pointing out that doctors are frightened because of the DEA raids of their colleagues' offices, claim, "We found out there are hundreds of doctors in prison in our country, without real legal evidence they did anything wrong. Just because they gave people like us a chance at pain relief with a legal narcotic. We are living scared. Any day now, our pain medicines can be stopped. The government bullies who started this disaster should be voted out." Also, **K.G.**, reported that "the guideline caused many innocent doctors to go to jail, others to restrict our pain drug. Mine went down from 135 tablets of hydrocodone 10 mg., down to only 90 tablets. I heard other doctors stopped being doctors altogether by retiring. They're scared."

Unwanted Steroid Injections A victim of the DEA onslaught against normally-prescribing physicians, **A.F.** says, "I had to find a new pain clinic. They switched me to steroid injections. Painful themselves. Don't work. Staff treats me like an addict, suspicious. Urine test, constant questions. Now my dose is so low it can't take my pain away."

Pharmacies Won't Fill Legal Opioid Prescriptions When **C.R.** took her prescription to her once-friendly local drug store, they refused to fill it and "recorded in my file that I was 'a drug-seeking patient'".

50 Million Suffering from Government Intrusion in Pain Patients' Lives

E.P. points out that 50 million pain patients are left to suffer because the government is worried about 2 million illicit drug addicts. "Many of us are ending our lives because our doctors no longer give us our pain meds in the dose amounts that worked for us for years."

Postponing Surgery because No Adequate Pain Relief is Given

D.S. needs back surgery but is putting it off indefinitely, despite its exigency, because his orthopedist told him he won't prescribe a narcotic except for only a few days after the operation. Knowing, because he's had these surgeries before, that the bad pain levels last much longer than that, he's put off the much needed operation. Meanwhile, his physical condition will deteriorate because of this postponement. The surgeon told him, "After the operation, take Tylenol." That decision by the orthopedist, even though he knows that bone healing, as well as muscle and other tissue healing, especially during required physiotherapy, will be quite painful and will extend far longer than merely a week. "Without surgery I have pain. With surgery the doctor won't relieve it. How long will I let myself survive?"

Predicting the Deaths of Chronic Pain Patients

About the intrusion of the federal government into pain management, particularly singling out HHS's CDC and its DOJ henchmen at the DEA, **N.R.** says, "They're killing chronic pain patients. They're hurting me by stopping my prescription hydrocodone that has worked well for years and years. And it's let me keep my job too. Now how will my family survive?" And, after 15 years on his methadone prescription, "They're tapering me," says **T.L.** "The amount is so low now, my pain never leaves. I keep thinking of suicide."

"My chronic condition means it's never going to heal," says **S.K.** And, "So don't rob me of my opioid. Though my pain never goes completely away, it keeps me comfortable. That's what pain doctors should want."

P.E. is upset about the role of PROP (see Chapter Twenty-One for more about this group) in this unfortunate anti-healthcare assault on chronic pain patients. She asserts, "There are riches to be made promoting the hundreds of anti-addiction clinics nationwide."

Especially, I say, if you can label chronic pain patients "addicts," force them off their reliable prescription opioids, then force them into one of the many Suboxone® (buprenorphine/naloxone) clinics around the country. They've proven this is the goal because they've requested and received permission to up their patient censuses greatly in the wake of this maelstrom sweeping away the equanimity of pain patients and the professions of caring physicians.

Cut off her hydrocodone, now bedridden and on Disability, for two decades, **L.V.**, a pediatric nurse, had been a pain patient. In nursing and medicine, she remembers, "Pain came to be called 'the fifth vital sign', my hydrocodone prescription really helped my long-standing intractable pain, so I could work and take care of my son." These days, she says, abruptly cut off from her opioid relief, and she's bedridden. No longer working. No longer a productive member of society. Depressed. Suicidal. Children Services has removed her son from her home. All that, and she's still abandoned by her physician and by our government. Still in constant pain!

S.T. asks, "With all we IPPs are being put through by people in Washington, D.C., we need doctors to step up and advocate for us."

Questioning the Authority of CDC Operatives to Harm So Many

W.G. is angry and wants to know why the only persons who were party to the drafting of the infamous 2016 *CDC Guideline* came from groups such as Workers Compensation Managers, Big Pharma, Employers, Prescription Drug Insurers; all groups with their own financial agendas, without a care for the suffering of patients in lifelong pain. He points out, the decisions in the fateful document, were narrowly crafted to be in accord with those special interest goals and have zero to do with American pain patients' best interests. "They literally stole our right to essential healthy medical care by stealing our pain medicines from us."

Lost Hope

It's terrible, as **E.S.M.** reports, that she was forced, cold turkey, off her opioid medication, forced to undergo 15 dorsal injections "which hurt and then made the pain worse. I can't trust doctors anymore. I feel hopeless." And, reporting his situation is dire, **D.G.**, formerly stable on his hydrocodone dosage that enabled him to stay at his job and enjoy family life, that his sudden under-dosing by a flippant clinic doctor, in response to the *CDC Guideline* has "sent me back to bed all day, lost me my job, put me on disability."

Anonymous Pain Physician Arrested. It's unconscionable. This long-time pain specialist was arrested, lost his medical license, all because he honorably treated pain appropriately for his chronic pain patients. A government "investigator," spurred on by a paranoid social worker whose daughter had died of illicit street fentanyl plus Xanax® (alprazolam) has been on a mission to target doctors writing legal prescriptions for opioid analgesics. This vengeful woman totally ignored the fact that her teenager had not died of a carefully manufactured prescription narcotic, but of an unknown quantity of grossly impure substances. And, also, had a companion had a rescue naloxone available, the girl's life could have been saved. All of that, despite having zero to do with what pain patients require and how responsibly they use their medications, this woman-on-a-crusade has managed to ruin Anonymous Physician's career and life, along with all the other empathic clinicians she has targeted. Will anybody stop this healthcare interference insanity? Says, **Anonymous Pain Physician**, "Thousands of patients have lost top doctors because of this individual who is fueled by government intruders in the patient-physician relationship."

Law and Legislators Should Protect Patients; Violations of Laws Protecting Disableds

K.W. warns that "The Disability Act is being violated when patients aren't given their pain prescriptions." And, "It's important to reach out to lawmakers and political leaders," says coach **H.J.**, "help them be a champion of chronic pain patients by giving them the ammunition to fight the good fight for us."

Dr. G.M. wants to "remind lawmakers the DEA is using the 'guideline' against doctors as well as against patients." And this woman, **Z.C.**, is fed up with politicians: "When I wrote them about my opioid being stopped they told me to go to rehab. No feelings." Still, **O.M.** spoke to his congressman and sees a glimmer of hope that things could change for the better: "Seems to be getting through but painfully slow so we keep suffering." And **L.L.** is sure it will take "radical action" for this "war on pain patients to change. But the majority of us are too crippled by pain to do mass protests and marches to Washington." Optimistic **P.D.**, a cancer patient says. "I think they're beginning to hear us. The lawmakers. The health agencies." Thus, he is hopeful despite no change in policy for 3 years since the *Guideline* tore through the fabric of American medical care.

L.B. exhorts pain suffers to **"Overrule the Feds and force your governors and other politicians to kill the laws that are killing us off. While thousands are dying by suicide because of no pain medicine laws, government sleeps."** And **N.C.** agrees, "Some government types could care less if we kill ourselves."

E.W. can't resist this prediction: "It'll be 20 years before any politician gets off their rears to do anything for pain sufferers. And doctors will now always fear being raided by the DEA and put in jail."

Contemplating Suicide A retired economics professor, **G.C.**, says, "I'm 85 with worsening pain, so losing my low dose morphine would kill the rest of my life. I'd like to live longer, but...." Then, a patient, who is living with untreated Addison's Disease and can't find a doctor to treat it, let alone offer any analgesic medication, **S.M.,** encourages other pain patients to "Hang in there. Stay strong. Don't give the CDC one more suicide to ignore." **T.H.** decries "Living in pain these last three years while the DEA, PROP and CDC murdered thousands whose only crime was living with pain. Suicide looks bright now." Also, here's how these government workers think, says **W.E.**, "Suicidal patients are expendable.

They taper down the list of patients on opioid prescriptions. The government wins by this diabolical Catch-22." **K.J.** Even with cancer, this patient says, "They won't give me real pain medicine. Steroids? No, don't want. Who should I sue for cruel and unusual punishment?"

Inadequate Doses, Wrong Narcotics Prescribed - Quality of Life Nil

W.B. reports, "One tramadol I got, instead of my hydrocodone. Could as well have been lemon drops. Did nothing for me. Before, the hydrocodone managed to keep me out of bed and doing my electrician job. Now I can barely walk to the kitchen for a coffee." **L.J.** says, "My job as a plumber is dead since the pain clinic dropped me to that 90MME low dose. In bed, calling politicians. Feeling hopeless."

Terminal Pain Patients Also Mistreated, DEA at Fault

F.G., an engineer, who has end-stage disease with almost constant bladder pain, reports that his doctor of ten years recently told him, "I am not allowed to prescribe what I know is best for my pain patients because of the CDC rules. My brother-in-law, also a doctor, was raided by the DEA."

Abandoned by their Pain Care Physicians to Despair

"Silencing a scream" is how **M.J.** describes his way of dealing with drastic tapering down of his opioid, without his permission. Feeling "abandoned" by his physician, and his below-pain-relieving pills not helping, "Despair is all I feel. Terror and despair."

Chapter Five

ON OxyCONTIN: Physicians Refute Vilification of Purdue Pharma

According to at-large Medscape writer, George D. Lundberg, MD, who lectured on the dangers of various drugs in 1970s California and about "the medical, advertising, and pharmaceutical industries hawking [of] Valium® (diazepam), Librium® (chlordiazepoxide), and like agents to a frail, gullible public," the Sackler brothers, Arthur Sackler, MD, Mortimer Sackler, MD, and Raymond Sackler, MD, principals of OxyContin® (extended-release oxycodone) manufacturer, Purdue Pharma, are sleazily responsible for much of the medical and human chaos currently swirling around two very divergent groups: addicts using illicit drugs and normal patients in pain taking prescribed opioids responsibly.

Note: Nowhere does Dr. Lundberg acknowledge the questionable prescribing of **Suboxone®** (buprenorphine/naloxone), a morphine analog product. Its **buprenorphine**, derived from the opioid alkaloid thebaine, is 25 to 40 times more potent and a longer lasting analgesic than morphine. It appears to act as a partial agonist at mu and kappa opioid receptors and as an antagonist at delta receptors supposedly salubrious for detoxing addicts, a medical indication which is currently highly questionable. (Read about the **"The Suboxone Hoax"** in Chapter 20.) What's worse is that Suboxone proponents (over the 17 years Suboxone has been falsely touted as a miracle detox agent) have forced into detox facilities Intractable Pain Patients, after nonconsensual *cold-turkeying*, to up their Suboxone prescribing censuses in Suboxone clinics across the country. Such unethical medical conduct continues despite the lack of evidence that this product actually produces pain relief for chronic pain. Perhaps its proponents forgot that its naloxone component could well cancel out the analgesic effect of the buprenorphine.

Conflation of Street Addicts' Self-Drugging Behaviors with Chronic Pain Patients' Normal Use of Prescription Narcotics

What Dr. Lundberg does not address (in his blanket dismissal of prescriptions for narcotic medications) is the conflation of Street Drug Addicts' behaviors – addictions, overdosings and deaths – with the legitimate prescribing of, and healthful, long-term use of narcotics by Intractable Pain Patients (IPPs). This widespread, inflammatory misinformation, by gossip-hungry nonmedical "journalists," who've been mixing street addicts into the same category as safely- and successfully-treated Intractable Pain Patients, as a result of the CDC's ill-designed and irresponsible 2016 *Guideline*, has created a nationwide hysteria leading to witch-hunts by DEA zealots targeting empathic pain-treating physicians, intimidating them into not treating pain patients at all.

Instead, Dr. Lundberg credits Dr. Arthur Sackler as "a creative marketing genius who virtually invented modern medical marketing [influencing] physicians to prescribe specific drugs via advertising and promotion, and was wildly successful." He goes on to lament that most of his income, as Editor of *JAMA (The Journal of the American Medical Association)* between 1982 and 1999, came indirectly from medical journal advertising "largely influenced by the methods of Arthur Sackler."

The Supposed Villain, OxyContin® (extended release oxycodone)

Dr. Lundberg goes on to excoriate the Purdue Pharma wealthy Sackler brothers and their descendants, as well as Big Pharma in general, lawmakers, and the FDA (Food and Drug Administration) for their impotence against a misperceived OxyContin® glut. Growing ultra-dramatic, he equates the Sacklers' activities with those of drug honcho, El Chapo.

Many physicians responded to this broadside. What follows are some excerpted commentaries.

Anesthesiologist Peter Lucas, MD: "I am so tired of the relentless vilifications of pharmaceutical companies. OxyContin has relieved the pain and suffering of countless patients....Drug reps must promote their drugs honestly according to the best science at that time....We have learned new things about narcotics. That does not render older promotional (and prescribing) activities as suddenly evil."

Psychiatrist David Behar, MD: "Pain patients are not overdosing. Addicts are, from Chinese fentanyl. It is available by the kilo on the regular web, for $3000."

Psychiatrist Paul Leber, MD: "Let's look at the facts. Opioids are legally marketed drug products. The therapeutic benefits of opioids are indisputable....Promoting a lawfully marketed drug product is not a crime; selling illegal narcotics is. George Lundberg surely is aware of the critical distinction."

Internist Jeffrey Rosen, MD: "In practicing addiction medicine, by far the amount of medical prescribing ending in addiction is very low down on the list. Most of my patients had issues predating the release of OxyContin®."

Obstetrician/Gynecologist Olu Ogunsanwo, MD: "How come we don't have recriminations of this decibel level about alcohol usage and its manufacturers?"

Nephrologist Subramanya Santhanam, MD: "I would compare advertisements for Alcohol and Tobacco, which we know are injurious to health....It is ludicrous to suggest that pharma industries are violating some form of ethical code and be silent on other products that cause equal, if not greater harm."

Family Medicine Practitioner Kurt Elward, MD: "...to equate Big Pharma with a murderous illegal drug lord is inappropriate. Their products were FDA-cleared. Their studies published in major, peer-reviewed journals like *JAMA*. The medical community, major specialty societies, NCQA [the National Committee for Quality Assurance] and the Feds all signed onto the "Fifth Vital Sign". [PAIN has been designated the Fifth Vital Sign, on a par with Pulse, Blood Pressure, Temperature, and Respirations.]

Finally, considering the burgeoning assignments of Intractable Pain Patients to Suboxone® clinics, for detox, instead of for narcotic analgesia, assuring a cash-cow influx of desperate pain victims (for whom this detox product is ineffective against their pain), note Dr. Kraus' warning about the greedy Suboxone proponents:

Anesthesiologist Don Kraus, MD: "Can you say 'Addiction Industry'. Can you say 'Suboxone Stock'?"

Chapter Six

The Epidemic of Death from Pain Patients' Reduced Health and Suicides Due to Physician Intimidation by Government

Doctors are running scared because of U.S. federal overreach. Thus, many have decided, actually have felt forced to retire to avoid gestapo-style scrutiny, DEA office raids, DEA seizing of patients private records, DEA phoning them with the temerity of discussing medication dosages and hinting at the danger these victim-doctors are in dare they prescribe appropriately for their Intractable Pain Patients.

Yes, There is definitely an epidemic that the Centers for Disease Control and Prevention (CDC) is, ironically, the cause of. It's an epidemic of death. Due to suicides of patients abandoned to zero narcotic analgesia after years, even decades, safely pain-relieved on such medications. Despite that glaring fact, the CDC has been aware of for the three years since it inflicted its ominous *Guideline* on America's severely ill pain patients and their clinicians, these stubborn miscreants continue to lack the decency and conscience to cancel this document in order to reverse all the horror it and they have wrought.

All this terrible torture of innocent pain patients due to an outright lie by government officials, bureaucrats without a heart. This fact counters all the misinformation they've created the national opioid hysteria about: While narcotic prescriptions have continued to decrease, illicit drug deaths continue to rise. Which means that prescription opiates and opioids are not the problem.

Despite that truth, the falsehood that drug addict deaths are from prescription narcotics, spewed forth to the media and metastasized far and wide to the public, continues to cause terrible damage to millions of American pain patients' lives, to their families, to our economy, and to the medical profession. And so, the phony CDC statistics and DEA oligarchic actions continue to invade patients' privacies, physicians' medical practices, imprison doctors in criminal jails, imprison once job-holding pain patients in homebound, often bedbound jails.

When do these high-and-mighty autocrats get toppled from their disastrous realms? Who in our nation will step forward and rescue these pain patients at death's door – from progressively deteriorating health, final decline, and death – many to suicide? And who will apologize to and rescue those clinicians whose ethical prescribing of narcotics for their pain-illness patients has landed them in prison? Who will apologize to them for ruining their careers and their lives? How very low America has stooped!

Don't Believe the 'Prescription Overdose' Lie

And, not only has the CDC fooled around with overdose death statistics, fooled around with pain patients lives by their nutty underdosing requirements of only 90MME (morphine milligram equivalents), fooled the DOJ and its DEA into persecuting and prosecuting pain management physicians, fooled journalists about who's really dying in the streets, they've criminally colluded with the DEA's negligence by diverting its attention from its interdiction and arresting duties, from the real perpetrators.

And the CDC (Centers for Disease Control and Prevention? Really?) has done zero to rehab and psychiatrically commit street drug addicts who are unable to make rational decisions about their own self-care. That's an epidemic they should be attending to. All the while, though, these so-called "disease preventers" have let flourish burgeoning populations of addicts, sick on adulterated fentanyl, on fentanylized heroin, and on assorted mixtures of impure benzodiazepines and alcohol. Not to mention the use of yet another morphine, purportedly "to detox" such addicts. Surprise! It's Suboxone® (buprenorphine/naloxone). (See Chapter 20, "The Suboxone Hoax".)

Baffling how the population of drug addicts keeps growing, and their death tolls keep rising, despite all the Suboxone® (buprenorphine/naloxone) available by prescription around the country. But that's an additional story which I discuss in greater detail in Chapter 21, "Hidden Agendas of Anti-Opioid Proponent$".

Right now, American pain patients are dropping dead like flies from suicides caused by the CDC's callousness and irresponsibility. These people's motives for torturing millions of Americans need to be investigated. Stat! Hint, "advisors" of the specifics in the 2016 *CDC Guideline* have had ties to Big Pharma, even more specifically to Indivior–a subsidiary of Reckitt Benckiser, manufacturer of Suboxone®–surprise, surprise! Astoundingly, adjudicated in July of 2019, in U.S. vs. Reckitt Benckiser for "false advertising" of Suboxone products, RB will pay America $1.4 billion.

Physicians for Responsible Empathic Prescribing (PREP) – That should be the name of an organization countering all these government scare tactics, demonstrating the determined, ethical and empathic actions physicians are sworn to by The Hippocratic Oath. Even society's highest regarded professionals, the physicians among us, are daily victimized by a deaf, dumb and intransigent autocracy based at HHS, the CDC, the DOJ and the DEA. Linked together in a diabolical cabal, determined to rout those patients too sick to fight back due to their life-limiting painful disabilities, just managing to hold a job, barely able to be sociable, unable to live full lives – from their modest equanimities, or kill them off due to suicides. How dare they live lives of quiet desperation, their pain somewhat modulated by prescription narcotic medication? How dare they? Such is the mindset of intellectually- and empathically-challenged cold turkeys at this alphabet soup of federal agencies.

Marilyn Singleton, MD, JD, writing as President of the Association of American Physicians and Sugeons, cautions the Chief Medical Officer of Health and Human Services, Vanila Singh, MD on March 15, 2019, referring to a Task Force convened to address the harsh results of the 2016 *CDC Guideline*: "...too often...past robotic, top-down policies resulted in harm to patients....Now, the current shift to deterrence is improperly punishing pain patients and those trying to care for them. That is why....restoring the primacy of individual patients' interests is key to solving the issues the task force is addressing."

"The report also makes another important observation...published in early 2018. 'Illicit fentanyl-related overdoses are now a leading cause of overdose deaths in the United States. Blaming doctors and pain patients for the surge in opioid deaths is misplaced and diverts resources from addressing the true culprits complicit in the increased deaths.' It is encouraging to see that the Task Force is acknowledging these facts."

Dr. Singleton goes on to point out ancillary problems patients encounter with their pharmacists and their health insurers: Both pharmacies and health insurance companies often steer patients away from alternative medicines; and insurers feel emboldened by CDC and DEA actions, refusing to reimburse patients or pay clinicians for alternative pain relief medications or physical treatments.

There are physician problems with Medicare which also limits or discourages critical pain treatments, narcotic analgesics and ancillary medications. Dr. Singleton suggests, in this letter, that "Steps could include granting Medicare beneficiaries more control over the funds for their care...."

The Nightmare of Invasive Drug Monitoring Programs (PDMPs)

"A final area of concern with the report, writes Dr. Singleton, "is the encouragement for expanding reliance on Prescription Drug Monitoring Programs." She points to a July 2018 report in the *Annals of Internal Medicine* which found "evidence that PDMP implementation either increases or decreases nonfatal or fatal overdoses is largely insufficient....' While the PDMP concept might seem like a helpful tool, extreme caution should be taken when infringing on patient privacy and the patient-physician relationship in this way, especially in light of abuse of the data. For instance, the California Medical Board is mining the data and cross-referencing with death certificates (the 'Death Certificates Project') to improperly initiate discipline against physicians who are doing their best to care for complex patients. **Bureaucrats should not be second-guessing patient care decisions in this manner, or in any manner."**

Dr. Singleton cautions Dr. Singh, the HHS and the CDC, with this statement: "In conclusion, we would like to reiterate our support for the report's emphasis that the needs of individual patients need to remain at the center of patient care decisions and that actions by third parties interfering in the patient-physician relationship need to be minimized and even eliminated."

Section II

PERIL:
The Painful Dangers of the 2016 CDC Guideline

Chapter Seven

Critique of the 2016 *CDC Guideline for Prescribing Opioids for Chronic Pain*

Introduction to the Critique

For at least the last 75 years, nurses and doctors, experienced on a day-to-day basis in the hospital care of variously-afflicted patients, and in the prescribing and administration of narcotics both orally and intramuscularly, have observed the excellent efficacy and value of drugs like the opiates Morphine sulfate and Codeine, and the opioid meperidine (Demerol®) - some of the narcotic class of hospital-prescribed analgesics - and their excellent capacities to subdue intolerable pain. However, because in the early part of this 21st Century, overdose deaths of illicit drug addicts were rising, alarming health officials of government agencies, something odd overtook common-sense thinking and obscured the substantive body of medical knowledge about pain and its amelioration well-embraced by specialist physicians in Pain Management for generations.

Generally, the pain management subspecialty is practiced by highly skilled anesthesiologists, physicians who know about pain mechanisms from rendering patients unconscious in the Operating Room, to "twilight" anesthesia states, and more. These specialists are skilled in treating Herpes zoster attacks (aka "shingles) and its aftermath, postherpetic neuralgia, a years-long, even lifelong, affliction that attacks various segments of the spinal cord producing severe pain in sites innervated by the viral-afflicted nerves. There are various medications to treat this horribly painful chronic illness, including opioids. Herpes zoster is but one example of a dire, pain-suffering illness that requires powerful analgesia. In Chapter One, I discuss other diseases, afflictions and injuries that also demand similar specific and strong narcotic care.

All of a sudden, in 2016 — despite extensive medical profession awareness of that awfully painful affliction, and of many other severe, unendingly painful disorders — illicit addict deaths had so unnerved the powers that be that, nonsensically, they, in the guise of government do-gooders, decided to dump sick-in-pain patients into the drug addict category, thereby ruining many chronic pain patients' lives by forcing the denial of opioid medications. Such untreated pain is still causing rapid declines in physical health leading to early deaths. These would be avoidable if such patients were allowed to continue on their usual opioid analgesic regimen.

Suicides due to Despair from Untreated Intractable Pain

Sadly, too, these severe restrictions on opioid medications, have been sending many pain-filled others on a journey out of this world by suicide due to despair of ever feeling relief. Such pain patients–who had managed to hold jobs, take care of their homes and families, because their narcotic analgesics allowed them some modicum of a quality of life and maneuverability–would now be confined to bed, unable to work, dependent on government funds (often on Disability) to scrape by. But always in insufferable pain because a handful of bureaucrats made a terrible, unempathetic decision to limit pharmaceutical manufacturing of narcotics, to cut patients' doses down sharply, and to reduce the number of times patients can take these low doses throughout their pain-filled days. And so, abrupt disruption of millions of pain patients' lives by the return of unrelieved pain continues to cause many to choose suicide.

And those horrendous happenings are occurring because poor-thinking committees, some with questionable "connections," perhaps even behind-the-scenes financial interests, decided to scare our country to death about an "opioid epidemic," elevating this concept into a hysteria that continues to grip our nation. Especially due to the feeding frenzy of media sharks out for a sensational "story," even if it's exaggerated or untrue altogether. Thus, the U.S. Department of Health and Human Services (HHS) via its extension, the Centers for Disease Control and Prevention (CDC) swept legitimate pain patients, long-stabilized on their prescription narcotics, into a crazy maelstrom of unrelated drug addict deaths due to adulterated-fentanyl and fentanylized-heroin.

That, even though these two groups of patients have always had entirely different medical problems and always require entirely different treatments to address them.

Barbarism in Medical Practice

Lately, scarily, this government insanity has extended even more illogically to Emergency Department patients in acute pain and needing "Stat!" relief. And to postoperative patients in acute pain from having had body parts cut, excised, skin sutured, faux body parts implanted, organs removed, etc. All denied a medically appropriate prescription narcotic, or offered an ineffective drug, like Tylenol® (acetaminophen), or nothing. Many surgeons now are telling patients they won't be given an appropriate painkiller postoperatively. As a result, many patients are postponing, not only elective surgeries, but essential surgeries. This is a national crime caused by clueless desk-warmers in government offices, far removed from genuine, clinical patient care, who constructed a misguided "guideline" that continues to mess up millions of pain patients' lives and keeps "murdering" many others whose untreated pain drives them to kill themselves.

Important Abbreviations for the Critique which follows:

ADL	Activities of Daily Living
AHRQ	Agency for Healthcare Research and Quality
BSC	Board of Scientific Counselors
CRPS	Complex Regional Pain Syndrome
DEA	U.S. Drug Enforcement Administration

DoD	U.S. Department of Defense
DOJ	U.S. Department of Justice
ER/LA	Extended Release/Long-Acting
FDA	U.S. Food and Drug Administration
HHS	U.S. Department of Health and Human Services
IPPs	Intractable Pain Patients
MME	Morphine Milligram Equivalents
NCIPC	National Center for Injury Prevention and Control
NIH	National Institutes of Health
NP	Nurse Practitioner
NSAID	Nonsteroidal Anti-Inflammatory Drug (e.g., Aspirin)
OD	Overdose
OGW	Opioid Guideline Workgroup
ORT	Opioid Risk Tool
OUD	Opioid Use Disorder
PA	Physician Assistant
PCP	Primary Care Physician
PDMP	Prescription Drug Monitoring Program
PNB	Peripheral Nerve Block
PRF	Pulse Radio-Frequency Lesioning
QOL	Quality of Life
SNB	Sympathetic Nerve Block
SRG	Stakeholder Review Group
TENS	Transcutaneous Electrical Nerve Stimulation
UDT	Urine Drug Test
VA	U.S. Department of Veterans Affairs
VHA	Veterans Health Administration

Critiquing the 2016 *CDC Guideline*

Well-Intentioned "Guideline" or Hidden No-Opioid Agenda?

I carefully read every nook and cranny of the *CDC Guideline for Prescribing Opioids for Chronic Pain* (from here on, I will refer to it as the 2016 *CDC Guideline*). In sum, it purports to "provide recommendations for primary care clinicians who are prescribing opioids for chronic pain outside of active cancer treatment, palliative care, and end-of-life care and addresses opioid prescribing from initiating, continuing, selection of which opioid, what dosage, duration of use, follow-up and discontinuing of such treatment". It further claims, "This guideline is intended to improve communication between clinicians and patients about the risks and benefits of opioid therapy for chronic pain, improve the safety and effectiveness of pain treatment, and reduce the risks associated with long-term opioid therapy...." Unfortunately, as will be elaborated upon further on in this book, what this "guideline" has perpetrated on Intractable Pain Patients (and even, now, on Acute Emergency Patients and Postoperative Patients) is denial of any narcotic analgesic prescriptions altogether. This without the consent of the IPP patient to taper or cold turkey off their long-time highly effective opioid painkiller. Such patients falling victim to abrupt tapering to sub-analgesic levels, sudden cold-turkeying to dangerous withdrawal illness and mortality risk. And many pain patients, hopeless about ever getting any pain relief whatsoever ever again, are still killing themselves. These are not the outcomes any nurse or doctor would ever inflict on a patient. But the CDC "expert" bureaucrats are behaving oblivious to these sufferings and deaths.

On the surface, the 2016 *CDC Guideline*, by whoever brought all its varied elements together, appears to reflect a genuine concern for the well-being of patients, which should be the primary focus for any registered nurse and medical doctor caring for patients in pain. But there are huge caveats implicit therein. For example, the following quote seems to describe the true intent of this Guideline: "Pain might go unrecognized [putting varied vulnerable patients like elderly, cognitively-challenged, and ethnic minorities] at risk for inadequate pain treatment." Also, persistent pain can be poorly controlled. This introduction goes on to appear to empathize with the many "consequences associated with chronic pain including limitations in complex activities, lost work productivity, reduced quality of life....emphasizing the importance of appropriate and compassionate patient care. Patients should receive appropriate pain treatment...."

Further, the CDC defines chronic pain as that lasting over 3 months or beyond normal tissue-healing time. And, according to this guideline, "...researchers estimate that 9.6-11.5 million adults, or approximately 3%-4% of the adult U.S. population, were prescribed long-term opioid therapy in 2005." It goes on to describe "OUD" (Opioid Use Disorder), a fancy, language-police name for "illicits addict" with its dire overdose and mortality risks. The latter having zero to do with the need for potent analgesia for chronic pain, and potent analgesia for severe, acute pain and for postop pain (when a surgeon's scalpel has a few hours earlier just cut through a patient's skin, into an organ, excised an organ or a tumor, implanted a heart valve, secured a hip replacement, etc. And for certain dental pain, like root canal surgery.

Professed Guideline Intentions and Seeming Concern for IPPs, but IPP Reality is Dire

Those 2016 *CDC Guideline* pronouncements fly in the face of cold reality. The rampant, sudden cold-turkeying, sudden tapering without patient consent, sudden dismissal of Intractable Pain Patients from clinical care, pharmacies refusing to fill legal narcotic prescriptions—written by those physicians, so far unscathed by DEA raiders, who are still willing to prescribe an opioid for them—and forced referrals of IPPs to rehab or Suboxone® (buprenorphine/naloxone) clinics (See Chapter 20, "The Suboxone Hoax"), all cause doubt about the weak retrospective *mea culpas* by the CDC.

To add insult to injury, more pain, suffering, time-wasting and expense – forced unnecessary doctor appointments, unnecessary urine tests for drugs, extra transportation costs and total life upheavals, further punish pain patients now viewed suspiciously, and labelled drug addicts. This is abhorrent, cruel and the height of medical malpractice. Not only are they now refused normal narcotic medications that have sustained them in a modicum of liveable life quality for years, often decades, they are now stigmatized, humiliated, abandoned, untreated. Excellent reasons to kill the ill-conceived 2016 *CDC Guideline*.

What the Guideline Purports to Accomplish vs. What the Guideline Perpetrates

It says, "This guideline provides recommendations for the prescribing of opioid pain medication by primary care clinicians for chronic pain (i.e., pain conditions that typically last more than 3 months or past the time of normal tissue healing) in outpatient settings outside of active cancer treatment, palliative care, and end-of-life care. Although **the guideline does not focus broadly on pain management**, appropriate use of long-term opioid therapy must be considered within the context of all pain management strategies...." By which, what is meant is use of other, less effective strategies and mild, over-the-counter drugs that barely nick intractable pain at all.

This has turned out to be a hustle of mixed up "meanings" by the CDC which has befuddled physicians at the frontlines of pain patient care. Even the CDC itself reports that PCPs are worried about the complexities of taking on the care of IPPs. And that all these proscriptions and procedures and excess paperwork and patient-opioid contracts complicate their primary medical practices and jeopardize the time they have to care for all their other patients who don't suffer intractable pain. Furthermore, the introduction to the guide professes to offer clarity where it obfuscates and implicitly accuses physicians of misprescribing. It does warn, however, of the extra dangers posed by co-prescribing of a benzodiazepine like Xanax® (alprazolam) with an opioid. The latter combination more risky, more likely to lead to overdosing and OD death.

Moreover, the 2016 *CDC Guideline* makes it clear that it's not to be adhered to by patients in treatment for cancer, in palliative care, and end-of-life care. It also bows to the expertise of anesthesiologists, dentists and hematologists in the judicious use of opioids in their specialty practices. Particularly, too, to the pain management of Sickle Cell Crises in the care of hematologists. Nonetheless, implicit by the militant tactics loosed upon narcotic-prescribing physicians in America these days,(See Section III, **POLICE STATE AMERICA** ...DEA invasions of narcotic-prescribing doctors' offices), bureaucrats, federal police, and even State politicos have morphed into maniacal militants, hunting down doctors treating pain patients, destroying their lifelong work, throwing them into legal debt, simply because they dared to be high-quality, ethical, empathic physicians to their suffering patients.

Questionable Affiliations of Unreliable "Experts" Condemn the Guideline's Recommendations

Reportedly, by the CDC itself, recommendations from various clinical, scientific and government experts "...focused on determining when to initiate or continue opioids for chronic pain; opioid selection, dosage, duration, follow-up, and discontinuation; and assessing risk and addressing harms of opioid use." For the Guideline's integrity, the CDC asserts, it initiated a tiered review process obtaining input from the general public and affected stakeholders. And, the CDC also claims to have generated input from a wide range of experts. The problem is, however, though these varied "experts" were vetted for any financial conflicts or questionable allegiances that could compromise their input and advice, there are some "experts," still in strong advisory positions (even some from a position of anti-opioid zealotry against opioid medications for pain patients) like Andrew Kolodny, MD and his co-zealots whose backgrounds are starkly questionable enough to have excluded them from participating in creating the 2016 *CDC Guideline* that has swiftly turned into a battering ram against pain-treating physicians and patients suffering pain. (See Chapter 21, "Hidden Agendas of Anti-Opioid Proponent$")

The pressure-full presence of PROP (Physicians for Responsible Opioid Prescribing) members, like Dr. Kolodny, Dr. Jane Ballantyne, and others, refutes the CDC's claim to a measure of neutrality or even fairness in assessing the pertinent issues and in recommending appropriate procedures and prescribing principles for Intractable Pain Patients.

Morphed into Mandate: Making Law While Pretending the Guideline is Only a Guideline

Various federal agencies reviewed the Guideline, as did the Stakeholders Review Group (SRG) which was made up of members of professional associations of those specialists which usually prescribe opioids such as Physical Medicine, Rehab, Pain Medicine and hospital groups focusing on pain management and opioid prescribing. The CDC claims to have taken all these varied replies from these varied "stakeholders" into consideration when evolving the Guideline. I doubt that, considering the searing results inflicted on the Intractable Pain Patient population (which makes up millions of Americans nationwide) since the Guideline was released to the public for physicians to implement.

The CDC Claims to have Elicited "Public Comment" to "guide" MDs

Published in the Federal Register (80 FR 77351), its principals requested public comment, the comment period ending January 13, 2016. The CDC claims to have received 4,350 general public comments from patients, doctors, medical organizations, academia, state and local governments and industry. Who knows how many more "comments" would've been sent to the CDC about the Guideline had its call for comments been broadly publicized (like it managed to do about the illicits overdose epidemic)? Really? CDC? You should've received hundreds of thousands, millions of comments had this somewhat covert plan been broadly broadcast.

They claim that "The OGW comprised clinicians, subject matter experts, and a patient representative, with the following perspectives represented: primary care, pain medicine, public health, behavioral health, substance abuse treatment, pharmacy, patients, and research. The CDC also claims that it further sought attributes of appropriate clinical and academic experience, caregiver perspectives and high scientific standing. It further claimed, in the introduction to their specific Guideline, that "The professional credentials and interests of OGW members were carefully reviewed to identify possible conflicts of interest such as financial relationships with industry (?Big Pharma?), intellectual preconceptions, or previously stated public positions. Only, says the CDC, those OGW members whose interests were determined to be minimal were selected. When an activity was perceived as having the potential to affect a specific aspect of the recommendations, the activity was disclosed, and the OGW member was recused from discussions related to that specific aspect of the recommendations, (e.g., urine testing and abuse-deterrent formulations). Additional input was sought from various specialties, from pediatrics to psychiatry to rehab, and from a family member who'd lost someone due to a narcotic overdose. Still, the CDC neglected to recuse Kolodny and his cohorts who clearly have a specific *PROPagenda*, and who work in addictions treatment, a specialty diametrically opposed to opioid relief for patients in pain.

Although this document declares that "Members of the public provided comments at this meeting [the BSC one on January 2016]," there is no discussion of how or if these citizens' concerns were ever taken into account at all. Even so, the pro vote was "unanimous".

Five Clinical Questions were Considered [KQ = Key Question]

KQ1 Opioid Efficacy in long-term use

KQ2 Opioid Risks

KQ3 Comparative Efficacy of ER/LA (Extended-Release or Long-Acting) opioids, dosages, placebos relative to kinds of and etiologies of pain

KQ4 Evaluation of risk-reducing strategies such as urinalysis for drugs, PDMP data, pill counts and abuse-deterrent formulations [The latter could be related to Big Pharma's promotion of naloxone-contaning detox drugs such as Suboxone® (buprenorphine/naloxone).]

KQ5 "The effects of prescribing opioid therapy versus not prescribing opioid therapy for acute pain on long-term use."

This one is definitely "key" because some of the effects have been SUICIDES.

As to the above, the CDC reports that its focus was on the efficacy of opioid therapy in long-term prescribing, greater than a year and on the therapeutic or other outcomes relative to each patient's pain, function and quality of life "to ensure that findings are relevant to patients with chronic pain and long-term opioid prescribing." There was no attempt to evaluate the already known uses and benefits of short-term opioid therapy.

More than a Century of Opioid Efficacy Ignored by the 2016 *CDC Guideline*

The introduction to the actual Guideline itself is dense with asserted clinical and research "proofs" such as "...evidence on long-term opioid therapy for chronic pain outside of end-of-life care remains limited, with insufficient evidence to determine long-term benefits versus no opioid therapy, though evidence suggests risk for serious harms that appear to be dose-dependent. [which] supplement findings from previous review of the effectiveness of opioids for adults with chronic noncancer pain." I say, "What?" Thus, on efficacy, for KQ1, the guideline introduction claims insufficient evidence for opioid efficacy, of course ignoring at least a century of analgesic effectiveness clinically with narcotic analgesics.

Then the KQ2 "harms" segment reports that the greatest risk for prescription opioid addiction is in pain patients who previously had an OUD, aka with a drug addiction. Depressed patients and those on any psychiatric medications are also at risk. Various potential side effects are listed which pale compared to non-opiate treatment and the suffering from nonstop pain.

As to KQ3 considerations, comparative efficacies, there's a complex discussion referencing long-acting or extended-release formulations and favoring methadone over morphine for presumed safety considerations. It goes on to disclose: "However, a new observational study found methadone associated with increased risk for overdose versus sustained-release morphine among Tennessee Medicaid patients." From this, combined with conflicting results from other studies, the CDC concludes that "The observed inconsistency in study findings suggests that risks of methadone might vary in different settings [and that] more research is needed to understand factors associated with safer methadone prescribing."

Very Disappointing Results of Poor Quality Studies on Tapering and Cold-Turkeying

Importantly, though, "...evidence on the comparative effectiveness of opioid tapering or discontinuation versus maintenance, and of different opioid tapering strategies, was limited to small, poor-quality studies." This latter is a huge red flag that should be a clear warning to clinicians who are cold-turkeying or tapering Intractable Pain Patients who've been stable, working, and living a semblance of a normal life along with their crippling disabilities, on long-term opioid medications that have modulated their pain so they can manage some QOL each day. And the CDC reports that ORTs cannot be relied upon because evidence of their value is "sparse".

Then, in the KQ4, risk-reducing strategies category, "No study evaluated the effectiveness of risk mitigation strategies [including patient education, urine drug tests, more frequent monitoring, pill counting or abuse-deterrent formulae which might demonstrate] improving outcomes related to overdose, addiction, abuse, or misuses."

As to the KQ5 concerns on any association between opioid analgesia for acute pain and that for chronic pain, the CDC asserts that there is no evidence that postop opioid therapy results in addiction.

Other Treatment Approaches for IPPs are Less Dependable than Opioids

The overture to this 2016 *CDC Guideline* mentions other possible treatments Intractable Pain Patients might benefit from. But please put the accent on the word "might". These include, as discussed in Chapter 2, psychotherapy, physiotherapy, NSAIDs (e.g., aspirin), acetaminophen, low-dose antidepressants for their known analgesic properties, and some anticonvulsants. Each of these categories, it must be stressed, holds potential financial gains for anyone who owns such businesses and/or products. So it's needless to point out why each of such entities would enjoy an extra boost of patients from the chronic pain market, heretofore inaccessible to them because a high percentage of Intractable Pain Patients are stabilized on their opiate or opioid formulation and may not need those other services or products. Ergo, an IPP stabilized on a long-term narcotic, living a reasonable quality of life, with an ability to hold down a job, must never be forced off what has been working successfully for them, in order to accommodate other financially-interested parties for their "therapies". Note, too, according to this 2016 *CDC Guideline*'s introduction, there are faults with so-called "alternative treatments" and lesser drugs: "CBT [cognitive-behavioral therapy] that trains patients in behavioral techniques and helps patients modify situational factors and cognitive processes that exacerbate pain has small positive effects on disability and catastrophic thinking." And, nonsteroidals like acetaminophen can negatively affect liver or kidney function in certain patients.

Co-Prescribing Opioids with Benzodiazepines or Other Psychoactive Drugs Can Be Problematic

When prescribing antianxiety medications (or other psychotropics) in conjunction with an opioid, drug purity and dosage accuracy are assured with clinician prescriptions of FDA-approved narcotics from a known pharmaceutical manufacturer. However, illicits drug deaths, often attributed to such combinations, have "hidden dimensions": Most are due to adulterated, excessively high-potency fentanyl or fentanylized heroin.

And many of these, at autopsy, have alcohol and other impure substances in their blood. Therefore, federal, state and municipal health agencies need to differentiate between illicit combinations upping opioid-related mortality rates and carefully document the vast statistical differences between those drug addict mortalities and, perhaps, accidental combinations by unschooled chronic pain patients and/or by MDs..unaware of the additive or cumulative effects of such combinations.

What the 2016 *CDC Guideline* says about that, "Regarding specific opioids and formulations... there are serious risks of ER/LA opioids, and the indication this class of medications is for management of pain severe enough to require daily, around-the-clock, long-term opioid treatment in patients for whom other treatment options are ineffective, not tolerated, or would be otherwise inadequate to provide sufficient management of pain."

Furthermore, the Guideline warns: "Regarding co-prescription of opioids with benzodiazepines, epidemiologic studies suggest that concurrent use of benzodiazepines and opioids might put patients at greater risk for potentially fatal overdoses. Three studies of fatal overdose deaths found evidence of concurrent benzodiazepine use in 31% -61% of decedents." Importantly, though, reader be alert to drug-seeking behavior—atypical for well-controlled intractable pain in opioid-treated pain patients—which the CDC reports "...those whose deaths were related to opioids were more likely to have obtained opioids from multiple physicians and pharmacies than decedents whose deaths were not related to opioids." It's important to be aware however, too, that certain patients are at greater risk from opioid harms. These include those with sleep disorders that affect oxygen intake, kidney or liver disease, the elderly more subject to falling, pregnant women, and those with psychiatric diagnoses including drug addicts.

Risks of UnderPrescribing: Inadequate Control of Pain

Harms to Intractable Pain Patients, the 2016 *CDC Guideline* acknowledges, could come from "...overestimation of risk, which could lead to inappropriate clinical decisions" such as underprescribing with inadequate pain control.

From the 2016 *CDC Guideline*, "Concerns have been raised that prescribing changes such as dose reduction might be associated with unintended negative consequences, such as patients seeking heroin or other illicitly obtained opioids....With the exception of a study noting an association between an abuse-deterrent formulation of OxyContin® and heroin use, showing that some patients in qualitative interviews reported switching to another opioid, including heroin, for many reasons, including cost and availability as well as ease of use." The 2016 *CDC Guideline* did not identify studies evaluating these potential outcomes.

The Case for Making Naloxone Widely Available

Importantly, according to the 2016 *CDC Guideline*, "...naloxone distribution through community-based programs providing prevention services for substance users has been demonstrated to be associated with decreased risk for opioid overdose death at the community level."

The Real Epidemic is DRUG ADDICTION TO ILLICITS

Therefore, according to the 2016 *CDC Guideline*, "Regarding the effectiveness of opioid use disorder treatments, methadone and buprenorphine for opioid use disorder have been found to increase retention in treatment and to decrease illicit opioid use among patients with opioid use disorder involving heroin....some studies suggest that effectiveness is enhanced when psychosocial treatments...are used in conjunction with medication-assisted therapy; for example, by reducing opioid misuse and increasing retention during maintenance therapy, and improving compliance after detoxification." It's important to note, here, that buprenorphine, the morphine component in Suboxone(R), has been diverted by some addicts in detox for sale to other addicts.

And that it's claimed detox benefit is now seriously questioned. (See Chapter 20, "The Suboxone Hoax".)

The CDC Demotes Physicians to Medical Kindergarten, Interferes with Quality Medical Practice and Harms Pain Patients

The 2016 *CDC Guideline* states, "Many physicians lack confidence in their ability to prescribe opioids safely, to predict or detect prescription drug abuse, and to discuss abuse with their patients. Although clinicians have reported favorable beliefs and attitudes about improvements in pain and quality of life attributed to opioids, most consider prescription drug abuse to be a 'moderate' or 'big' problem in their community, and large proportions are 'very' concerned about opioid addiction and death."

Inconceivably, time-consuming procedures for doctors and their patients include the PDMPs, urine tests, electronic medical records and the stress on clinicians' practices, overburdened with these cumbersome, time-eating requirements, interfering with the care of non-pain patients in their practices. The CDC, in effect, claims that doctors are overworked and undereducated. The latter is an insult to these high-quality physicians. The former is caused by CDC- and DEA-imposed mountains of needless paperwork, spying by DEA police on patients' prescriptions, even on other medications unrelated to pain care, via the PDMPs, and the brazen federal and state government interferences, in pain patient care and opioid prescribing, by nonmedical bureaucrats. How did these unthinking rules-and-regulations interlopers manage to impose this document of stupidity, the 2016 *CDC Guideline*, on American patients in pain and on their diligently empathic, knowledgeably prescribing physicians?

The CDC on the U.S. Economic Burden of Pain Patients' Opioid Treatments

"Risk mitigation," asserts the 2016 *CDC Guideline*, can be expensive to the economic well-being of the country. Which includes urine testing for drugs (as though pain patients are secretly addicts), and far too many other procedures. Costs, reported since 2010, have been between $20 billion and $55 billion for strategies monitoring "drug abuse". In 2012, in contrast, "expenses for outpatient prescription opioids" were a mere $9 billion.

It appears to me that mitigating pain can, not only help Intractable Pain Patients, but will also minimize economic pressures from the healthcare segment that treats pain effectively. And, by providing naloxone to street addicts and their companions, overdosing catastrophes and mortalities can be prevented.

Finally: The Infamous "RECOMMENDATIONS": The takeaway from the Notorious 2016 *CDC Guideline*

As CDC operatives would later claim, the meat of their 2016 *CDC Guideline* was merely meant as a "recommendation" and was really only aimed at primary care clinicians who (apparently, nonmedical federal bureaucrats presume) are medically-educationally deficient and unschooled in pharmaceuticals and in the general knowledge of, and treatment of, various forms of pain. Therefore, their brazen assumptions wrong, they relied heavily on vested interests. Those, in the persons of powerful anti-opioid zealots feeding the "recommendations" with a thinly-veiled agenda promoting an alternative opioid (Suboxone® (buprenorphine/naloxone) used in the detox of drug addicts and, since the 2016 *CDC Guideline*, being forcibly imposed, by ripping chronic pain patients away from their well-working, nonaddictive medication regimens.

The 2016 *CDC Guideline* Focuses on Three Key Issues

One: Determining when to initiate or continue opioids for chronic pain

Two: Opioid selection, dosage, duration, follow-up and discontinuation

Three: Assessing risk and addressing harms of opioid use within these three categories are the **"Recommendations"**:

Prescribers should only provide opioid therapy if pain and function criteria outweigh opioid risks. (Of course, that makes good sense with any medication, i.e., antibiotics, some people are allergic, etc.). "Patients with pain should receive treatment that provides the greatest benefits relative to risks." Duh! This section goes on to extol alternative nonpharmacologic therapies as adjuvant, not instead of, narcotic relief for pain, despite the fact that earlier in this same document, the CDC does not report superior benefits with these approaches, nor do they guarantee pain relief. In fact, the varied methodologies mentioned seem to be suggesting that professionals ought to divert the pain patient's attention from directly quelling the pain to unguaranteed methods or lesser-analgesic methods... just to avoid narcotic prescribing. Although they do mention some, only some, of the kinds of lifelong conditions that produce intractable pain, i.e., osteoarthritis, low back pain, fibromyalgia, and rheumatoid arthritis.

The 2016 *CDC Guideline* "Recommendations" Zealously Pushes an Anything-but-Opioid Regimen

This section of the 2016 *CDC Guideline* goes on to report that various nonopioid pharmaceuticals may help, including a wide array of unexpected classes of drugs whose primary indications have nothing to do with analgesia (pain relief). These include certain anticonvulsants like Lyrica® (pregabalin) or Neurontin® (gabapentin) recommended for diabetic neuropathy and for postherpetic neuralgia (the aftermath of a severely painful acute attack that often lasts a year, Herpes zoster aka foolishly named "shingles). Both latter drugs, as well as Tegretol® (carbamazepine) can also treat neuropathic pain.

Surprisingly, psychiatric drugs like the categories of tricyclic antidepressants, such as Elavil® (amitriptyline), and the SNRIs (serotonin and norepinephrine reuptake inhibitors) like Wellbutrin® (bupropion), and the SSRIs (serotonin selective reuptake inhibitors) like Zoloft® (sertraline) provide effective analgesia for neuropathic pain disorders, such as diabetic neuropathy and postherpetic neuralgia, but at much, much lower doses than would be effective for the treatment of any psychiatric disorders.

The 2016 *CDC Guideline* cautions, however, that when it comes to the use of NSAIDs (nonsteroidal anti-inflammatory drugs), like Aspirin (acetylsalicylic acid), Advil ® (ibuprofen) and Motrin ® (ibuprofen), these also have their limitations and dangers. Acetaminophen is liver toxic. And most of these NSAIDs can cause blood-thinning leading to bleeding, cardiovascular events, gastritis, and potentially gastric ulcers with the danger of gastric hemorrhage.

A Crazy Statement Buried in these CDC Opioid-Prescribing "Recommendations"

"Although opioids can reduce pain during short-term use [there was] insufficient evidence to determine whether pain relief is sustained and whether function or quality of life improves with long-term therapy." This assertion flies in the face of millions of Intractable Pain Patients who are stabilized, to some level of comfort and function, of relief, so they can keep their jobs, leave their beds, physically ambulate better, are able to participate socially and experience various levels and modicums of a quality of life impossible without their decades-long efficacious prescription narcotic medications.

There is a long-winded CDC instruction demonstrating the CDC's bias toward everything else, despite their own expressed recognition of their limitations, reported in this, their own document – again, physiotherapy, psychotherapy, NSAIDs – anything but what's been working for the Intractable Pain Patient all along. The CDC's blatant bias against effective opioids with lifelong benefits to desperate patients is glaring.

Scaring Intractable Pain Patients Off Well-Working Narcotics

While this document frequently mentions the problems that excessive, unrelenting pain causes, which can trigger emotional and social consequences that result in sadness, depression, hopelessness, as a so-called "guideline," it nevertheless persists in downplaying, or negating altogether, the long-term analgesic value of opioid pain relief. Thus creeps in the first hint of the "recommendations" bias: "...clinicians should consider working with patients to taper and discontinue opioids...."

Then, there is a long section instructing pain-managing physicians on how to scare Intractable Pain Patients about the opioids they are on. And, of course, instruction about having naloxone on hand for overdose reversal.

Furthermore, the 2016 *CDC Guideline* recommends immediate-release opioids instead of ER/LA (extended-release/long-acting). ER/LA opioids include methadone, transdermal fentanyl and extended-release versions of other opioids such as oxycodone, oxymorphone, hydrocodone, and morphine. ER/LA formulations are deemed more risky for overdose occurrences than immediate-release opioids.

The FDA (Food and Drug Administration) Chimes in

The FDA, which oversees the use of all prescription drugs marketed to Americans, from scientific discovery to animal studies, to clinical studies, to labeling, to marketing practices, in 2014 recommended that ER/LA "opioids be reserved for 'management of pain severe enough to require daily, around-the-clock, long-term opioid treatment" when all other treatment options are ineffective or untolerated.

Here again, the *2016 CDC Guideline* Hassles Doctors without Surcease

Furthermore, cardiac function should be monitored for patients on methadone and only physicians familiar with the characteristics of methadone as well as of transdermal fentanyl should prescribe these. Duh! Start with the lowest effective dose of whatever opioid you prescribe, the CDC "recommendations" exhort. Doctors know this! And, again, despite living and breathing evidence in Intractable Pain Patients of long-term efficacy, the CDC again exhorts physicians with onerous, detailed instructions about every minute aspect of opioid therapy for long-term pain that is sure to discourage any prescriber, however empathic, from taking on these challenging patients. That's because of the impositions on their office time, added professional concerns, and their concerns about the chronic pain patient. Not to mention the looming cloud, in many doctors' minds: "What are the consequences if I take excellent care of my pain patients, but I don't adhere to these opioid-prescribing minutiae?"

More Onerous "Recommendations" from the 2016 *CDC Guideline:* Tapering

Physicians are implored to taper opioids in patients on high-dose, long-term use: "For patients who agree to taper opioids to lower dosages, clinicians should collaborate with the patient on a tapering plan." Such patients, the 2016 *CDC Guideline* goes on, "...may require very slow opioid tapers as well as pauses in the taper to allow gradual accommodation to lower opioid dosages." But, despite this admonition, what's actually occurring, as a result of the presumption that this mere "guideline" is law, is utter abandonment of such patients altogether, abrupt *cold-turkeying* with denial of further medical care, and tapering without patients' permissions and without consideration for the reduced or lost analgesic efficacy of the lower opioid dosages. The latter often leading to reversal of a reasonable quality of life, regular employment, and well-controlled pain to a life of despair, unemployment, and often bedridden-ness.

Despite It's Professed "Intent," the 2016 *CDC Guideline:* Continues as a Guillotine Against Pain Patients and Pain-Treating Clinicians

The 2016 *CDC Guideline* is onerous in the minutiae it echoes repeatedly throughout the document. Any physician, or other prescribing professional (e.g., Nurse Practitioner, Physician Assistant) could spend a lifetime mastering these insufferable details which, in truth, amount to this admonition and implied threat:

[The following is my version of the effect the 2016 CDC Guideline has had on clinicians since its publication 3 years ago.]

"If you don't refuse opioids to new patients with intractable pain and if you don't taper or cold-turkey those who have been successfully living reasonable qualities of life on an opioid and have been using it responsibly, only as prescribed and safely, you could risk losing your professional license, and thus your beloved career in healthcare practice." Add to that, increasingly, the frequent news stories of doctors' offices being invaded by Drug Enforcement Administration (DEA) gestapo-behaving government police, and you have a sense of what this 2016 *CDC Guideline* has morphed into in the national mind and in the medical mind. And of what it has inflicted on Intractable Pain Patients and their empathic physicians.

Thus, this 2016 *CDC Guideline* document – taken as a sort of "bible" by many physicians, pain clinics, hospitals, emergency departments, surgeons, dentists, health insurers, prescription drug insurers and pharmacists – has ruined once-stabilized pain patients' lives, has caused proliferating suicides by patients despairing of ever being relieved of their once, opioid-well-treated pain, has fostered invasions of patients' private health records (normally HIPAA-protected) with illegal searches via PDMPs, has falsely prosecuted and imprisoned thousands of American clinicians for the awful crime of properly treating pain patients with time-proven opioid medications.

The 2016 *CDC Guideline* is Not Really about Pain Patients' Well-Being

It's always, in the formation of the panels who finagled the 2016 *CDC Guideline* into existence, been about illicits drug addicts and the diversion from attention on deaths from adulterated fentanyl and fentanylized heroin, and the national hysteria this scare-tactic engendered. It's never been about the well-being of all varieties of pain patients, acute, dental, surgical, emergency, chronic, cancer. Thus, it goes on to detail certain specifics relevant to cautions in pregnancy, in the elderly, and in addiction.

The Glaring Mistake: Drug Addicts Mixed in with Intractable Pain Patients

Several sections of the 2016 *CDC Guideline* further focus on an entirely different patient population, addicts. Situating this group of ill patients within the same diagnostic demographic as Intractable Pain Patients is unconscionable and blurs the clear distinction between these two groups – clinically, socially, therapeutically.

Thus, this 2016 *CDC Guideline* has managed to stigmatize non-addicted Intractable Pain Patients—who've theretofore, before the "recommendations," been successfully modulating their pain with their prescription opioids—by conflating illicit drug overdoses with therapeutic successes via long-term opioid treatment.

The only positive in all of this is the caution to avoid prescribing benzodiazpines, such as Valium® (diazepam), together with opioids because of the known risks including mortal overdosings.

NET FEARSOME RESULTS OF THE 2016 *CDC GUIDELINE*

1. Fearful MDs....who, heretofore, successfully managed severe pain for their patients
2. Chronic Pain Patients...Untreated, unbearable, nonstop pain
3. Health Insurers and Drug Insurers...Denial of coverage for opioids and other treatments
4. Pharmacies...illegally refusing to fill legitimate opioid prescriptions
5. Intractable Pain Patients...scorned as "drug seekers" in ER, in pain clinics, in Drug Stores
6. SUICIDES of patients suffering unbearable, untreated pain.

Whatever happened, Doctors (note: many of the 2016 *CDC Guideline* contributors are physicians) to "PRIMUM NON NOCERE"...FIRST DO NO HARM?

The 2016 *CDC Guideline* Coup de Gras, "Low Quality Evidence" Afflicting Pain Patients and their Physicians

Significantly, the 2016 *CDC Guideline* sums itself up like so: "This guideline provides recommendations that are based on the best available evidence that was interpreted and informed by expert opinion. **The clinical scientific evidence informing the recommendations is low in quality.** To inform future guideline development, more research is necessary to fill in critical evidence gaps....CDC will revisit this guideline as new evidence becomes available to determine when evidence gaps have been sufficiently closed to warrant an update of the guideline."

With that, Intractable Pain Patients are the scapegoats of, perhaps some well-meaning, but overall confused scientists and clinicians who contributed to the misconstruction of the misguided 2016 *CDC Guideline*. Confused because they ignorantly chose to interweave patients with one distinct disease, addiction, with the unrelated patient group living (and many now suiciding) with Intractable Pain.

Chapter Eight

Conflation Nation: Patients Needing Pain Relief Differ from Addicts Seeking a "High"

Pain has usually been viewed as a symptom that points to an illness, an injury, a genetic abnormality. Lately, expert pain management clinicians have come to agree that pain should be viewed as a pathology in itself, a disease entity that requires vigorous medical attention and specific analgesic treatment that effectively subdues it. What's more, as mentioned earlier, in the current medical lexicon, Pain is the fifth vital sign added to the time-honored other four: Pulse, Temperature, Blood Pressure and Respirations.

Intractable Pain Patients are Not Drug Addicts

With these simple facts in mind about pain, it's essential to note that neither drug addiction nor alcoholism relate in any way to chronic pain. Nor do pain patients' need to stop the severe, crippling pain that hurts terribly physically, that kills family and social life, forcing the pain patient to be unemployed, and thus, often, crushing emotional stability.

Too Many Journalists have Spread Fallacies about Prescription Painkillers

The widespread fear of legally-prescribed narcotics is not generated from the medical community of physicians, registered nurses and other experienced and knowledgeable clinicians.

Instead, irresponsibly, journalists on a quest for a sensational story have allowed themselves to be flummoxed by anti-narcotic zealots, who comprise a small coterie of special interests. (See Chapter 21, "Hidden Agendas of Anti-Opioid Proponent$".) Sadly, leaders of this group are physicians, some even psychiatrists. You'd think they'd know better. And you'd think they'd want to ameliorate physical pain so it wouldn't escalate to emotional pain, despair and suicides, the latter which has been occurring since the onslaught of the *Guideline*. Instead, unfortunately, this little band of professionals, who had undue influence on the drafting of the CDC's folly, appears immune to the sufferings of patients in pain, to their deteriorating overall health and early deaths when pain goes unrelieved. And unmoved by their suicides when they can no longer endure the physical agony their painful conditions put them through.

The PROPaganda Machine: From Opioid Hearsay to Opioid Hysteria The group, PROP (Physicians for Responsible Opioid Prescribing) is discussed in Chapter 21. Because of the confounding stubbornness of this tiny band of extremists against narcotic pain care, programs like CBS TV's *60 Minutes* recently, and publications across the country, have been emboldened to broadcast and publish these extremists' implicit mantra: "Normal pain patients on opioid analgesics are the same as drug addicts on illicit drugs." And, because of this fallacy, four terrible, glaring happenings have ensued since the unfortunate inception of the 2016 *CDC Guideline*:

1. Patients suffering ordinary levels of pain - acute, ER, postsurgical and dental pain are now denied prescription narcotics and told to manage on an NSAID.
2. Long-term, lifelong Intractable Pain Patients are rapidly tapered with dire effects, or worse yet, suddenly cold-turkeyed with unconscionable effects, or they are severely under-dosed with no relief whatsoever.

3. Drug addicts hooked on illicits continue to access dangerous impure substances, easy prey for dealers, left to fend for themselves without supervision by a negligent DEA and HHS, which should remand them to treatment.
4. Perfectly innocent physicians and other prescribing clinicians have been raided with patients records illegally seized, have been persecuted, prosecuted, and imprisoned. Hundreds of these professionals, across America, are languishing in jail, their assets seized, their lives ruined because of gestapo-DEA tactics, illegal in this democracy, but overlooked by Congress which appears to have, by default, given the DOJ-DEA cabal *carte blanche* with zero oversight to rein in their brazen activities against doctors and pain patients.

Therefore, what has ensued, from the misreporting by medically-naive journalists, who continue to prop up the nonsense spewed by anti-opioid proponents, is the conflation of the problem of addicts dying of adulterated fentanyl or fentanylized heroin with Intractable Pain Patients long-stabilized on their prescription narcotics.

The conflation, thus, has fed back to Gestapo-style DEA raids of physicians' practices (further feeding certain journalists' frenzies), stealing (the DEA calls it "confiscating") doctors' assets, giving ominous "warnings" to legitimate MDs who know medicine, to cease prescribing certain dosages. Like these federal police know medicine? They went to medical school? They know Central Nervous System neurology so they can decide medicinal dosages?

The truth is that 99%, or more, of pain patients prescribed opioid analgesics for long-term or lifelong use never become addicts. The comparable truth is that most addicts acquired their addictions illicitly, not by a physician's prescription.

American Viewpoints are Skewed to Punish Patients in Pain ...and the Impotence of HHS and the DEA against Illicits

Other than cautioning IPPs on a narcotic painkiller to keep one's medicine under lock and key, there's nothing else a pain patient can do to safeguard these medicines. All Americans, therefore, must take the focus off pain patients and, instead, scrutinize the DEA's impotence against illicit imports, street dealers and obvious street-wandering addicts they should, instead, escort straight to a detox facility.

Blaming Pharmaceutical Manufacturers for Drug Addicts' Deaths is Ridiculous.

And suing them is worse because those lost millions could have gone to fresh Research and Development of new medicines to save lives. Citizens should be aware that the FDA signs off on all the science and advertising for every prescription drug. It's up to the FDA to add additional warnings if necessary to the package insert greatly detailing the characteristics of every prescription medication. With any prescription medication marketed: (1) The FDA scrutinizes the science before permitting marketing, (2) The FDA monitors all medical journal advertising and advertising to the public of a drug (3) The FDA removes a dangerous or problematic drug from the market. The volume of lawsuits by federal, state, county and municipal prosecutors may reflect why our medication prices are so high. Many state attorneys-general and federal attorneys appear to enjoy a "feeding frenzy" against pharmaceutical companies, forgetting that they manufacture the antibiotics that save us from bacterial pneumonia, the corticoids that treat asthma, the adrenalin that reverses anaphylaxis, the insulin that keeps diabetics alive, and so forth. They're just killing the opportunities for further research and development of new and better drugs that will help even more stricken patients.

The Trajectory of Tragedy: How the Media have Worsened Life for Pain Patients

Starting immediately, journalists need to be honest, not biased. And get all the facts before disseminating stories that could have a horrible impact on the millions of American pain patients. Right now, this is precisely what the American media's promotion of opioid hysteria and opiophobia has visited on millions of Americans in pain:

- Zero pain relief
- Housebound
- Return to Bedriddenness
- Loss of Employment
- Quality of Life Destroyed
- Despair
- Suicide

Blaming Innocent Pain Patients for Illicit Street-Drug Deaths

False ideas about prescribed painkillers ignores the truth that overdose deaths rarely result from diversion of prescription opioids to the street. Thus, some researchers, responding to the 2016 *CDC Guideline* called its declarations "pseudoscience". In fact, several scientists report that many narcotic fatalities occurred due to methadone or a mixture of a narcotic plus a benzodiazepine (BZD), like Valium® (diazepam) or Xanax® (alprazolam), a class of drugs used in psychiatry to treat anxiety, also known as anxiolytics.

Federal agencies like HHS, CDC, DOJ and DEA, and overstimulated journalists from the American news media, have failed to accurately report the rates of such mixed drug-taking behavior (which also occur with adulterated fentanyl and fentanylized heroin) that would accurately reflect the true cause of the epidemic of stated deaths: Greater numbers of overdose fatalities occur in people taking a BZD with an opioid.

Reported by the National Forensic Laboratory System in 2016, these BZDs most often turned out to be Ativan® (lorazepam), Xanax® (alprazolam), and Klonopin® (clonazepam). Also, alcohol, frequently an additive among addicts, is a mortal danger when used with narcotics. This was demonstrated in cases where, in combination, it was found postmortem with hydrocodone (the generic name of Vicodin® and several other brands), or morphine, or oxycodone (Percodan®, OxyContin® or other brands).

Heroin Metabolizes to Morphine

Always bear in mind, though, that morphine is a metabolite of heroin, first as 6-monoacetylmorphine. If this fact is absent from the consciousness of public health officials, forensic pathologists, and CDC tabulators, for example, they will carelessly attribute these deaths to prescription morphine. Thus escalating to paranoia the false notion that narcotic-prescribing physicians are fueling street fatalities. And the hysteria that Intractable Pain Patients have somehow lost track of their legitimate morphine medications, that their medicine cabinets have been robbed, their contents "diverted to the street". And so goes the canard that opioid prescriptions for Intractable Pain Patients (IPPs) – and, lately, even for postsurgical, acute ER and dental patients – are responsible for the abnormal behaviors of drug addicts using illicits and, thus, for their untimely deaths.

False, too, is the belief by people in power, particularly at the CDC and DOJ/DEA, that prescription narcotics launch people to heroin use. This is known to be rare.

Poisons: The Truth about Illicit Fentanyl and Heroin

Fentanyl deaths are due to tainted fentanyl which, itself, is often more powerful than prescribed fentanyl. Tragically, street fentanyl is sold in pill form which makes it even more highly dangerous, lethal. In fact, it's illegal to sell prescription fentanyl in any but dermal (skin) patches, or lolly pop forms because those allow for slow absorption for pain relief. Fentanyl by pill kills because it acts too rapidly when swallowed. Also, suppliers and dealers have been adding overly potent fentanyl to heroin with deadly results. One wonders how they expect to boost their profits, these dealers, when they're providing a one-time extra high all the way to the Great Beyond for their clueless customers.

It's imperative, also, to point out that the CDC's "statistics" on morphine deaths have been grossly exaggerated or are false altogether. Morphine has been used for decades and decades in acute pain care and palliative care. Safely!

Heroin Metabolizes to Morphine, Skewing Morphine Death Statistics

Therefore, the CDC, by skewing the truth about prescription narcotic analgesics, has distorted the clinical picture of the cause of the much hyped "opioid epidemic".

Heroin, even without a dash of fentanyl added, can be lethal. Note that it's Chemistry 101 for medical clinicians to know that 6-monoacetylmorphine is what's found in the blood, at autopsy, of a heroin overdoser. But, unconscionably, these deaths have been recorded by forensic pathologists, and subsequently by CDC statistics-creators as "morphine deaths," resulting in the inflation of morphine fatalities and in the severe government overreach into the healthcare of both chronic and acute pain patients. And in the militarized raiding of pain management specialists and other physicians offices who dare to care responsibly for their patients in pain.

More Painful Perspectives on the 2016 *CDC Guideline*

Though most of the doomed document's instructions were related to common medical protocols for efficacy and safety, several questionable admonitions are inherent in disputed contents of the *Guideline*. The American Medical Association, as well as oncologic organizations, professional pain associations, and IPPs' organizations raised many issues regarding their specific and dire concerns.

Thus, criticisms abound from these variously focused parties who've come to realize why the birth of this faulty *Guideline* was in the hands of questionable doulas within the Guideline Development Group (GDG). Because, sorrily, that group's priorities were ill-formed. Their emphasis, instead of on patient care and well-being, was on cost controls and concerns for special interests. I'll elaborate on the latter, later, in Chapter 21, "Hidden Agendas of Anti-Opioid Proponent$".

The needs of patients in pain appears to have disappeared from the GDG's awareness. Nonetheless, as nurses and doctors, we know that the patient comes first. That's why they've come to us to help them. Because we have specific knowledge and skills that can help them. And we should have a healthy helping of empathy, or we don't belong in these professions.

Conflating Unrelated Patient Groups Causes Needless Suffering

Addicts overdosing and dying on illicit drugs are markedly different from pain patients. Therefore, the 2016 *CDC Guideline*'s poorly thought-out and narrowly-viewed major therapeutic issues impacting the lives of millions of IPPs deserves much more comprehensive and expansive views of the issues. And requires approaches with the primary objective of keeping the focus on medical relief of intractable pain – and on its related sufferings, acute ER, postop and dental pain. All four of these, traditionally well-handled patient groups, are currently being sacrificed, stripped of their healthcare rights to pain relief. Which is due to the muddled co-mingling of ideas about addicts' deaths from so-called "recreational" drug use all mixed in with normal IPPs with various incurable conditions whose pain is unbearable and which requires narcotic management.

Objections to the 2016 *CDC Guideline* by the Washington Legal Foundation

Out-of-balance "recommendations" drip poisonously from a document supposedly constructed to help millions of patients in pain, but skewed to focus on illicit drug deaths unrelated to pain patient care. Thus, in 2015, before it could take effect, the Washington Legal Foundation requested the proposed *Guideline* be scrapped and redrawn to include pain patient treatment assurances, that medically-accurate protocols for appropriate prescription narcotic analgesics would continue. This was that foundation's worry, then. Their lawyers had been justifiably concerned (as the current opioid hysteria has borne out) about the following problems with the CDC's original draft:

- That persons drafting it were known to favor strong anti-prescribing for pain patients
- That there was nondisclosure, then, of the group's principals' credentials
- That alternative ideas for the *Guideline* were never encouraged, nor adversaries invited to participate in the development of them
- That there were definite conflicts of interest, specifically since the only two purported pain medical doctors were PROP (Physicians for Responsible Opioid Prescribing) members who are vehemently anti-opioid for pain-suffering patients. (See Chapters 20, "The Suboxone Hoax" and Chapter 21, "Hidden Agendas of Anti-Opioid Proponent$".)

Furthermore, one was a consultant to a law firm suing a narcotic manufacturer, and was paid handsomely for this consultancy work. Seems like a cabal of PROP members, including its leader, slithered its way into this working group and had undue influence in the drafting of the 2016 *CDC Guideline.*

Sadly, with the Guideline's anti-pain-patient rhetoric, its one-sided GDG were hell-bent on publishing their misguided document. So they did. Despite everything sensible that made sense to everyone but them. They did this, though many in the entire group are physicians, it seems to me with limited consciences. Empathy lacking for real-life-suffering IPPs.

Thus, the 2016 *CDC Guideline* misguided other chomping-at-the-bit, but medically-ignorant parties – such as most legislators, officials of various agencies, and the DOJ-DEA cabal – which have moved forward with it, implementing it as though it were law, not merely a guideline. Thus this fateful document morphed into fiat.

As fiat, what were masked as "recommendations" have been elevated to federal commandments, law that, if not adhered to, will send Drug Enforcement Administration gestapo invading doctors' offices, prosecuting prescribing physicians, intimidating pharmacies, accusing and stigmatizing normal pain patients as addicts.

Conflating Patients in Pain with Illicit Drug Users

Despite facts, the fiction constricting the treatment of genuine pain sufferers from decades-long, successful prescription narcotic analgesic therapy, arises from that faulty document, misconceived before its birth, warned against by empathic others in law and medicine. And by the huge population of pain-suffering patients. All predicated on the hysterical conflation of illicits addicts' poor choices in their lives that could lead to overdosings and deaths (but which naloxone will reverse in most cases) with the innocents, IPPs who've no recourse but their prescription narcotic analgesics. Of course, there's always suicide, which far too many have opted for and completed in the face of an empathy-less CDC, DOJ, DEA and the zealous anti-opioid adherents.

American Streets Rife with Chinese and Mexican Illicit Drugs

Known is that it's adulterated fentanyl and fentanyl-laced heroin which have become epidemic in American streets. The hysteria, engendered by the exaggerations and hubris of the original GDG, has ignored these facts and propagated erroneous thinking and fear in the media which has infected the public mind, distorting the truth well-known by medical professionals and patients in pain. The victims? Again, IPPs, and now also ER-, postsurgical- , and dental patients. For, recent studies affirm that any existing epidemic does not involve innocent pain patients at all, but happens illicitly, in users of street narcotics concomitantly with benzodiazepines.

Powerful DEA Curtails Legal Narcotic Supplies, Further Harming Pain Patients

Moreso, DEA mandates have reduced availability of prescription narcotic analgesics, shrinking the legal supply, limiting what normal pain patients require for equanimity and some basic quality of life. Now, far too many IPPs are negatively judged by a once caring healthcare system. Hostile attitudes toward them abound. So, in addition to their physical suffering, they must now fend off painful judgments, mean and bullying behaviors never before seen in the supposed empathic healthcare professions. It appears the chain of connection between patient, doctor and regulators has been chopped up, amputated really. No longer can pain patients rely on quality, optimum care and relief of their sufferings.

Zealots against Narcotic Prescribing: Sadly, Some are Physicians

Viewing patients in lifelong pain as one thing, a block of opioid-seeking junkies, has turned some physicians into zealots opposing any treatments that include opioid prescribing. This, despite evidence in many, many cases that IPPs have been on their narcotic medications for decades without self-harm, allowing them some measure of normalcy in family life and work.

We must wonder why these same zealots are unfazed by the Tobacco Epidemic. How come this nation still permits the sale of lethal substances in the forms of cigarettes, cigars, chewing tobacco? And the Alcohol Epidemic. This nation still permits alcohol sales, despite its ruination of imbibers' lives and brains, its destruction of families and the deaths on our highways due to drunk driving. Of course, lets ban food because of the Obesity Epidemic which is widespread (*sic*).

Controlling Severe Pain Still Relies on Centuries-Old Opiates and Opioids

Nothing in the physician's armamentarium, not even interventions like back surgeries, for instance, though often eliminating the pain-causing pathology, surprisingly often does not eliminate the pain generated by the brain habituated to sending pain signals despite the removal of the causative body part. Nor do implantables, Yoga, massage, psychotherapy, etc., measure up to the predictable relief form one's prescription narcotic analgesic.

Ergo, the war on accessibility of prescription opioids for IPPs will not alter the truth, nor will it alter the behaviors of illicit opioid users which costs so many of them their lives. It's time for the CDC to admit its mistake in drafting a so-called "guideline" from a decidedly biased perspective (worrying about saving illicit drug users while sacrificing, to suffering and suicide, innocent pain patients) with zero input from pro-pain-patient pain specialists, nor from burgeoning pain patient groups clamoring for their human rights to live with the least amount of physical suffering as their medicine will allow.

Time to focus separate resources of interdiction, prosecution and imprisonment for suppliers and dealers. And medical resources for illicit drug users by remanding them to detox, to medical and psychosocial recovery.

Time to restore prescription narcotics to IPPs in high enough doses to be truly analgesic, as they were experiencing before this government-fueled insanity. And, also, time to stop denying postoperative patients appropriate narcotics for surgical pain. Time to stop denying acute Emergency Department patients appropriate opioids for their pain. Time to leave dentists alone to prescribe what they know is narcotic-appropriate after certain dental procedures. And, finally, it's time to abandon the CDC's folly, the 2016 *Guideline*. It's caused nothing but tragedies as the following chapters will describe.

Chapter Nine

Dangerous Under-Dosages, Forced-Taperings, and Sudden *Cold-Turkeyings*

Today, millions of Americans in pain are being medically violated: (1) Without warning, chronic pain patients are placed on scientifically unfounded under-dosings of long-time effective prescription opioid medications; or (2) These patients are being rapidly tapered off their dependable opioid analgesics causing great physical and emotional harm as their bodies try to adjust swiftly to drastic medication cuts; or (3) Many such patients are simply being unethically *cold-turkeyed* off their prescription opioid analgesics without recourse, without follow-up resources, without America's healthcare system protecting these unfortunate souls.

Suicide Their Only Option"

Upon the clueless onslaught of the 2016 *CDC Guideline*, more than 66% of 2300 patients surveyed had their prescription narcotic dosages lowered or ended altogether, and without their permission! After which, due to unrelenting, untreated pain , many admitted they were bent on suicide once they realized their doctors seriously meant to continue reducing their opioid dosages or cut them off these analgesics altogether.

Apparently, neither the DEA police raiding pain doctors' practices, nor doctors themselves, were aware that the "Guideline" did not have the force of law. They didn't know it was just a "recommendation" (as CDC operatives would later stress). Thus, once doctors felt disempowered by this federal document, their pain patients reported that they began being embarrassed at their pain clinics, labelled "drug seekers," forced to make extra doctor appointments for urine tests, and many were dropped from treatment altogether. As a result of the latter, many lifelong pain patients were forced to relocate from their home states in order to get appropriate pain treatment.

Patients soon became aware of their physicians' fears of DEA raids, medical license revocations, and increasing imprisonments across America of pain management clinicians. And, as some of their own doctors were arrested and jailed, they were abandoned by the beleaguered medical profession as a whole. Because no other doctors would accept their patients for pain care.

All that despite the fact that, the CDC now claims, its 2016 Guideline was meant only for Primary Care Physicians. Nonetheless, DOJ/DEA operatives have continued, to this day, to clamp down on all doctors, even erudite, experienced, excellent pain specialists, who have the temerity to dare to prescribe appropriate narcotics in patient-specific dosages.

Thus, reportedly of the surveyed group, 70% of thousands of these pain patients had been forcibly tapered or cold-turkeyed altogether, leaving them to deal, alone, with dire narcotic analgesia-dependent symptoms plus their, now, untreated pain. Half of these surveyed responders live with constant thoughts of killing themselves.

Deteriorating Life Quality

Quality of life benefits, that appropriate narcotic prescriptions previously provided, are lost. Now, the rule for IPPs is Homebound, Bedridden, Despair. Where, formerly, they could be employed, socialize a bit, manage some kind of an acceptable existence, now they are frozen in pain, in fear of more pain.

Even Pharmacies are Emboldened to Cancel Opioid Prescriptions

Suddenly discharged from pain treatment by their physicians who're being intimidated by the DEA – the reenactors for the behind-the-scenes

CDC perpetrators – these patients, who've never evidenced addictive misuse of their narcotic analgesics are suffering, grievously. Egregiously, even many of those still getting low doses of their pain prescriptions, often can't get their prescriptions filled by pharmacies which have also misinterpreted the CDC's document as mandate, and which are also being intimidated by the DEA-gone-wild tactics.

Painful, Expensive Procedures as Alternatives to Well-Working Opioids

This story darkens even more when you realize that 41% of surveyed chronic pain patients said their doctors, instead, were attempting to coerce them to submit to questionable implants and painful surgeries instead of letting them have their usual painkillers at their usual well-working dosages. Upon refusing such invasive procedures, these patients report being dropped from their pain care altogether. Their doctors' fears are now palpable and are reflected in their abandoned patients' desperate status – nowhere to turn, no doctor to help, life becomes unbearable.

And all those painful, amoral actions targeting these suffering millions continue to occur, long after the 2016 *CDC Guideline* struck down common sense, because of Federal government cold turkeys who invented opiophobia and opioid hysteria by conflating addicts' illicit drug over-dosings and deaths with normal patients requiring lifelong narcotic pain relief.

Worse, Stefan Kertesz, MD has pointed out that if the pain patient, forced off long-term opioid pain relief, develops emotional symptoms like anxiety, stress, despair, certain zealots against prescription narcotics seek to diagnose them anew as "Opioid Use Disorder" in order to treat them with Suboxone® (buprenorphine/naloxone), Which, Dr. Kertesz stresses "is not supported by diagnostic criteria for addiction". (See Chapters 20 and 21 to understand the *sub rosa* financial motives for anti-opioid crusaders claiming pain patients are "addicts".)

Physicians Abandon Pain Patients as DEA Spying Turns Pain Care into a Nightmare:

Physicians prescribing appropriately for IPPs in dosages individualized for each patient's unique pain condition, began receiving letters from the spying Prescription Drug Monitoring Programs (PDMPs) of their states. Suddenly, for example, a pain patient long stabilized on 400MME (morphine milligram equivalents) per day of his/her opioid, who the DEA insists must be cut to a mere50MME per day, were soon forced to at least a maximum of only 90MME per day.

Spasms, out-of-the-blue sharp pains, unrelenting suffering from various pain conditions, none of millions of patients' algesias put a dent in the poor judgment of nonmedical government officials at the Department of Justice, the Drug Enforcement Administration nor among the HHS/CDC perpetrators of this medical disaster afflicting innocent pain patients.

Because of the threats by DEA spies and aware of DEA gestapo-style raids, many physicians and pain clinics have been rendering IPPs *personae non grata*, cutting these innocent patients off from medical help altogether, gutting their foundations of some percentage of a tolerable quality of life. Highly ethical doctors continue to turn desperate pain patients away from care due to these DEA tactics. They can't afford to have their licenses revoked, their assets illegally confiscated by government goons, all their other patients abandoned, their own families paying a high price, as they are persecuted, prosecuted and imprisoned for a questionable and obscure cause, "conspiracy". Hundreds of clinicians, nationwide, are victims of this nazi-istic outrage.

Enter, Medicare and Medicaid with Added Restrictions on Pain Care

And, not to be outdone, Medicare and Medicaid have been chiming in with all manner of restrictions, not only on prescription narcotics for pain patients, but also on alternative treatments that may, in some cases, provide some ameliorative benefits. So, now, narcotic analgesic prescriptions are killed by these additional government agencies.

Suicide Instead of Painful Torture

One dedicated pain specialist reports that his pain patients "contemplate suicide" when faced with the swift removal of their trusty opioid analgesic. A horrible catch-22: frightened clinicians have to choose between their fears of government overreach into their practices and prosecution for simply prescribing opioids appropriately. And then imprisonment. Is this America? Government bullies harming legitimate patients and doctors, intimidating our entire country? Turning healthcare into Hell on Earth.

A Commentary in a 2018 issue in Pain Medicine Calls for "Urgent Action on Forced Opioid Tapering"

Hundreds of physicians, nurses, other clinicians and scientists signed this plea: "We [are] deeply concerned about forced opioid tapering in patients receiving long-term prescription opioid therapy for chronic pain. This is a large-scale humanitarian issue. Our specific concerns involve: rapid, forced opioid tapering among outpatients; mandated opioid tapers that require aggressive opioid dose reductions over a defined period, even when that period is an extended one." To access the details of this professional plea and the pages and pages of signatories to its principles, please visit **https://academic.oup.com/painmedicine/advance-article/abstract/doi/10.1093/pm/pny228/5218985**

Chapter Ten

Early Warnings from Physicians and Other Health Professionals Against the 2016 *CDC Guideline*

There has always been – for at least a century – empathic nursing and medical attention, care and appropriate sufficient medication for patients in pain. Until 2016, when all hell broke loose, attacking the proper prescriptions for Intractable Pain Patients – now also blasting its extremist proscriptions deep into the acute pain arenas of operating theaters, emergency departments and dental facilities all over this nation as an almost comic follow-up to a bad idea, the *CDC Guideline*.

Narcotic? Opiate? Opioid, you say? My God, it's a downright sin to prescribe an on-target medication in dosages sufficient enough to adequately manage the severely excruciating, unremitting pain of the many and varied diseases, conditions, injuries and congenital deformities that millions of Americans suffer.

A Nightmare World of Moral Pontifications

Along comes a bureaucratic body, tucked comfortably away in neat Atlanta, Georgia offices, even more comfortable with microscopic minutiae embedded in rules and regulations they invent – loosing, on pain-sick millions, poorly thought-out "recommendations" without regard to the real human beings their myopic policies would mortally affect. And soon these myopes, red-faced, feel compelled to defend this ill-born document.

Blaming Pain Patients' and their Prescription Opioids for Illicit Drug Deaths

Astigmatically, or with thinly-veiled intent, participants in the unfortunate construction of the 2016 *CDC Guideline* completely destroyed the truth about two major public health issues:

1. Drug Addiction with escalating overdose deaths
2. Painful Pathologies requiring prescription narcotics

Suddenly, upon release of the biased *Guideline* (See Chapter Seven), wrongfully motivated journalists in print, broadcast and internet media, all over our country were publicizing the so-called "opioid epidemic".

Pain Patients become Pariahs: Millions in Lifelong Pain, Thousands Commit Suicide

Just as suddenly, patients suffering conditions of lifelong, unrelenting pain, many of whom had been successfully managed for years, often decades, with individually prescribed dosages of specific opioids, were now *personae non grata* at pain clinics. No more empathy. No more analgesic medication. No more doctors willing to care for them. No more livable lives. Only despair. Suicide.

Perversion of Healthy Paincare Protocols Hides DEA Impotence Against Illicit-Drug Deaths

Simultaneously, hundreds of physicians and other prescribing clinicians all over America were being (and are still being) haunted by DEA spies, dogged by DOJ prosecutors. The DEA police reading patients' medical records, warning doctors by phone what and how much they can't prescribe, raiding their practices. The DOJ prosecuting and jailing them. Nor did the CDC bureaucrats, who created this mess, intercede to get the DOJ/DEA over-reactors to back off.

Opiohysteria, whipped up by the misguidance and by DOJ-DEA intent, divert public focus away from illicit drug deaths.

As described from various perspectives throughout this book, the climbing opioid deaths are of users of illicit, adulterated fentanyl or fentanylized heroin, often co-present in the postmortem blood of addicts along with alcohol and/or benzodiazepines - antianxiety drugs like Xanax® (alprazolam), Valium® (diazepam) and Librium® (chlordiazepoxide). None of which relate to narcotic analgesics prescribed for pain!

Therefore, this holocaust (characterized this drastically because of the unjustness of government overreach causing denial of pain care to American millions) extinguishing proper healthcare for pain patients, extinguishing still others by suicide, must stop NOW! In medicine, the word for an immediate urgent action to be taken RIGHT NOW is STAT! The 2016 *CDC Guideline* must be killed STAT!

Note: So far, though drastic reductions in normal narcotic prescriptions forcibly occurred due to government intruders in confidential pain care; though pain patients are suffering mercilessly; though more and more pain physicians are being raided and incarcerated, the rate of illicit-drug deaths continues to rise alarmingly.

And that is where federal and state health policy and policing efforts should be focusing. On interdiction, prosecution and detox. Confiscate the Chinese, Mexican and Internet illegal imports! Prosecute the sellers and dealers! Remand drug addict patients to detox and psychiatric care because they can't make sane decisions for their own health! Those are your jobs HHS/CDC and DOJ/DEA. Do them! Stat!

Oncologist and American Medical Association President, Barbara L. McAneny, MD Reports on One Victimized Cancer Patient

AMA President, Barbara L. McAneny, MD, an oncologist, speaking to physician attendees at the November 10, 2018 AMA Interim Meeting in National Harbor, Maryland, related this sorrowful story of patient care gone awry by meddling secondary parties whose financial and/or political interests clash with traditionally excellent medical care.

One of Dr. McAneny's metastatic prostate cancer patients, with "ca in his bones, now", was doing well on chemotherapy. He'd been on two opioid doses daily and needed more to quell his pain. So she upped his prescription to three daily doses. He then took this prescription to his pharmacy, whereupon the pharmacist searched the state's Prescription Drug Monitoring Program (PDMP), noted years of narcotic prescriptions, decided the patient was a "drug seeker," and wouldn't fill Dr. McAneny's prescription.

Her Cancer Patient Attempted Suicide, She Felt She had Failed Him

Now, not only does this patient have cancer metastasized to the bones, the pain of which is modulated by the narcotic Dr. McAneny prescribed, but he's also been shamed and sent home without his painkiller. Feeling ashamed, embarrassed, at home he shortly thereafter attempted suicide and, thankfully, was saved by an ER physician. Then, after a week's hospitalization, Dr. McAneny "got his pain under control on the exact regimen I'd prescribed him as an outpatient."

While the CDC and DEA have drummed up hysteria about drug addict over-dosings, Dr. McAneny stated, "My patient nearly died of an under-dose." She reports apologizing to her patient in the hospital and told her doctor-audience, "I felt I failed him....the frustration of knowing what the patient needs and having the healthcare system get in the way and prevent that care....too often the healthcare system gets in the way of actual health care."

Referring to many diverse healthcare system problems, in addition to the imposition of the unfortunate 2016 *CDC Guideline* fall-out, she affirmed: "Health care runs on our licenses, so we have the power to fix it. When doctors work together, for the good of patients, we are unstoppable."

Finally, Dr. McAneny reminds her physician-audience, "Sooner or later, we are patients. And patients need doctors." Implying that everyone needs empathic physicians who can deliver patient care unhampered by foolish restrictions.

To paraphrase only one professional (telling me his opinion in early 2019), whose anonymity I am protecting against DEA intrusion: All these federal and state employees at the culpable health and police agencies, who've generated the widespread unmedicated sufferings of millions of chronic pain patients, pushing many to suicide, should be arrested and tried for murder.

Objections to the "Guideline" by Doctors, Nurses and Other Health Professionals

According to Health Professionals for Patients in Pain – HP3 **https://healthprofessionalsforpatientsinpain.org** there have been distressingly unfounded suspicions of real pain patients. And there are disastrous, ongoing barriers to appropriate pain care for millions of pain sufferers. What's more, there are also forced *cold-turkeyings* with forced "referrals" to Suboxone® (buprenorphine/naloxone) detox clinics. However, since the naloxone component of Suboxone would interfere with any analgesic properties of its buprenorphine component, its unlikely pain patients would find any pain relief therefrom, as such detoured pain patients have reported.

Misdiagnosing normal pain patients as addicts, forcing them off their well-working prescription narcotics, and shoveling them, like so many Nazi holocaust victims, into the maelstrom of the addiction detox population where they definitely do not belong, is a medical outrage. It's torture. It's criminal. The American government ought to be ashamed of this herding-like-cattle of innocent pain patients, into sick places where they do not belong, because some unscrupulous officials have financial interests in Suboxone®. (See Chapter 20, "The Suboxone Hoax".)

2018 American Medical Association Resolutions against the *CDC Guideline*

- Resolved...that some patients with acute or chronic pain can benefit from taking opioids at greater dosages than recommended by the CDC Guidelines for Prescribing Opioids for chronic pain and that such care may be medically necessary and appropriate.

- Resolved that our AMA advocate against the misapplication of the CDC Guidelines for Prescribing Opioids by pharmacists, health insurers, pharmacy benefit managers, legislatures, and governmental and private regulatory bodies in ways that prevent or limit access to opioid analgesia.
- Resolved...that no entity should use MME [morphine milligram equivalents] thresholds as anything more than guidance, and physicians should not be subject to professional discipline, loss of board certification, loss of clinical privileges, criminal prosecution, civil liability, or other penalties or practice limitations solely for prescribing opioids at a quantitative level above the MME thresholds found in the CDC Guidelines for Prescribing Opioids.

The fact that the distinguished AMA organization had to even construct these resolutions glaringly broadcasts the CDC's impotence against the misuse of its ill-fated "Guideline".

Government Operatives, Unlicensed to Practice Medicine, Continue to Cause Suffering, Sorrow and Suicides

Though untreated, under-treated and mistreated Intractable Pain Patients (IPPs) are suiciding in droves rather than suffering excruciating minute-by-minute daily pain, our dilatory federal government agencies still haven't gotten their acts together after three long-suffering years under the ominous shadow of the misguided 2016 *CDC Guideline.* This prolonged inhuman cruelty continues from the combined lock-step actions and inactions of the Department of Health and Human Services (HHS) and its subsidiary, the Centers for Disease Control and Prevention (CDC). A terrible government infliction, enforced against IPPs and their narcotic analgesic prescribing physicians, by their allies in this injustice, the Department of Justice (DOJ) and its Drug Enforcement Administration (DEA) gestapo-behaving police.

It's like a stubborn two-year-old resisting being toilet trained. The outcome is inevitable but continues to be resisted. Inexplicably.

Undoubtedly, CDC bureaucrats are more than a little embarrassed by their poorly-conceived document of so-called "recommendations". But not embarrassed enough to scrap it in order to save pain patients' lives from suicide. In order to save other pain patients from lives of screaming hell with a zero quality of life.

Why aren't Congressional Senators and Representatives Demanding Accountability from the DOJ and its DEA?

Inexplicably, far-removed members of Congress appear oblivious to these nationwide patient and physician tragedies caused by the intransigent DOJ-DEA cabal. So unconcerned are they that no legal entity exists to protect excellent physicians from DOJ-DEA spies on normal narcotic prescribing, from gestapo-style raids, arrests and prosecutions. Nor from flagrant eclipsing of patients' human rights and violations of their HIPAA privacy protections–illegalities these miscreants openly practice without anyone to answer to. Why?

(There's a groundswell building in America. Organizations. Groups. Medical Professionals. Patients. Attorneys. Critical mass is arriving. And the voting booth is beckoning. Soon medical practice and prescribing will be returned to physicians. Soon pain patients will have their normal opioid medications, at their normal dosage levels, restored. Soon blinders-wearing congress members will be replaced by empathic souls who understand how badly pain hurts, how dangerous it is to have police (DEA) and lawyers (DOJ) practicing medicine, how important it is to immunize physicians from police actions absent clear and present proofs. Especially since such past and current DOJ/DEA actions against pain patients and their doctors have, thus far, been largely without merit. Pain patients have been, everywhere, gathering and pleading for help from some courageous political leaders. But, they're suffering and can't wait any longer. They're a voting bloc of 50,000,000.)

DOJ-DEA Threats also Intimidate Pharmacies and Health Insurers

As if such overreaching federal intrusions on clinicians and patients weren't egregious enough, these persecutory actions have infiltrated two other key players in this national debacle: American Pharmacies and American Health Insurers. Because of looming DOJ-DEA threats, other intimidations, and the ominous state Prescription Drug Monitoring Programs (PDMPs), where government thugs can illegally raid patients' HIPAA-confidential medical records, pharmacies refuse to fill legal narcotic prescriptions and insurers refuse to pay for legally prescribed opioids. Add to that outrageous anti-patient behavior, it has become popular for pharmacies to label normal pain patients as "drug seekers" merely based on the fact they've been successfully treated for years, even decades, with prescription narcotic analgesics.

Far Too Many Suicides after Opioid Medication Stopped

This 50-year-old female, so physically damaged due to a bus crash when she was 21, had been stabilized on her narcotic prescription medication for 29 years. So she'd been able to work, marry, have some friends, live. But when that *Guideline* happened, she was *cold-turkeyed* by her frightened pain specialist, who'd been intimidated by the growing threatening actions of the DOJ/DEA against pain-medicine-prescribing physicians. With no alternative, her daughter said, "I found her dead in bed a week after her doctor stopped prescribing her narcotic. She left a note. She took an overdose of sleeping pills."

According to Stefan Kertesz, MD, a medical professor at the University of Alabama in Birmingham, over-dosings and suicides are to be expected where pain patients are destabilized by forcible cutting off of their opioid medications.

According to Thomas F. Kline, MD, PhD, a once Harvard Medical School Program Administrator, and a Pain Management Physician, IPPs are being forced off a centuries-old beneficial analgesic – the opiate, morphine – and its analogs the semi-synthetic and synthetic opioids. The results are disastrous as Dr. Kline demonstrates with his growing list of obituaries of desperate in-pain patients, who saw suicide as the only way out of excruciating pain. The details are at his site. **https://medium.com/@ThomasKlineMD/thomas-kline-in-the-media-bbfc876a0b59**

Unfortunate Victims of Myopic Federal and State Prescription Opioid Restrictions

Despite the federal insanity, diverting public and legislative attention away from the illicit street drug problem, prescriptions for opioids dropped 10% in 2017, while deaths due to street fentanyl and street heroin have soared over the past decade.

Nevermind common sense. Nevermind facts and statistics. The misguided 2016 *CDC Guideline* still impelled 20 states to legislate prescription painkillers to be prescribed at below-analgesic levels. And, a most egregious participant in this torture of its IPPs is the State of Oregon whose legislators seek to force Medicaid patients' pain prescriptions down to NO OPIOID MEDICATION AT ALL.

There is no comprehensive compilation of all the suicides of patients left bereft of appropriate prescription narcotic treatment of their lifelong pain; however, researchers at the Department of Veterans Affairs report that **veterans cut off from their opioid medications commit suicide up to four times more frequently than those still on opioids prescribed for their pain.**

DOJ-DEA also Created a Dire Shortage of Opioid Medications

These agencies have the power to limit the supply of legal narcotics to pharmacies, diminishing their ability to fill such prescriptions even if they're inclined to do the right thing for their patients. Now, even cancer and hospice patients can't get their appropriate narcotic analgesic dosages. Not to mention how all this horrible attack on sick people has affected acute ER pain patients, postsurgical pain patients, and dental pain patients. All of these normal paincare exigencies have been brought to a virtual standstill while DOJ-DEA and HHS-CDC operatives force physicians to under-prescribe dosages of opioids, to cold-turkey patients off opioids without their consent, and to unethically prescribe Tylenol® (acetaminophen), aspirin or nothing for severe and excruciating pain experiences.

Aside: Can you imagine cutting down on a patient's anti-epileptic medications so seizures will increase in number, patients will fall, hit their heads, may die during a seizure? Or reducing insulin dosage to where hyperglycemia can't be controlled? Or decreasing an antibiotic dosage to where it can't fight the bacterium it is meant to eradicate? Or prescribing schizophrenics lowered antipsychotic doses so they will still hear the voices the correct higher dose would have eliminated?

Then, why is it okay to force IPPs into extremis? Excruciating, unremitting pain with the only solution being suicide? This is the Federal government's solution to illicit street drug deaths? This is various State governments' solution to illegal street drug mortalities? If so, where are the consciences of all the participants in this government fiasco, in this horrific government-made medical disaster?

Empaths Still Fighting the *CDC Guideline* for Patients' Rights to their Opioids

On May 6, 2019, Sean Mackey, M.D., PhD, Chief of the Division of Pain Medicine and Redlich Professor at Stanford University, sent an imperative request to key Oregon legislators and to the president of the Oregon Health Authority, Dana Hargunani, MD, MPH. Also Director of the Stanford Systems Neuroscience and Pain Laboratory, Department of Anesthesiology, Perioperative and Pain Medicine, Neurosciences and Neurology, Dr. Mackey is a staunch pain patient advocate. Thus, in this letter, he urged the Oregon Health Authority's Health Evidence Review Committee (HERC) to reject its proposal for mandatory opioid tapering of Medicaid patients.

He goes on to remind these key individuals of his prior communication to HERC on March 7, 2019, that was signed by more than a hundred "leaders in pain and addictive medicine, health policy, and patient advocacy – that "raised grave concerns about the lack of scientific evidence backing Oregon's opioid tapering proposal" as well as zero arrangements for patient safety.

In this letter, Dr. Mackey further points out, "Alarmed by reports of mandated opioid tapering, these public health authorities have all clarified that patients on long-term opioid therapy should not be subjected to mandated opioid tapering policies or practices":

- U.S. Centers for Disease Control and Prevention [ironically, in a later modification of its "recommendations"]
- U.S. Food and Drug Administration
- The American Medical Association
- The U.S. Surgeon General

Recent Calls to Cease and Desist ALL Mandated Opioid Taperings
Due to the dangers to pain patients of risks and harms, three hundred medical and other health professionals signed and agreed with CDC's Director, Robert Redfield, M.D., who expressed alarm at "non-consensual opioid tapering or dose reductions due to misapplications" of the 2016 *CDC Guideline.*

Underdosing of Morphine Milligram Equivalents (MMEs)
Dr. Mackey's letter also points out the inflexibility of "the CDC's dosage recommendations" which forced long-term opioid treatments down to 90 or 50MME or even lower. He reminds this letter's recipients that clinicians need to be making clinical medication decisions based on each individual patient's needs and diagnosis. One of Dr. Mackey's final statements in this letter is prophetic: "The Guidelines have been misapplied so widely that it will be a challenge to undo the damage".

Recipients of this "cry for help for patients in pain" letter included:
Norman E. Sharpless, MD, Acting Commissioner, FDA Robert R. Redfield, MD, Director, CDC Alex Azar, Secretary, HHS Vanila M. Singh, MD, Chair HHS Inter-Agency Pain Task Force Shari M. Ling, MD, Deputy Chief Medical Officer, Ctrs for Medicare & Medicaid Patrice A. Harris, MD, President-elect, American Medical Association, Chair AMA Opioid Task Force Tim Lamer, MD, President, American Academy of Pain Medicine

Section III

POLICE STATE AMERICA

Chapter Eleven

DEA Gestapo Actions Destroy Physicians' Careers and Pain Patients' Lives

Emboldened by the medically intrusive 2016 *CDC Guideline*, DEA operatives have deputized themselves with greater powers to raid innocent doctors' medical practices even more invasively than they've been doing all over America for at least two decades. These incursions keep occurring with nary a whisper from opiohysterical journalists about these onslaughts on innocent narcotic-prescribing doctors. Where is the "free press"? Who speaks for abandoned pain patients? Who speaks for wrongfully imprisoned physicians?

As a pain patient, what you'll experience as a result of one of these federal police invasions is beyond lamentable. One day you're at your pain management physician's office for your scheduled exam, and to refill your pain medicine prescription. But, unlike all your previous pain doctor appointments, in barge dark-uniformed invaders, scaring patients to death, intimidating office staff, barking demands at your doctor, grabbing file folders, handcuffing your empathic doctor, leaving you without your exam, without your prescription refill, without recourse. Abandoned without pain relief.

By what Constitutional right do these goons give themselves permission to place the medical community under siege, to rob patients of their high-quality clinicians? By what right, do they dare to interfere with the medical care and pain relief of millions upon millions of pain-suffering Americans?

DEA Police Seize and Spy on Confidential Medical Records

Several states have implemented a system called the Prescription Drug Monitoring Program (PDMP) which tracks all medications each patient is prescribed. These also include your medications prescribed for disorders other than pain. In other words, anyone reading your PDMP record will know everything about you medically, and who knows what else is included in these records? What happened to patients' HIPAA (the Health Insurance Portability and Accountability Act) rights? HIPAA is supposed to provide strict privacy protections for patients, which no one is allowed to violate. So, how does the DEA come to invade this deep into patients' lives? Especially, with these confidentiality assurances for American patients, you'd think only clinicians would have access to these records to help them understand each patient's history, diagnosis, treatments, and medication needs. But, no! This PDMP system allows facile access to meddling federal police and other DOJ-intimidated entities readily allowed to delve into your healthcare histories and medications without your permission.

Not only that, during DEA raids of your doctors' offices, these feds carry away boxes and boxes of your physicians' charts about your current healthcare. As a result, once intimidated or arrested, your doctor's practice shut down, you've no current health records to bring to any new physician still brave enough to prescribe your usual opioid medication.

DEA Spies "WARN" Physicians by Phone to Lower Patients' Opioid Dosages

Listen to these few examples of telephoned intrusions–in too many physicians' workdays by DEA spies who've accessed their state's PDMP–told to me in confidential interviews:

Dr. L.C. told me: "One day, when my office was busy with many sick patients, about ten percent there for pain management care, my nurse hands me the phone. It's a Drug Enforcement agent saying, 'Doctor, you keep prescribing more than the Guideline's rule of no more than 90 morphine milligram equivalents of [Mr. Smith's] narcotic. We're tracking your prescribing activities through the PDMP!' His voice sounded threatening. For the first time in my career, I felt fearful of being a dutiful doctor."

Dr. B.R., almost whispering, hesitatingly reported to me: "I'm wrapping up my workday, making notes on the day's patients in their EMRs (Electronic Medical Records), when the phone rings. A cold, calm male voice informs me that the DEA is monitoring my 'over-prescribing' of hydromorphone for two of my patients, one with cancer, the other with a crippling congenital condition. He told me, 'There are serious consequences if you don't lower the doses.' Then he hung up. I was never so angry in my life. Who gave the DEA permission to spy on doctors? What right have they to make medical decisions for my patients? How dare the DEA intrude on patient care, read patients' records, and scare doctors to death?"

One final example of the many intimidating phone calls reported to me: Dr. E.K., reluctant to speak with me at all, in process of closing her pain management practice and moving with her family to Canada, was almost weeping as she related how the DEA-raiding of her medical practice was preceded by this phone call: "'Doctor: You are prescribing too many opioids in too-high doses which our agency prosecutes doctors for.' Thereafter, speaking with my husband, also a physician, who was aware of other colleagues imprisoned for practicing good pain care medicine, we decided this isn't America anymore. So we're leaving the country. I feel so bad for my patients. How will they survive this? Doctors are now too frightened to take good care of them and prescribe the correct narcotic analgesic in the dosages their conditions require."

The DEA Invades Pain Care Physicians' Family Dwellings as Well as their Offices

It's about time all Americans stood up and told the powers that be that we won't stand for this gestapo state any longer. Look at this one scary example of what Nazi America is doing to our wonderful physicians who only went to medical school to take excellent, empathic care of all of us.

A highly-knowledgeable, dedicated physician is raided and arrested by the DEA, his assets seized. The year the ill-conceived *CDC Guideline* was inflicted on America, Monroe, Michigan pain management clinician, Lesly Pompy, M.D. was under siege by DEA operatives. The latter shamefully bolstered by city and state police, rendering the onslaught even more fearsome. It was September 26, 2016. (Note that such outrages are still being perpetrated against innocent doctors to this day.) These government operatives have zero accountability for their illegal actions. No one questions them. They operate *carte-blanche* and our legislators are clueless about these attacks on our nation's physicians. As I write this in September of 2019, Dr. Pompy is still being victimized by these miscreant feds. They had his MD license revoked while he awaits adjudication of his case, still not resolved. They seized his assets. In the meantime, he's trying to, at least, get an EMT (Emergency Medical Technician) license so he can use his medical skills to help patients and feed his family. But no. Government functionaries are maliciously delaying anything positive he can do while awaiting a trial on charges he knows he'll be acquitted of. (See the reference to Dr. Pompy's case, below, in the discussion of Dr. Linda Cheek's Doctors of Courage.)

It's crucial to note Dr. Pompy's impeccable credentials: 1) A New York Medical College Medical Degree, 2) A University of South Florida Masters in Business Administration, and 3) a Madonna University Master of Science Degree. Significantly, he is Board Certified in Anesthesiology, the field of medicine from which most pain specialists emerge. Which is because these particular physicians have unique expertise in varied states of consciousness and pain sensations, and in various procedures to modify consciousness and pain.

Here's what happened: One day, without warning, state police invaded Dr. Lesly Pompy's legitimate medical practice. There, they confiscated his patients' private medical records. They also took possession of his personal and family assets, from his home and office. These

Hitlerian tactics were coldly executed that fateful day in September 2016 with police, unschooled in things medical, tallying up his legal narcotic prescriptions and making ridiculous judgments about the volume of his pain patient prescriptions over the many years Dr. Pompy has been practicing medicine legitimately, empathically, and ethically.

Here are some of Dr. Pompy's patients' reactions to this police-state disruption in their medical care:

~ "He helped my dad for 15 years to keep the pain low enough so he could work."

~ "Without Dr. Pompy, I'd have killed myself, it hurts so bad. Now what?"

~ "When other doctors gave up on me, Dr. Pompy carefully examined me and chose the best pain medicine I've ever had."

~ "I was there when the cops broke into Dr. Pompy's office. Frightened me. I cried because I'll never find such a kind doctor again who figured out the exact right dose for my pain."

~ "My husband was hurt on his job and was helped with pain medicine by Dr. Pompy. Years later, my spine bones were causing pain and Dr. Pompy chose the best pain reliever for me. What will we do without him?"

Those were only tiny samplings of the broad array of patients with congenital conditions producing constant pain, with post-injury lifelong pain, and with post-surgical unrelenting pain, who've expressed their shock and distress to me at the mistreatment of Dr. Pompy and the despair of no longer having their beloved physician taking care of them.

One patient even pointed to this admonition from the Declaration of Independence as applicable to America's plight, today, with the DOJ-DEA gone amok: **Jefferson on the right to change one's government (1776)—That whenever any Form of Government becomes destructive of these ends, it is the right of the People to alter or to**

abolish it, and to institute new Government, laying its foundation on such principles, and organizing its powers in such form, as to them shall seem most likely to effect their Safety and Happiness.

Amen! I say, we need to abolish the Drug Enforcement Administration, as they are structured today, for the unscrupulous and mafia-like tactics they've been using for decades against innocent American physicians. Intrusions which have totally disrupted normal medical care of their charges, which are continuing to injure millions of Intractable Pain Patients, sending thousands of them to the finality of suicide.

As they are currently structured, and as they currently sidestep all sanity and compassionate human behavior with their harmful actions, we don't need them. We must focus new eyes on what the public really needs. We deserve real consciences embedded in such agencies that are supposed to benefit we citizens. Regrouping, anew, with true senses of responsibility, we need to expel the current malfunctioning operatives in both the DOJ and its DEA who have come to the delusional belief that they grasp the depth and nuances of medical practice in general, and the erudite specifics of pain management in particular. And, because these draconian actions by them reek of unscrupulous motivations, the DOJ-DEA smells of corruption and should be investigated by Congress.

All American Physicians Must Fight this DOJ-DEA Outrage: Visit Doctors of Courage

To witness the unbelievable numbers of innocent physicians, other clinicians and pain clinic owners who've been raided, all their assets "confiscated" (stolen by the DOJ so they've no money to hire lawyers), smeared in the media, arrested, prosecuted and imprisoned by this rogue DOJ-DEA cabal, visit Linda Cheek, M.D. website **https://doctorsofcourage.org**

Significantly, reports Dr. Cheek, a higher-dose opioid-prescribing doctor was used as a so-called "expert" witness against Dr. Pompy, which demonstrates the capriciousness and slithery unprofessional conduct of the DOJ's tactics. At present, Dr. Pompy is in professional limbo, still awaiting judicial proceedings while he, his family, and his patients languish – as the Department of *In*justice slogs through its misapplications of the law. Even his application to qualify as an EMT continues to be capriciously mishandled and delayed. Note too: Even Dr. Cheek, this pioneer of justice for pain management doctors, was imprisoned for two years, yet another medical victim of storm trooper DEA thugs and hitlerite DOJ injustice.

As our nation decries other governments' crimes against their own innocent citizens, who will speak up for these American medical giants withering away in prison, with real criminals, for the "horrendous crime" of rendering high quality medical care to suffering pain patients?

A Reminder to the DEA: Your Only Jobs are Interdiction of Illicits, Prosecution of Dealers, Remanding of Illicits Addicts to Detox

If you focus on these illicit problems: interdicting adulterated fentanyl, fentanylized heroin (often ingested with ethanol and anxiolytics such as diverted benzodiazepines); on Mexican, Chinese and Internet drug imports; on arresting dealers; and on transporting addicts all the way to detox facilities - you'll have plenty of legitimate policing activities to keep you busy. Now, get out of the lives of patients in pain and stop killing quality medical practices!

Chapter Twelve

Brilliant, Compassionate Pain Specialist, Forest Tennant, MD Targeted and Sidelined by Out-of-Control DOJ/DEA Incursions

Yet another super-qualified, excellent physician has been forced to make a life-altering decision that impacts him, his wife and family, and his chronic pain patients who've relied on his excellent medical care for decades. He retired–having felt under duress to do so–on April 1, 2018. Sadly, this scientifically-erudite, well-published expert chose to close his Los Angeles pain management practice after intrusive (though fruitless) onslaughts by DEA rogues, on behalf of DOJ prosecutors, whose *carte blanche* tactics match Hitler's and Stalin's. The latter, the evil fall-out of the poorly-conceived 2016 *CDC Guideline.*

Not long after that infamous document was loosed on unsuspecting America, Dr. Tennant's home and office were targeted by the DEA because medically-ignorant DOJ/DEA operatives couldn't distinguish between drug pushers and physicians who know what they're doing. Who know, intimately, what dosages, no matter how high when necessary, of opioid analgesics are necessary to quell the pain of each individual patient.

Imagine this: Your distinguished physician, Dr. Tennant, is served with a search warrant accusing him of "drug trafficking," despite his reputation as a scientist as well as a skilled treating physician in the specialized field of pain management medicine. Physicians, like Dr. Tennant, consider constant pain a disease in itself. And, when it's not treated, or when its inadequately treated (with lower-than-adequate opioid dosings), the patient's overall health deteriorates, life quality vanishes, and premature death occurs.

(As a reminder of the complexities of painful conditions and their usually successful treatments with prescription opioids, see Section I where pain, pain conditions, and their treatments are elaborated.)

Dr. Tennant Accepted the Most Challenging Cases

Some of Dr. Tennant's patients suffered intractable pain from incurable genetic diseases or permanent damage from injuries. Others were victims of poor post-surgical outcomes. Because of these complex cases, in addition to direct patient diagnosis and care, Dr. Tennant did research to advance scientific knowledge in the potential of hormonal help that might reduce narcotic needs for pain patients. Also, he was involved in the search for enzymes, via genetic testing, that could clarify differences in opioid level absorption.

Ominous Results of this Siege Against this Blameless Doctor

Because of such unfounded government invasion of such high-quality physicians, other doctors all around these United States, are quaking in fear of losing their licenses, their assets, their freedom – of being imprisoned despite being faultless. Merely because they want to practice excellent medicine by prescribing narcotic analgesics for patients in pain, at dosages appropriate for each individual's condition. Just imagine, a federal government bloc, a cabal allied to take doctors down, no matter that they've done nothing but take good care of their sick patients. Quivering fear. That's the state these rogue entities – DOJ/DEA – have left America's physicians in. And their patients are quivering, too, because of excruciating, untreated pain. Still others fearlessly enter suicide mode to escape never-ending suffering.

Criminal Federal Operatives Prosecute Doctors, Persecute Patients

Criminally, some operatives of the clueless DOJ/DEA assert that they can't worry about those innocent physicians prescribing correctly for their patients. That these onslaughts, sieges, arrests and imprisonments – no matter that the vast majority of clinicians are innocent of any wrongdoing – "serve as a deterrent". Such an idiotic pronouncement. Such, even in the wake of these DOJ/DEA tsunamis on the innocent. Even after causing unjustly terminated medical careers. Even though there are innocent MDs...spitefully prosecuted, unjustly imprisoned. Even though there are pain patients no longer with any physician to examine them, take care of them, to prescribe their narcotic analgesic for them. Even though such patients are suiciding in droves, at an alarming rate. And that is a genocide that these malevolent DOJ/DEA actions are perpetrating on innocents.

Untreated, Unendurable Pain Leads to Suicides

A Helena, Montana paincare physician, Mark Ibsen, MD, had his suspended medical license reversed back to active by a judge during a withering 5-year onslaught by his medical board starting in 2016. At the reversal, the judge ruled that the Montana Board of Medical Examiners had deprived Dr. Ibsen of due process and had made numerous errors. Despite this reversal, at 63, he closed his medical practice. As a result, three of his patients suicided. This in a state where 35% of suicides are by chronic pain patients.

DEA Agents Vandalize Dr. Tennant's Home after his Defense Testimony for another Doctor

Only a day after testifying, for the defense, in an out-of-state trial of yet another DEA-victimized pain-treating physician, wrongfully accused of two overdose deaths, Dr. Tennant and his wife arrived back in California, their front door kicked in by DEA invaders. Despite the fact that nothing incriminating was found during such mindless DEA intrusions into Dr. Tennant's home and office, the clueless feds argued that the high doses of narcotics he was prescribing for some patients must be because these patients were selling them and giving him kickbacks. That, despite the fact that there was never any evidence of injury nor overdosing by any of his patients. Which didn't halt the DOJ/DEA's determination to ruin his life's work. Nor did these rogue federals care that they'd also victimized his patients thereby.

American Government Agents of the DOJ/DEA Target Pain Patients and Paincare Physicians

Despite his innocence and ultimate exoneration of all the false, fraudulently concocted charges the DOJ/DEA manufactured against him, reports Dr. Tennant, they were determined to ruin his excellent reputation in order to intimidate all of America's other opioid-prescribing physicians. Thus, he warns America: It's not just him they're targeting, "They're targeting pain patients." They're disregarding legal regulations, causing abandonment of medical and scientific standards. Furthermore, he points out that the DOJ/DEA "will decide who can get opioids and how much. I'm worried about every pain patient, not just mine."

Apparently, too, these government goons lie, having rigged a phony collusion with a pharmacy that filled Dr. Tennant's patients' prescriptions. Yet, Dr. Tennant had no financial partnership (as the phony feds invented) with any druggist, asserting at the time, "My clinic is more like a charity". And, though in his seventies, he hadn't chosen to retire because he wanted to continue treating his many patients who depended on his pain-relieving care, many of whom were on palliative treatment with but a year left to live.

A Hero Doctor with Innovative Approaches to Pain Care

Dr. Tennant, over his career, evolved treatment regimens for such intransigent pain conditions as Ehlers-Danlos Syndrome, Adhesive Arachnoiditis and RSD (Reflex Sympathetic Dystrophy). And, in addition to narcotic analgesics for these conditions, he'd developed protocols that include hormones and anti-inflammatory drugs which can reduce the dosages of required opioids.

DOJ/DEA Operatives Care Nothing about Pain Patients Sufferings and Suicides

Recognizing his singular status in the paincare specialty community, Dr. Tennant declared that he'd never prescribed incorrectly nor excessively. He did decry what he feels about the DOJ/DEA war-against-pain-patients onslaughts: That these government agencies are conscienceless about pain patients' sufferings and suicides. Furthermore, he points out that if they can take a blameless doctor like him down, no doctor will ever again prescribe narcotics, no matter how badly their patients are suffering. "I think," he said in a TV interview the year he was raided, "there needs to be an outcry".

The DEA will not return patients' medical charts and prescription records they've "confiscated", refusing to return these to the doctor despite his exoneration of any wrongdoing. As a result of this infantile recalcitrance, in order to get any further treatment for their pain, Dr. Tennant's former patients were forced to go through the trouble and embarrassment (non-medical people reading their private information) of pleading with DEA authorities for their records so their next doctor can provide the ongoing pain care that they desperately need.

DOJ/DEA Tactics Rob Intractable Pain Patients of their Beloved Dr. Tennant

On April 1, 2018, the knell fell for beloved Dr. Tennant's severely hurting patients. His lawyers advised him to get out of the DOJ's bull's eye. His own personal doctor advised, too, that that was best, considering the pressures of an out-of-control federal mob posing as protectors of vulnerable citizens. Like stubborn four-year-olds–despite Dr. Tennant's innocence and with zero criminal charges against him–the DEA refused to drop his case. Feeling in limbo and unwilling to under-dose or mistreat his patients in pain, he chose to retire. Though 77, that hadn't been his plan because he loved his patients like they were family.

In response to Dr. Tennant's retiring, many of his patients and colleagues lauded him and shamed the DOJ/DEA for their autocratic destruction of Dr. Tennant's blemishless practice of medicine. One patient commented on this loss of a great physician as "a crime. We are fighting a genocide against pain patients by out-of-whack federal employees who act as though they are God." Another, on the loss of his pain care due to the closing of Dr. Tennant's practice, asked, "What was that thing Hitler did when he rose to power? Got rid of the sick and mentally and physically disabled. Or they were just murdered."

Today, in our America, the murderers are DOJ/DEA rogue operatives indicting and imprisoning innocent physicians, condemning pain patients to never-ending pain or to ending it all in suicides.

Chapter Thirteen

Ominous Overreach of the Department of Justice

Plight of Pain Patients and their Doctors: Victims of the DOJ

Since the 2016 *CDC Guideline* was thrust upon our unsuspecting healthcare system, this is what's been happening to patients in pain all over the country: They're suffering. Uncared for. Ignored. Treated like junkies, like criminals. Forced to beg for minuscule amounts of their prescription narcotic analgesics which, formerly in their correct dosages, kept at least some of their pain at bay for years, often decades – without addiction! And those years of such appropriate medical treatment allowed many to remain employed, pay taxes, take care of their families, maintain at least a modicum of social interactions.

Ominously though, with the advent of federal government intrusion into pain patients' lives and into their physicians' practices, all that humanity has come to a screeching halt. Following is only a small sampling of some of the thousands of stories shared by suffering pain patients – trapped in a government maze of bureaucratic hubris, and opiate and opioid ignorance – criminalized and bullied into nonconsensual tapering or outright *cold-turkeying*, many resorting to suicide. These few stories exemplify what millions of Intractable Pain Patients have been enduring for the three years since the 2016 *CDC Guideline* was imposed.

One patient, I call L.F., with a severe neurologic condition that is progressively worsening told me he'd been stabilized on his narcotic analgesic since 1999, able to ambulate, to keep working as a carpenter, and gratefully partaking in family life. Without his painkiller, he is home-bound, bedridden. I quote him: "Thoughts of suicide...it hurts so bad. Before, I had a life. Now, I'm dead." Another pain sufferer, I'll call her T.Z., was able to get around using a walker, engage with nature, socialize with neighbors. Now, she too is stuck at home, stuck most of the day in bed. She said, "Without my pain medicine, I'm a vegetable." And a retired teacher, I name A.V., reported, "The shooting pain in my legs and back never stop...can't sleep. My doctor won't make any more appointments to see me. He's afraid of the DEA.

MDs are Invaded, Raided, Degraded, Ruined because the DOJ Conflates Drug Addicts with Pain Patients

Because of the DOJ's conflation of two markedly different illness categories, our blinders-wearing Department of Justice is torturing pain patients and their doctors.

Category One: Millions of Intractable Pain Patients (IPPs) are entitled to various normal narcotic analgesic prescription regimens. That's because some 50 million Americans, a large percent being IPPs, are suffering some level of pain as you read this. But out-of-control DOJ/DEA onslaughts, nationwide, against faultless physicians – raiding them, intimidating them, confiscating their life's' earnings, imprisoning them – have shuttered many doctors' clinics and left pain patients without physicians, without their essential opioid painkillers. As a result, in addition to the millions left suffering, countless others have been choosing suicide. That's why I've come to call these enmeshed federal conglomerates HHS/CDC-DOJ/DEA a feelingless cabal "Cold Turkeys".

Category Two: Illicits Drug Addicts, Traffickers, Dealers are, unfortunately, in the inner operations of the DOJ/DOE – subjects of factual obfuscations, mendacious falsehoods, and a purposeful "hands-off" – due to thinly-veiled collusions with "advisor" parties who have conflicting fiduciary interests (See Section VI, "PERPETRATORS".), counter to the best interests of both drug addicts and pain patients.

Thus, because the 2016 *CDC Guideline* slanted its "recommendations," in admonitions that caused clinicians to stop prescribing opioids for pain patients, too often to abandon their care altogether, this served the errant DOJ/DEA by averting the nation's attention away from these glaring national disgraces:

1. The sloppy, bungling job the DOJ/DEA is doing about drug traffickers and dealers, about the illicit chemicals that "somehow" find their way, from China, Mexico and the Internet into the post-mortem blood of addicts.
2. The diversion of national attention from the feeble job our federal alphabet soup of "health" agencies – NIH, HHS, CDC – is doing to treat and rehabilitate users of dangerous illicit substances. It's known, despite rehab facilities and Suboxone® (buprenorphine/naloxone) clinics nationwide, treatment to recovery appears nebulous in many such patients, with frequent relapses and unpredictable outcomes. Could it be this "legal morphine" is not helping addicts? (See Chapter 20, "The Suboxone Hoax".)
3. DOJ and DEA operatives practicing medicine without a license. What do these rogue raiders know about anatomy, physiology, the Central Nervous System (CNS, Brain and Spinal Cord), neurology, biochemistry, pharmacology? And what do these mini-minds know about conditions that produce excruciating pain? And what about the variations in metabolism of opioids in different human bodies? That would explain the varieties of dosages that different patients require to quell their sufferings. But, no! DOJ "geniuses" have unilaterally decided on the medical care of all pain patients. And being know-it-alls, they're dead-set (emphasis on "dead') on pushing dosages way below the already "recommended" too low 90MME (morphine milligram equivalents) that often won't alleviate severe levels of pain. None of them regrets these pernicious

> impositions. None of them feel sorrow for the multiple suicides due to their imbecilic directives that forced IPPs off their usual prescription narcotic medication. None of them takes responsibility for these death-dealing results.

It's time to remember the practice of medicine is to care for ALL the people in our country. If this were about tuberculosis, there'd be forced quarantining because this contagious disease spreads from person to person via the afflicted patient's cough. Therefore, consider this: Treatment for drug addicts should be mandatory for their own protection and for the protection of society in general. This is because escalating substance addiction often leads to property and personal crimes, sometimes to murder. And because, there are facilities that exist to provide useful psychological and medical tools to help these patients to remission.

That said, here's a clarification of the vast difference between the two groups of patients I've been referring to:

1. **Pain Suffering Patients** – those in severe, unrelenting pain, plus others needing acute, short-term narcotic analgesics
2. **Drug Addicted Patients** – those who, due to genetic, psychological or experimental reasons are drug addicts

These two must be viewed and treated as distinctly separate entities. Sadly, the 2016 *CDC Guideline* fails this criterion. All the while, these years since its misguided inception, pain patients are suffering and suiciding. MayDay! S.O.S.!

Help! Patients in pain need their prescription opioids STAT!

We Must Treat Patients in Pain Differently than We Treat Drug Addicts

Because of the current widespread EPIDEMIC OF PAIN, pain once well-controlled on legal prescription opioid medications, due to capitol blunders that have been multiplying exponentially, the DOJ must immediately reverse its misguided trajectory. Stat!

DOJ: Halt your spying on patients' confidential health records. Halt your intimidations and imprisonments of innocent doctors.

Halt your threatening phone calls and insinuating letters to innocent clinicians. Do your job against illicit drugs, and their transactors, and see that addicts get into rehab. You, DOJ, have the legal recourse to remand these patients to treatment to prevent the overdose deaths you are blaming on pain management physicians and pain-suffering patients.

The fact that drug rehab is "voluntary" is senseless. When patients, in this case illicits addicts, are too physically and mentally sick to make healthy decisions for themselves, remanding them to a medical, psychiatric and/or rehab facility should be mandatory – not only for their well-being, but for society's.

To take the pressure off themselves for their failings in curbing illicit drug overdose deaths, and their impotence against escalating rogue fentanyl and fentanylized heroin imports, federal officials have created a catch-22 agenda of draconian proportions and a colossus of human suffering. The misery inflicted on pain patients these ominous three years since the Guideline has been circulated, because of the collision between these two entirely different groups of patients, has been a conflation manufactured out of unholy cloth, a focus irresponsibly torn away from common sense and quality medical practice.

Opioid Expert, Josh Bloom, PhD, Chastises Anyone Still Unmoved by Real Pain

Writing at his website in December 2018, referring to the tragic DOJ/DEA crackdown on normal narcotic prescribing for chronic pain patients, Dr. Josh Bloom, Director of Chemical and Pharmaceutical Sciences of the American Council on Science and Health (ACSH) and an expert on the opioid crisis asserted that, even a Shakespeare tragedy could not match "the tragedy...imposed on this country by self-appointed drug experts, bureaucrats, self-serving politicians, and various other fools. It's that bad. And it was largely preventable."

Dr. Bloom further blasts the CDC for "sticking its nose where it shouldn't have" and *PROPagenda* PROP (See Chapter 21, "Hidden Agendas of Anti-Opioid Proponent$.) for "creating a mess we will not be getting out of anytime soon". You can read the vast writings of Dr. Bloom and his blastings aimed at this war against pain patients and their doctors at this site: **https://www.acsh.org**

Family Physician, Kenny Lin, M.D. Speaks Up for Pain Patients Needing Prescription Opioids

Kenny Lin, M.D. points out that moderate to severe pain is suffered by 25 million of our citizens, while opioid medications are prescribed for 5 million to 8 million of these sufferers. Still, he cautions against adopting "inflexible dosing limits" and policies denying opioid therapy altogether, claiming that doctors and pharmacies which do so have "caused substantial harm to patients." He reminds his fellow physicians that "forced tapering and patient abandonment is unethical".

Dr. Lin's Plea to Physicians Who've Stopped Prescribing Narcotics

Having "inherited" long-term opioid therapy patients, left doctorless when their physicians retired or no longer prescribe opioids, Dr. Lin requests complete medical records of such patients. This helps their transition to a colleague's care by providing documentation of the intractable pain diagnosis, other physical and emotional ailments, what triggers their pain experiences and "other medications or interventions that have and have not helped," plus reasons for higher or lower doses of their narcotics.

Dr. Lin Wants to Rid Medical Practice of the Minutiae Imposed by the *Guideline*

About the 2016 *CDC Guideline*, Dr. Lin reminds anyone reading it that "legislation or payer requirements for a one-size-fits-all approach to acute or chronic pain are inappropriate and potentially harmful." He further decries CDC mandates tracking every minute interaction between doctors and pain patients, stating, "For example, although care teams should access PDMP data periodically, making it mandatory to check the PDMP prior to every single interaction involving an opioid prescription creates [unnecessary, time-consuming] burdens for medical practices." Finally, he asserts that criminalizing and stigmatizing pain patients on prescription opioids, and applying these same negatives against pain management practices must stop! You can read Dr. Lin's pro-pain-patient articles at **commonsensemd.blogspot.com**

DOJ Loose Cannons Boast about Destroying Paincare Doctors' Lives

Since January of 2017, boasted their June 2018 press release, the Department of Justice aggressively prosecuted about 200 clinicians and 220 other healthcare professionals. Emphasis on the word "aggressively". Thus, with no legal process to check their runaway, illegitimate incursions (with the DEA acting as their militia arm), the DOJ is committed to destroying the lives and careers of medical professionals who have the unmitigated nerve to dutifully prescribe narcotic analgesics for their suffering pain patients – and in doses individualized, based on their diagnoses and on each one's inherent opioid-absorption metabolics. And so, the clueless, medically-ignorant, DOJ's DEA operatives barge into the lives and healthcare work of dedicated physicians and their staffs, ripping professionals away from the patients who need them, leaving chronic pain patients bereft of follow-up care and abandoned without their regular, well-working legal prescription opioids.

Aggressive Nationwide DOJ/DEA Attacks Cause Doctors to Abandon Pain Patients

Here are some examples of the severe impositions on, and persecutions of, blameless clinicians and their pain patients by DOJ bureaucrats and DEA police:

1. Arrests of doctors who'd prescribed a narcotic for pain, but, unbeknownst to them, a patient may have sold some of their medication to an addict.

2. Severe, time-stealing from quality medical practices by requiring endless procedures inappropriate for pain patients (stigmatizing them as "addicts") such as pill counting, urine testing, and extra doctor appointments, expensive for both patients and insurers.
3. Mistreating patients as though they are drug addicts by labeling them "drug seekers".
4. Demands that doctors taper patients off their painkillers – though most of these physicians are not practicing "addiction medicine" and are not trained in the signs, symptoms and dangers of withdrawal.

Note: Pain Patients Experience Pain Relief. Addicts Experience "Highs".

Though pain patients will experience symptoms of withdrawal when suddenly or too-rapidly tapered off their prescription narcotic, they are not addicts. They never chase "highs". Their bodies and brains are simply adapted to the chemical that has somewhat, never completely, relieved their pain for years and years, maintaining them in enough relief so they can keep their jobs, socialize, prepare meals, and avoid being bedridden, miserable and headed toward suicide. This natural adaptation to the effect of a patient's narcotic analgesic is known as being "dependent". Which is different than addiction.

The DOJ is Relentless Against Quality Pain Relief

Despite cautions by the American Medical Association (AMA) and the American Cancer Society (ACS) against the 2016 *CDC Guideline*'s nitpicking constrictions on normal narcotic prescribing, the DOJ remains relentless against adequate pain relief for millions of suffering Americans. That, in spite of, the AMA's warning to the CDC that too much scientific evidence is lacking in that document, strongly challenging its *raison d'etre.*

The DOJ's Erroneous Federal Crackdown Empowers State Legislators to Worsen Opioid Restrictions

At the time of this writing, due to the widespread misapplication of, the 2016 *CDC Guideline*, Oregon, the most stringent state government-enforcer of the questionable CDC "recommendations," is planning to impose a stringent 90-day prescribing limit on opioid medications for Medicaid patients. As a result, this emboldened the Medicaid system to stop covering opioid prescriptions altogether for these unfortunate, low-income patients. (See my extensive critique of all aspects of the 2016 *CDC Guideline* in Chapter 7.)

North Carolina Pain Patient Advocate, Thomas Kline, M.D., PhD Opposes the Guideline, Risks Scrutiny by Vindictive DOJ Operatives

Speaking of the drastic, and widespread, misapplications of the 2016 *CDC Guideline*, Dr. Thomas Kline told an interviewer that he'd suddenly realized "...the CDC was going to sit in my office and tell me how to prescribe pain medicines, instead of tracking Zika." That reference, of course, referring to the CDC's real job – tracking and preventing infectious and toxic epidemics and pandemics.

In this case, of course, the "epidemic" the CDC should be working with the DOJ/DEA about is that of drug addict mortalities caused by adulterated fentanyl and fentanylized heroin along with illicit antianxiety drugs and alcohol. That's the real drug misuse mortality epidemic – not innocent pain patients using their prescribed narcotic analgesics properly.

Hero, Dr. Kline, refuses to taper any of his pain patients off their therapeutically effectively, well-working prescription narcotics. You can be uplifted (though saddened by the patient-suicides he reports) by Dr. Kline's pro-pain-patient articles and interviews at **https://medium.com/@ThomasKlineMD**

Relentlessly Smug, the DOJ Boasts about its Nefarious "Take-downs" of Health Professionals,

In its 2018 report, entitled "Healthcare Enforcement Year in Review," the DOJ lauds its own tyrannical actions. I ask, "How in the world are these clowns 'enforcing healthcare' when they're mangling it to death? When they're rendering American physicians impotent to provide quality pain management?"

Furthermore, in an early 2019 announcement on its anti-opioid goals and on its prosecutions and imprisonments, the DOJ pridefully reported on the entrapments, prosecutions and imprisonments of physicians, nurses and pharmacists. And they seemed gleeful that those convicted got lengthy prison terms.

No wonder pain patients can't get their prescription narcotics anymore. Boastfully, DOJ operatives-gone-amok managed to snare 601 professionals of whom 162 were charged with prescribing opioids. Duh! That's their job in providing medical care for patients with pain diagnoses. You treat them with the appropriate opioid at the appropriate dosage for their painful illness and the manner in which their bodies metabolize opioids.

Unrestrained, Boastful DOJ Prosecutors Intimidate Pharmacists

The DOJ's sieges on Healthcare Providers also Intimidate Pharmacy Corporations. CVS Caremark, for example, and even Medicare Part D are also subjecting pain victims to drastic prescription narcotic reductions. For example, unashamedly, the DOJ reported that, on February 8, 2019, it served a TRO (Temporary Restraining Order) on two drugstores and its three pharmacists, preventing their dispensing of all controlled substances. This, they puffed up their empty chests about, was an action based on the PIL (Prescription Interdiction and Litigation) Task Force (funny how many "task forces," negatively affecting Americans, are run by do-nothing-good committees) purported "to address the opioid epidemic." That, in direct counterpoint to what their essential focus should be – on the illicit street drug deaths of drug addicts. Not on sick-in-pain patients and their well-qualified physicians and pharmacists.

These DOJ insipids continue to display abnormal pride in ruining hundreds and hundreds of health professionals' lives and careers, and in creating a climate of such fear and intimidation in America that most pain patients can't access normal narcotic analgesic treatment ever again. As a result, such pain patients are dropping dead sooner due to deteriorating health from sudden cold-turkeying and untreated pain. Others are suiciding out of despair of ever again receiving adequate medical care for their pain. This is a medical nightmare, glaringly huge, unbelievably ignored by, or ignorantly misrepresented by too many in the media. Too many, that is, who don't dig for the facts about our government DOJ/DEA gone amok against our excellent physicians and against the sick in pain.

DOJ "Opioid Warning Letters" Meant to Intimidate Paincare Doctors

The DOJ, these non-physicians, have unilaterally decided to persecute clinicians prescribing narcotic analgesics for patients suffering conditions of lifelong pain. Clearly, they've taken this uneducated position and this amoral stance, rather than focus on arresting dealers, on confiscating Chinese, Mexican and Internet illicits, and on remanding illicits addicts to detox. Though that's where their focus should be, the DOJ is bent on diverting the public's attention away from their failures in those crucial areas by targeting healthcare professionals, thereby leaving a trail of misery in their wake of raided and imprisoned high-quality physicians, other clinicians, and now pharmacists. And a maelstrom of severely suffering pain patients without their opioid medicines, some going on to failing health and early deaths; others choosing suicide.

Good going, guys. You at the DOJ can rack up hundreds and hundreds of notches on your gung-ho gestapo belts for the dead pain patients you've left in your wake. Your clueless insurgencies into intricate medical affairs you have zero knowledge of has forced scores and scores of pain patients, who'd have loved to live longer, onto an early journey into eternity.

Imagine: You're an Innocent Doctor and You Just Received an Ominous DOJ "Opioid Warning Letter"

This is insanity. Imagine, a DOJ lawyer or a DEA policeman, non-physicians, ordering your doctor to lower dosages of your insulin, your penicillin, your antiepileptic, or your antipsychotic medication. If diabetic, you'd have a dangerous hyperglycemic crisis; if you've an infection, it'd worsen; if epileptic, you'd have more seizures; and if schizophrenic, you'd suffer hearing those voices again. Yet, these law-school and police-academy graduates give themselves permission to prescribe medications. Shouldn't these dangerous clowns be imprisoned for practicing medicine without a license?

As to appropriate paincare, physicians and other prescribing clinicians, know what they're doing in each individual pain patient's case. Thus, though every drug can have some negative side effects, risk-to-benefit ratios are considered by these well-educated professionals when they prescribe anything, not only painkillers. And dosages, though often uniform among many medicines for all patients, in the case of pain management, one size does not fit all. Differences, in pain intensities and durations, and in the individual ways each patient's body metabolizes specific opioids, mean that doctors must tailor their dosages individually. As a result, some patients need higher doses than others. And some need their narcotics more often throughout their day.

On top of all the intimidations generated by the DOJ and it's DEA, MDs now have to worry about these missives. Sadly, and with added expense and time-loss, doctors receiving such intrusive letters are advised to seek legal counsel immediately. Otherwise, you're being set up by the DOJ for whatever they wish to perpetrate against you. This is the fallout from an unchecked federal agency that appears to be run by conscienceless autocrats.

The Department of Justice should back off! Stop interfering in the doctor-patient relationship. Stop intimidating and raiding medical practices. Stop prosecuting and imprisoning innocent

clinicians. It's not your job to practice medicine. Because telling physicians what, when, and how much they can prescribe is practicing medicine without a license. So you at the DOJ need to be prosecuted for impersonating physicians all over this country. Remember your real job is to catch criminals via legal processes.

Thus far, you at the DOJ have failed in that duty, When it comes to the millions of American pain patients and the physicians they depend upon for their care, you at the DOJ have failed our whole country. How your entanglements in down-the-rabbit-hole laws, admonishments, warnings, even threats, raids, spying via PDMPs on patients' confidential medical records, and intimidating blameless physicians are meant to cure the still-uncontained, ever-rising deaths of those addicted to illicit fentanyl, fentanylized-heroin, and, sadly, assorted mixtures of other nonprescribed drugs and alcohol is a mystery to me and millions of baffled innocent in-pain citizens. Addicts using illicits are your true targets. Remand those sick patients to detox. Interdict illicit drug imports. You know they're arriving from the Internet, from Mexico and from China. And vigorously locate and prosecute suppliers and dealers. Those are your duties that, when handled responsibly, will lower the death statistics of opioid addicts.

Due to Lawless DOJ Tactics, from New York to Los Angeles, Pain Doctors are Retiring, Pain Patients are Dying

Unconscionable DOJ actions–forcing patients in pain to give up their well-working opioid analgesics, forcing doctors to meet some ridiculous fictitious dosage diminishments that are too low for pain relief, destroying millions of IPPs' lives, and being okay with the growing numbers of suicides due to despair of ever being pain-free–these are not okay.

According to the Health Law & Business section of Bloomberg Law on February 4, 2019 **https:/news.bloomberglaw.com** it is questionable whether the DOJ has the right to "warn" doctors with such presumptive letters. Too, it's obvious these "warning letters" are meant to frighten doctors, to intimidate them into unethically lowering necessary dosages of narcotic analgesics, to alarm prescribers about the viability of their hard-won careers. Writers of that Bloomberg Law article advise doctors who receive such DOJ "warning letters" to "retain counsel and conduct a review of your prescribing practices.... given the uncertainty and high stakes involved...inaction is too great a risk." No wonder doctors all over America feel forced to stop taking care of patients in pain. No wonder ethical, empathic physicians are abandoning Hippocrates' *Primum Non Nocere!*

Stop the War on Pain Patients and their Physicians

Let us hope that there's some ethical soul at the DOJ, some fearless empath, who can influence this run-amok agency to refocus on the real opioid epidemic, the illicits in the streets. And, hands off medical practitioners who are doing nothing wrong. Otherwise, the DOJ will keep causing the ever-increasing epidemic, which the CDC should do everything to prevent – PAIN PATIENT SUICIDES. Stop, DOJ. Stat! And that means, "It's an emergency. Stop immediately!"

Section iv

POLICE STATES: Pain Sufferings, Physician Imprisonments, Suicides

Chapter Fourteen

Our Federal Government Weaponized the Word "Opioid" Emboldening Most States to Kill Pain Prescriptions

With a venal, strategically-plotted publicity campaign, based on their various clueless or nefarious intentions, Health and Human Services with its CDC, plus the Department of Justice with its Drug Enforcement Administration, loosed on unsuspecting Americans a barrage of statistics lies, and unabated nonsense conflating illicit drug abusers with normal patients requiring legally-prescribed narcotics for their pain. Thus, firing up the public with skewed news blitzes, these federal loose cannons planted The Big Lie in the minds of Americans: that prescription narcotics are the cause of drug addicts overdosing and dying. That, despite these facts:

1. Illicit drug deaths continue to increase drastically even as there has been a significant decrease in narcotic drug prescriptions over several years.
2. Most street drug deaths are due to adulterated fentanyl or fentanylized heroin, neither of which are prescribed for pain patients.
3. Postmortem blood, from heroin overdosers, contains 6-monoacetylMORPHINE, the metabolite of heroin.
4. These heroin deaths have been unethically recorded as "morphine deaths". Then slyly, by the CDC, attributed to prescription

morphine when reporting "opioid death statistics," tilting naive journalists and the public toward demonizing prescription opioids and the pain patients who need them.

5. A high percentage of illicit drug deaths are caused by illegal combinations, including various benzodiazepines, like Xanax® (alprazolam) - antianxiety chemicals - and/or alcohol.

Thus, that Federal propaganda, spread far and wide all over America, crept into multi-levels of our society, inflicting its baseless hogwash on pain experts, pain patients and their families, pain clinics, pharmacies, healthcare professionals at all levels, on Emergency Room acute pain patients, on Postsurgical patients in pain in the ICU and thereafter, and on Dental Patients. Thus, these inexcusable federal untruths have turned our United States into a dungeon of horror for the known existing 50 million pain patients. Add to that, all the other kinds of short-term, but no less unbearable pain patients who are also now being told to take aspirin or acetaminophen or nothing.

Truths Hidden from the Public by Federal Officials and the Media

These truths have been systematically ignored, or deliberately misreported, by our federal health and drug policing agencies. Their unremitting goal appears to be diversion of America's attention from the real guilty parties – illicits suppliers, dealers, importers – and from sick addicts using illicits who should be in detox as patients. These truths have gone almost completely unreported, or downplayed by even esteemed journalists who Americans rely on to hold government accountable for its actions and their effects on citizens.

Oregon, the State Most Restrictive of Opioid Prescriptions

It is widely known, by Oregonian pain experts, by Oregonian pain patient advocates, and by pain patients across the nation, that Oregon, among all our states, is leading the pack of wolves at the door of pain-wounded lives and their doctors. Strangely, or perhaps to be expected (See Chapter 21, "Hidden Agendas of Anti-Opioid Proponent$" to learn more about this group), Dr. Andrew Kolodny's clan of questionable contributors to the doomed 2016 *CDC Guideline*, inserted itself into Oregon's assaultive legislative process against Intractable Pain Patients and their physicians. Thus insinuating themselves into Oregon's pain-guidance-related Tapering Workgroup, they made false assertions, as pointed out by distinguished paincare expert, Stephen E. Nadeau, M.D..

[The Brandeis-Associated, misguided anti-opioid zealots, who temporarily transplanted themselves into Oregon to inflict their wrongheadedness on already over-legislated opioid prescribing in that state, included Dr. Kolodny, Dr. Jane Ballantyne, Dr. Anna Lembke, Roger Chou and Paul Coelho. Bravely, however, Dr. Nadeau roundly disputed their "Tapering Guidance and Tools".]

Pain Management Expert, Stephen E. Nadeau, M.D. Challenges Oregon's "Tapering Workgroup"

On January 16, 2019, at **http://paindr.com**, Dr. Jeffrey Fudin hosted the guest blog "Opioids and Politics" by neurologist and cognitive neuroscientist Stephen E. Nadeau, M.D., Professor of Neurology at the University of Florida College of Medicine and Associate Chief of Staff for Research at Malcom Randall VA Medical Center, Gainesville, Florida.

Since 1982, Dr. Nadeau has specialized in the care of chronic nonmalignant pain patients. Significantly, he is also Senior Research Advisor to the Alliance for the Treatment of Intractable Pain (ATIP). In his blog, discussed below, Dr. Nadeau was responding to assertions of The Oregon Pain Guidance Clinical Advisory Group, Tapering Workgroup's dicta in "Tapering Guidance and Tools"

Does Tapering Chronic Pain Patients Ever Make Sense?

At the outset, Dr. Nadeau disputes the group's assertion that tapering opioids for chronic pain patients is needed, pointing out the twin debacles of decreased employment and increased healthcare costs for patients deprived of their well-working narcotic analgesics. He further declares that research evidence demonstrates the effectiveness of prescription opioid regimens over the long term for such sufferers. And he points to the evidence of "lost productivity" when such patients, deprived of their narcotic pain relievers, become housebound, often bedbound, therefore unemployable. The pressure on our economy in escalating healthcare costs and lost job productivity is between $560 to $635 billion annually, he further emphasizes.

Dr. Nadeau also insists that there is "good clinical practice" evidence that "opioids are highly effective in the treatment of nonmalignant pain," a benefit sustainable for years, he asserts, paralleling his clinical pain management experience. He also addresses the true statistics, contrary to the faux allusion by both federal and Oregonian bureaucrats, of potential misuse of prescription opiates and opioids.

Thus, in this guest blog, Dr. Nadeau points out the very low rates of yearly deaths due to chronic opioid use - 0.08%, 0.25%, or 0.5% annually, depending on dosages ranging from less than 200 MMED (milligram equivalents of morphine a day) to more than 400 morphine milligram equivalents daily. Comparatively, he emphasizes, the risk rate for negative effects equates to those risk-to-benefit ratios seen with medications for protection against Cerebrovascular Accidents (CVAs aka Strokes) and Atrial Fibrillation. This comparatively low risk rate, he insists, is justified for the kinds of pain that never go away and often worsen with time.

Dr. Nadeau, therefore, disputes the Ballantyne et al. claim that long-term, high dose opioids are ineffective and unsafe. Adamantly, he asserts, "These claims are not supported by scientific evidence." He further counters the wrong-headedness of the 2016 *CDC Guideline*, which the "Tapering Workgroup" relied on for its misinformation. He further decries that group's apparent notion that "one dose fits all," which is not to exceed 90MMED. His proof is that randomized controlled trials have shown "a 13-fold variability in dose requirements" attributable to varying pain intensities, varied liver metabolism genetics and inherited Central Nervous system differences, including nociceptor (neuronal endings signaling pain) transduction. That is my quick overview of this vital report. Read more of Dr. Nadeau's retort to the taperers at Dr. Fudin's **http://paindr.com**

And, Dr. Nadeau refutes the falsehood that restricting prescription opioids saves addicts' lives. Importantly, Dr. Nadeau emphasizes that deaths from illicit drugs far exceed those from prescribed narcotics, saying, "The very idea that constraining prescription opioids in the clinic is somehow going to solve the still-growing crisis in the streets begs credulity."

With those brave assertions–in this climate of federal overreach, of depriving pain patients of their appropriate medications, and of entrapping fine physicians who dare to do the right thing for their pain patients – Dr. Nadeau presents a must-do list. It dares to counter the federal misinformation spewed by the HHS/CDC and the DOJ/DEA, which puts every American physician at risk of professional license revocation, of having their medical practices and clinics raided, of indiscriminate access to their patients' HIPAA-protected medical records, and of incurring outrageous legal expenses to protect themselves, their livelihoods and their patients. Additionally, on some flimsy, indefensible illogic, targeted doctors are accused of a nebulous activity, "conspiracy," which the DOJ isn't required to prove, setting innocent clinicians up for imprisonment. Thousands, so far, across the country have been so invaded. Therefore, Dr. Nadeau demands:

1. The 2016 *CDC Guideline* must be revised to reflect the true data!
2. Government must not interfere in patients' pain care by physicians!
3. Add intensive training in pain management in medical school and in CMEs! (Continuing Medical Education programs)
4. Government can help greatly, too, by providing anti-addiction services!
5. And, I'm sure Dr. Nadeau would agree to this added directive; Government must switch its wrongful focus – from intractable pain patients, their physicians and their narcotic dosages – to

their real jobs: Interdiction of the Chinese, Mexican and Internet imports of deadly illicits; Prosecution of dealers; and remanding to detox of illicits addicts.

Dr. Nadeau is one of several brave physicians speaking out, in this federally threatening climate, against such onslaughts drummed up by a shrill anti-opioid minority, whose motives are not inherently meant to benefit pain patients. Some are even dead-set (*sic*) on the expanded prescribing of Suboxone® (buprenorphine/naloxone)—used for detoxing addicts - by adding suddenly cold-turkeyed pain patients to the lucrative patient censuses at Suboxone ® treatment centers. (See Chapter 20, "The Suboxone Hoax".)

As Oregon Goes in the Opioid War Against Pain Patients, So Goes the Nation

Not only has Oregon been hell-bent on denying narcotic pain care to Medicaid patients suffering intractable pain, the Oregon Health Authority (OHA) has the nerve to condescend to hold hearings of the Health Evidence Review Commission (HERC). The kind of "hearings" where nobody in power listens to the expert physicians, nor to the suffering patients, nor to the silenced cries of pain patients killed by suicide. Why call them "hearings" when your intention is to be deaf to voluble human screams of pain?

Compounding these never-ending-talkings, which have become common around the country, some even convened by the CDC which calls them "task forces," is the fact that zero happens beyond talk. Maddening because, again, they talk-talk-talk, accomplish nothing, keep the misguided *Guideline* intact with all its malignant fall-out, killing off innocent patients, causing others years of suffering since its inception, and ruining the careers and lives of thousands of innocent physicians and other caring clinicians.

And, because both pain patients and their empathic pain specialists are forced to hesitate, even cower, in the face of these never-before-in-America Gestapo tactics, birthed by the 2016 *CDC Guideline*, Oregonians, doctors, pain patients, journalists seem to genuflect in front of these sadists who have been okay with the concept of under-dosing of prescription narcotic medications, all the way to zero MMEs (Morphine Milligram Equivalents) of narcotics to severely suffering patients in pain.

Zero has been accomplished by convenings of talk-a-thons. Therefore, everyone concerned should stop applauding the nothing-but-talk feelinglessness of burgeoning "task forces" run by Federal and State bureaucrats who are burying, in mere blah-blah and paperwork, quality medical practices with storm trooper tactics, and burying pain patients, too, by condemning them to suicide.

Chapter Fifteen

States of Never-ending Pain

It isn't possible, in this one chapter, to lay out before you, the reader, the actual number of human-suffering stories from every single pain-sufferer denied their prescription opioids in every state and every city in America. That would take at least two more volumes of the personal reports of millions of Americans, now bereft of their medically-appropriate medications, left to suffer because of an ignorant government sweeping, like a tsunami, throughout our nation, whipping up a hysterical tide of opiophobia, via the automaton actions of DEA operatives, intimidating doctors nationwide.

Therefore, I will only present, here, the most representative sufferings of pain patients from all around our country, caused by the ineptitude of HHS/CDC bureaucrats and the gestapo-like invasions of the DOJ's puppet operatives in the DEA.

As you experience these Americans' pain-filled lives, their wishes for their own deaths, and some reports of actual suicides due to unbearable, ongoing pain, I ask you to multiply what is being described by all our fifty states and by thousands of our cities, towns and villages. Because the DOJ and its DEA, determinedly, have reached their venal claws into every nook and cranny of our medical system, impinging on patients' pain care, life quality, and on their very lives. Suicides abound and are ongoing by patients who had preferred to stay alive. But their unrelieved pain made their lives unbearable. Who, among these federal agency leaders, will take responsibility for these inhumane consequences of their, if not evil, then clueless Keystone Kop behaviors that have killed so many and are causing so very many others to suffer needlessly? Because, these deaths are murders caused by neglectful government incompetence at the least. Or by deliberate human rights violations of international prohibitions against torture and killings of innocents.

Therefore, please read these abbreviated pain patient reports with the realization that each represents hundreds of thousands of others in similar, medically-negligent circumstances.

And, after you've absorbed some of these painful experiences, contact whichever legislators you can to get the DOJ/DEA out of pain care medical practice. Then impress on your state's Board of Medicine the imperativeness of standing by all your doctors and defending all your DEA-raided physicians. Demand that they don't abandon their fine member-physicians by lowering their professional standards to match the unconscionable behaviors of the DEA police.

Millions of Pain Patients are Frightened their Doctors will Stop their Pain-Relieving Opioids

Opiophobia in Enid, Oklahoma: This retired Physician Assistant and sufferer of severe spinal pain, since injuring himself moving a patient in a body cast, calls for "an in-depth investigation of the DEA for invading good pain doctors' offices...all because of completely unrelated illegal street narcotics."

Daily Pain in Duluth, Minnesota: A piano teacher, suffering Sickle Cell Disease with periodic Sickle Cell Crises, was accused of being "a drug seeker" in the ER before her hematologist arrived to prescribe an intravenous opiate to be started STAT. Which means "NOW". "IMMEDIATELY!" (See Section I to learn about severely painful Sickle Cell Disease.)

Perpetual Pain in Philadelphia: If it weren't for this young woman's years of prescription opioid medicine, her severe migraines would have kept her from graduating college. But, now, "With the DOJ prosecuting my doctor, I can't find a new one to help me so I just lost my job as a computer programmer because I need to lie down in a dark room when the headaches attack me." She wonders, "Why is Pennsylvania letting the federal government tell our doctors how to prescribe medicines we need?"

Torture from Trigeminal Neuralgia in Chattanooga, Tennessee: A 57-year-old grandmother, crying to me on the phone, told me, "My neuralgia condition is terrible if I didn't have my pain medicine. Also, I had three failed hip surgeries. For 10 years my pain was controlled with my opioid until my doctor force-tapered me. Pain is very bad in my head and hips. I lost my job. Too many sick days in bed."

***Cold-Turkeyed* in Estes Park, Colorado**: Once a beauty queen in pageants, now a retired chemist, this diabetic bemoans the abrupt deprivation of her prescription oxycodone, telling me, "...because my pain doctor said the government is rationing pain medicines. He's afraid he'll lose his medical license because of the Federal Police."

Fearing Constant Pain in New Orleans, Louisiana: This 40-year-old says, "I no longer wake up and get breakfast, go to my job at the call center. All I can do, now that my doctor stopped my pain medicine, is roll of bed into my wheelchair. My back pain is excruciating. I just made my will out and am ready to write my final note."

Pharmacy Refuses Opioid Prescription in Peoria: A middle-aged woman, suffering with a terminal case of Interstitial Cystitis (See Section I to learn about this very painful, lifelong condition) recently went to her long-time pharmacist to pick up her prescribed narcotic pills. He told her, reports her husband, "The DEA says you're a drug seeker so I can't fill your prescription. That night," her husband told me in an email, "she shot herself to death with my police weapon".

Forced Injections and Painful Implants in Gary, Indiana: "The DEA and Indiana officials cause me worse pain than from my chronic illness," said this former fashion designer. Their regulations forced her doctor to inject into her spine and also place an implant there. Neither helped. "I hurt worse than before all this," she wept to her social worker. "I'd rather be dead than in bed all day in pain."

Third Degree Burns from Coerced Electrotherapy in Baltimore: The rush to comply with the specious opiophobic dictates of the DOJ/DEA police-run-amok caused this 47-year-old truck driver to suffer third degree burns from forced substitution of electrotherapy instead of his usual opioid that had kept him at his job for over 15 years. "I'm now ready to die. Life hurts." He told me, "I can't help my family anymore. No one cares. The government doesn't care about us."

Because HHS/CDC and DOJ/DEA Overreach is Depriving Americans of Prescription Narcotics

THERE ARE ONLY 3 PAIN PATIENT TYPES LEFT:

1. Contemplating Suicide.

2. Dying prematurely from physical sequelae of Untreated Pain.

3. Suiciding due to Unending Torturous Pain.

Unrelenting Pain in Orel, Utah: Weeps this housewife, suffering trigeminal neuralgia, "I almost died from withdrawal and return of my pain when my doctor was scared by a DEA raid of his partner's office. I know other patients who did die, " she kept crying to me, "they killed themselves."

Kidney Misery in Kalamazoo, Michigan: One 28-year-old man with nephrolithiasis reports, "My kidney stone was passing as I was in the ER. Waiting for the urologist, the ER doctor refused to prescribe a painkiller. I couldn't help screaming as the stone moved. When the specialist came, he said I should have been give a narcotic because this is one of the worst kinds of pain anyone can have." As an R.N., this horrible anti-patient treatment by the ER doctor makes me want to throw up. Not only in empathy with this patient, but aware this is only one egregious example of how the rogue actions of DEA operatives have infected physicians with such fear of prescribing exactly the painkiller they know is needed for known excruciating pain. Such as a kidney stone trying to squeeze its bruising way down the narrow sliver of ureter leading into the bladder. See? Now, even a one-dose injection of a prescription narcotic in a medically-acute one-time emergency is being stampeded out of existence by the overreach of DOJ/DEA intrusions into complex medical situations they know zero about.

Another Miserable Kidney Case in Ames, Iowa: This case further illustrates the added pain inflicted on nephrolithiasis patients when a stone is scraping and cutting its way down a ureter in this police-state environment. Another kidney stone patient reports getting merely a minuscule, non-analgesic dose of Dilaudid. Then being abruptly discharged from the hospital, still in pain, but abandoned by the physicians there, who wouldn't prescribe any painkiller for him while he was recovering from this attack. He lives in fear of when the next stone starts its painful ureteral trip.

Abandoned in Pain in Birmingham, Alabama: In my email survey, this chronic pain patient told me, "My neurological disorder was hurting much less for 18 years on my stable methadone doses. Suddenly, my prescription was cut to only 25% of what helped me. No pain relief whatsoever. Now I know why many pain patients get their final help from Doctors Smith and Weston!"

Copeless and Angry with Pain in Darien, Connecticut: This patient, suffering severe vertebral crippling and pain was so rapidly tapered off her hydrocodone, that she was, effectively, cold-turkeyed. So her pain clinic sent her to a Suboxone ® (buprenorphine/naloxone) prescribing facility with the diagnosis of "addict". She cries out, "A pox on all the political bootlickers...and on all the DEA police derriere-kissers." (See Chapter 20, "The Suboxone Hoax".)

Plea for Pain Pills in Plano, Texas: This secretary pleads, "I suffer chronic back pain. Please don't steal my ability to keep my job by cutting off my codeine."

Nightmarish Pain in New York, New York: This medically-abandoned man, even feeling intimidated about sending me this email, wrote, "I was forced off my hydrocodone for my inherited painful disease. Now my life is a living hell. Where do I turn for relief? I am seriously about to buy a gun." When I received this message, I contacted a suicide hotline and asked them to please help him.

Illicit Drugs a Last Recourse in Chicago, Illinois: The last resort for this actor with escalating neuropathies, he says, was to buy street drugs because, "otherwise, I will kill myself. And my wife just had our first child, a baby boy. Why is our government doing this to us?" Why, indeed.

Hellish Daily Suffering in Honolulu, Hawaii: "I am hurting beyond words," says this dance teacher. She's stuck in bed, lost her studio job, is on disability. All because her doctor was raided by the government. "No wonder," she laments, "the suicide rate has jumped in all fifty states at the same time our doctors stopped prescribing our painkillers."

Choosing Death Instead of Pain in Lexington, Kentucky: This patient's opioid prescription was reduced swiftly by 75%. The remaining 25% didn't touch her severe neurogenic pain. As she seriously plans to kill herself, she warns, "This country is imploding from lack of compassion and loss of common sense. Not long after expressing this, her family reported to me, she put a plastic bag over her head and was found dead by her teenage son.

Pain-suffering Farmer in California Wine Country: She, a hardworking female farmer, emailed me that her degenerative spinal disc disease pain had been successfully relieved much of these 23 years because of her prescription opioid. But, when her pain doctor forced a reduction to only the 90MME (Morphine Milligram Equivalents) the CDC recommended, she said, "My pain returned with a vengeance. I had to quit working, sell the farm, stay in bed all day. My doctor is too scared to raise my doses. I'm so scared. Too old to hang out in alleys buying street drugs. From now on, death looks welcoming."

Neglected Painful Injury in Newark, New Jersey: It was an accident. A truck hit his car ten years ago and he ended up with CRPS (Complex Regional Pain Syndrome). "My body was mangled," he told me, "and my pain medicine is the only thing that keeps me sane, walking, and able to do some freelance computer work at home. But, with the new restrictions, my doctor told me he's worried about, I am terrified my medicine will be stopped. I'll be lost if this happens."

Pain Management Paranoia in Portland, Oregon: This Oregonian feels beleaguered by "the irrational paranoia of so many medical professionals since the CDC 'recommendations' came out." He adds that his 17 years on hydrocodone never caused addiction. And, "I pray my doctor isn't scared enough to retire and leave me in pain because I'll lose my high-tech job."

Hopelessly Hurting in Honolulu, Hawaii: This middle-aged grandfather decries "the appalling lack of compassion and common sense that has infected medical practice since the CDC's recommendations." His crippling spinal disease, without his prescription opioid, means "I'm confined to my wheelchair all day, when I'm not in bed. Before my doctor stopped writing pain medicine prescriptions, I worked as a self-employed carpenter and, most days, my pain was pretty well-controlled. Now, I may as well be dead because I can't work or enjoy my family."

Too Bad, Take Tylenol for Trigeminal Neuralgia in Tallahassee, Florida: "You need to suck it up," sneered a practical nurse at a pain clinic to this mother of five. That said when this patient's doctor began to discontinue his treatment of pain patients altogether. "Shame on America!" That is what this woman said when she burst into tears from fear of never getting pain relief ever again. "With awful pain like that, how will I take care of my children," she moaned on the phone to me.

Dependency on Pain Relief, Not Addiction in Arlington, Virginia: This Sickle Cell Disease patient stresses how severe her lifelong pain is from her genetic disease. And, at only 23, she points out that "We are not addicts. But we depend on our opioids to reduce our pain. We know nothing can take it all away, but our opioids help us. I am not an addict, but I depend on my doctor's prescriptions for pain relief. Just like I depend on my insulin for my diabetes."

Worrying with Intolerable Pain in Wichita, Kansas: This Kansan lady, reporting how well her prescription opioid had quelled her 17 years of unrelenting pain, until the 2016 CDC Guideline burst her bubble of a somewhat livable life, told me how she could hold a job, play with her grandchildren, enjoy a little time with friends. But, since her medication has been cut, she said, "My life has declined 98%. I no longer can work." And her home of 32 years is now in foreclosure. "The pain is so bad, I isolate in my room so as not to scare my family...my life went from being engaged and happy...to barely existing, and living in a torturing hell...this is not living."

Hurting All Day Long in Helena, Montana: The end of his teaching job, says this gentleman, came when his pain medicine was abruptly stopped by his doctor. He insisted that "Opioid treatment should be on a case by case basis and be up to the prescribing doctor who should not feel threatened to lose his/her license...being bedridden shouldn't be the only option for intractable pain victims. That's inhumane torture when there's medicine that can bring relief."

Frightened at Losing Prescription Hydrocodone in Pensacola, Florida: With chronic fibromyalgia pain, it's frightening that non-experts are writing policy that will affect many, many thousands of us....There's no evidence to support removing stable patients from pain management treatment that works for us....Please stop punishing pain."

Burning Pain in Biloxi, Mississippi: Says this fed-up patient, "Taking aim at innocent pain patients while ignoring real needs to police illegal street drugs, angers me. I wonder how come these people, who do not suffer chronic pain, want to inflict more pain on us patients. Yet they continue to ignore the real crisis...the illegal heroin and fentanyl, the real killers."

Severe Suffering in St. Paul, Minnesota: This middle-aged grocer pleads, "Please consider the human lives made better taking opiate medications. It's made it possible for me to work and take care of my family. Without these life-saving medicines, I'll have to depend on government programs to feed and support us. Then I'll feel shame on top of pain."

Vibrating Pain in Lynchburg, Virginia: "I have so much nerve pain," says this former gym teacher, "I could scream. Which I do...when I'm alone in the house. That's because the DEA raided my doctor's office, took him away. He was very caring, giving me my narcotic prescriptions regularly for over 12 years. I could train a whole bunch of kids in sports. Now, I lie in bed all day, depressed. No other doctor will help me. I'm thinking of ending this life of pain."

Frightening Shooting Pains in Framingham, Massachusetts: Crushing osteoarthritis limited this artist's life and work until her pain specialist prescribed a life-altering opioid, "to take the edge off the pain, to allow me to make my paintings. A blessing for 32 years, my doctor has now 'retired' because someone from the DEA phoned him. Warned him about giving too much pain medicine." She goes on that, "Decisions to initiate, maintain and discontinue opioids should be made between the patient and the doctor, not by government agencies."

Under-Dosing Opioids Prolongs Suffering in Orem, Utah: This lawyer, with lifelong spinal disease, escalating pain, and newly *cold-turkeyed* off his reliable, pain-relieving prescription narcotic, declares: "Something's wrong with the DOJ/DEA raiding pain physicians all over

America, locking them up on untrue charges, when they should be going after the illegal drug imports and the drug dealers." The sad thing now, because of these wrong-focused government incursions, pain patients are so gravely under-dosed that some are driven to seek relief from those very street drugs. This man reminds the government entities perpetuating this patient abuse, as a result of his forced suffering, "Karma has a way of catching up with you. You're all just one sudden illness away from being in our shoes." I'm sure he was implying, "Then, where will you turn to for your opioid relief when there is no doctor left who is willing to prescribe these for anyone, ever again?"

Untreated Chemotherapy-Induced Neuropathy in Chillicothe, Ohio: Treated with chemo for her cancer, an awful side-effect was an unrelenting neuropathy (See Section I for a discussion of neuropathy). On her prescription opioid, she could easily work as a supermarket manager. "Suddenly," she emailed me, "my oncologist said he was afraid of losing his license because of DEA raids around the country. He told me he'd no longer prescribe my narcotic. Now, I can't work. Can't walk or stand. The cancer is tamed so I thought I'd be able to feel better. Now I'm in bed all day. This is no life."

Severe, Lifelong Pain in Suffern, New York: This freelance photographer has been in lifelong pain, since childhood, from multiple surgeries. Going from "annoying to debilitating". Magnetic Resonance Imagings (MRIs) and Computerized Axial Tomography (CAT) Scans demonstrated the steady progression of this pain-producing condition. And none of the array of ancillary treatments (See Section I for a discussion of these) such as Yoga, physiotherapy, NSAIDs (nonsteroidal anti-inflammatory drugs, like aspirin) nor psychotherapy minimized the pain of this sufferer, who said, "I live in fear of having my medicine taken away....I had to get to the point of being suicidal before my doctor realized how bad my pain was and stopped fighting me about the meds."

Collapsed Spine with Severe Pain in Nome, Alaska: My father screamed, daily in pain, from progressive rheumatoid arthritis." The only thing that helped him calm down, eat, rest a little, said his daughter, "was his narcotic pain-reliever prescribed by his very compassionate geriatrician." His collapsed spine finally caused his deterioration. But, she reports, "I'll always love his kind doctor for doing his best to keep my dad as comfortable as possible and to even, at times, enjoy his grandchildren."

Hard-to-Manage Pain in Harrisburg, Pennsylvania: This RN, only able to do hospital work because of the pain relief from her OxyContin, points out that "Dependence doesn't equal addiction." Her pain clinic forces, on her and other pain patients, pill counts, urinalyses...plus she gets insinuations from some professionals there that she's "a drug-seeking addict". If her medication is stopped and the pain returns, she wrote to me, "I'll have to go to the streets for relief."

On the Verge of Suicide from Excruciating Pain in Dallas: Once a hockey player, this pain-sidelined athlete, diagnosed with arachnoiditis with severe neuropathy, says that suicide is ever-present on his mind because his doctor cut his prescription narcotic by 60%. " I did not consent to this forced taper. It's like being raped, by my doctor and by my government. I've tried all other physical, mental health and "woo-hoo" Oriental therapies but none have relieved my pain like my narcotic...at the right dose. He chastises those who don't suffer pain yet feel free to make laws restricting narcotic analgesic dosages. He thinks they'll change their stances when they or a close family member suffers an illness or injury that produces never-ending pain like his.

Doctor on the Verge of Suicide from Untreated Pain in Chicago: This MD groaned, telling me, "As a physician myself, I'm ashamed of the way our government has beaten down American doctors to where they're shaking in their boots if a patient needs a narcotic prescribed for pain". She'd gone through everything else before requesting her colleague's well-working prescription opioid for her lifelong Interstitial Cystitis (See Section I where this dire condition is discussed)....Injections, chiropractors, stimulation, all alternatives – but none of those helped. Only her narcotic could be relied upon. "Now, that even my doctor, a colleague, won't prescribe for me anymore, I'm ready to leave this planet. Maybe on Mars I'll be treated as kindly as Earthlings treat their pets."

Doctor Dying in Pain in Danbury, Connecticut: I was able to go to the gym and run my small dermatology practice," said this MD on a moderate opioid dose for 15 years. His neurologist, who had diagnosed his Multiple Sclerosis, worked closely to help him as his MS progressed. But, "He recently retired because he couldn't, with a clear conscience, mistreat his pain patients by lowering their meds too low to control their pain." Sounding very depressed, he told me, "I have nothing to live for, now. In addition to my mobility problems, I'm in bed all day because of my pain."

Crying with Unrelenting Pain in Charlotte, North Carolina: "Without my prescription oxycodone, I would not be walking. With it, I work full-time and manage my home and family. Why would anyone want to take that away because there are drug abusers out there?" She goes on to plead, "Please make them hear our cries for help."

Painful Consequences for Many in Portland, Maine: This pain patient advocate asserts, "What's being done to chronic pain patients is inhumane and has no medical or scientific basis....the risks of opioids for chronic pain patients are minimal compared to the stress chronic pain puts on the body. People who refuse to recognize the medicinal benefits of opioids are living in an alternate universe, completely based on fiction and extremist propaganda."

Suicidal: Forced to Move to Another State for Pain Care: Simply, this woman said, "I was cut off from my meds cold turkey. After a year and a half of suffering, I wanted to kill myself. I finally had to relocate to another state for my pain care."

Another, Forced, Out-of-State Move for Pain Care: "In October of 2018, my pain had gone untreated for five months. I finally had to live away from my longtime home, in another state, to get my pain medicine...to save my life," sobs this patient who misses her family.

Terrible Pain Forced on Innocent Patients, Including Children: This sad woman reports, "I watched my husband die in pain and I watch my two kids struggle daily with pain caused by the same disease my husband had. They deserve access to prescription narcotic painkillers."

Severe, Multiple-Disease Suffering in Suffern, New York: For 23 years, this restaurant owner has managed to run her thriving Italian dining business, while being its chef for most of that time. All that involvement despite her daily wrestling with fibromyalgia, Crohn's Disease and myofacial migraine pain. Her doctor's prescription for her opioid painreliever dependably lessened much, not all, of her pain – but enough so she could work and put a nest egg away for her grandchildren. Now, she says, "I'm having an impossible time finding a doctor willing to even see me. My pain is too severe to work. I'm selling my restaurant. Things need to change. No one should have to live like this in constant pain."

Jarring Nerve Pain in Jersey City, New Jersey: Both a clinical researcher in neuroscience and a chronic pain sufferer, this professor declares, "Chronic pain patients are treated like drug-seeking criminals. We would not treat the family pet the way we are treating patients in severe daily pain. I'm ready to call it quits. What's the use of living this life of torture?"

Acknowledging Some Compassionate Doctors in Brooklyn, New York: Another Intractable Pain Patient sent me this direct message on Twitter: "My heartfelt thanks to all the bold, compassionate doctors who stand up in support of those of us suffering greatly due to noncancer chronic pain, including me from Ehlers Danlos Syndrome," a disease among Dr. Forest Tennant's top four most painful conditions. (See Chapter 12 for more about the courage of Forest Tennant,

MD) An incurable genetic disorder, this woman's pain worsens as time passes. Thus, she pleads, "It is cruelty to forcibly taper a patient who had been successfully stabilized, whose heart problems had finally gone away because they'd been due to unmanaged pain. But, since my pain doctor retired, no new doctor will treat my pain. And, now I have to have my cardiologist come to my home often. I'm very sad and hope some brave doctors will change what's being done to us."

Brain and Spinal Surgeries Painful Aftermath in Beaumont, Montana: This patient pleads with the powers that be, "I worked full-time due to my opioid prescription. Now I'm in bed. Please restore the doctor-patient relationship. My other option is suicide."

Terrible Pain in Taos, New Mexico: Our doctors and pharmacists are making pain patients suffer horribly from incurable pain," says this now bedridden professional golfer. "I pray this country gets back to allowing doctors to treat patients with incurable chronic unmanaged pain soon, before we lose more souls to suicide in this government war against pain patients, because I'm suffering...."

Paradox for Pain Docs in Oregon: Death with Dignity Okay – Life with Pain Relief Not Okay

One survey in May of 2019 uncovered that 80% of pain patients, whose prescription opioids had been discontinued, reported their lives were worsening, and that 38% were planning suicides. Additionally, 70% of clinicians, this survey found, feared prosecution for prescribing narcotic analgesics. Of these, 33% stopped accepting pain patients for care, and another 20% retired from medical practice altogether. The unchecked power of our overreaching "justice" system is killing quality medical care along with the killings of pain patients by suicides. Apparently, this Oregonian points out, "Euthanasia is legal in our state for a compassionate end to life. Yet, suffering unmedicated, in severe pain, is completely acceptable to our state politicians. Horrific government stupidity," cries this Sickle Cell Disease patient.

Mark Ibsen, M.D., Great Pain Expert, Speaks out in Helena, Montana:

Distressed by how non-physician government operatives have adulterated medical practice in this era of fervent opiophobia, pain specialist Dr. Mark Ibsen remarked recently, "Attorneys General practicing medicine without a license? I'm looking for anyone, ACLU, AMA, Disability Rights organizations, to sue them." Referring to these state lawyers who seem comfortable with deciding on opioid dosages, and even demanding that physicians stick to the low 90MME (Morphine Milligram Equivalents) and even as low as merely 50MME a day, Dr. Ibsen instructs, "This is like picking the appropriate amount of gas for trips to various destinations....How about 'enough to get you there?'" Finally, he asserts, "We can't allow politicians to set medical policy."

The End of Quality Medical Care in America?

Probably, after reading those real-life accounts of what pain patients are suffering all over America, you've experienced one of two reactions – tearfulness and anger. I know how you feel. As an R.N., I'm outraged by the cruelty inflicted on pain-suffering patients all over our country. This is not good medical practice. Not good nursing practice. Not good pharmacy practice. This is Unhealth-care. See? Even these professions are harmed by this Federal and State war on normal pain prescriptions of opioid analgesics. Imagine as a nurse, you're forced to tell your patient that "your doctor can't give you any more painkiller medicine". Imagine as a pharmacist, the DEA forces you to eye every pain patient suspiciously and to not fill legal opioid prescriptions. Imagine you're a physician who has just been arrested for normal narcotic prescribing for your patients in pain. This is the death of *Primum Non Nocere*. Hippocrates weeps.

Pharmacy Problems: Unfilled Prescriptions

Pharmacy Fails Pain Patient in Ogden, Utah: "My wife's chain drug store won't fill her Tramadol prescription. Her severe neuropain was safely treated with it for 18 years," reports this realtor. She would go out with him and work at her job in a flower shop. Now, he says, "She's in bed all day. Me? My life is also worse now. We have been talking about a pact so we both go together if it comes to that."

Pharmacy Refuses Prescription Refill in Phoenix, Arizona: This man suffered a crushed spine three decades ago and had to retire on pain medicine. "My extended-release opioid was miraculous, taking all my pain away. No euphoria. Just pain relief," he reports. But, last week his drug store for 15 years said they'd no longer fill his opioid prescription. "No other pharmacy will help me. This is our heartless government at work against pain patients. I'm desperate for help."

CVS and Walgreens Targeted by Florida's Opiophobia

In April 2019, **floridatrend.com** reported on the severe militancy of Florida's newest Attorney General, Ashley Moody, against major pharmacy corporations. One embattled issue is over Florida's PDMP (Prescription Drug Monitoring Program) – a centralized database of patients' medical records where physicians and pharmacists report their narcotic prescription activities – which the DEA has access to in many states, despite HIPAA confidentiality protections.

Many Other State Attorneys Disrupt Normal Opioid Prescribing

Note: Florida's attorney general attacking pharmacies is only one example of what's being perpetrated all over our country by many other state attorneys-general against what should be the smooth workings of our American healthcare system, with physicians prescribing what patients require to get them well or keep them comfortable, pharmacists filling their legal prescriptions, and patients receiving their medicines in peace, without suspicious glares by today's DEA-spied-on pharmacists. Without having to leave a drugstore minus one's desperately needed narcotic analgesic.

No Pharmacy or Manufacturer of Medicines is Safe from Accusatory Litigation by State Attorneys-General

The prior Florida Attorney General, Pam Bondi, sued manufacturers and distributors of prescription narcotics, including Johnson & Johnson, Janssen, and Purdue Pharma...and just before leaving office, Attorney General Bondi sued Walgreens and CVS (a combined total of 1500 drugstores in Florida), accusing them of not safeguarding their opioids and rushing as many out to the public as possible.

An Outrage Against Manufacturers and Dispensers of Vital Analgesics for Pain-Suffering Americans

Combined with the Drug Manufacturer defendants in the current Florida State attack on everything opioid, it must be remembered that – think of a strobe effect across our nation – other states' attorneys-general plus hundreds of American towns and cities are suing these faultless companies, which often agree to "settlements" rather than waste more time and money in court.

Lawmakers Stooping to the Ridiculous: Indemnification for "Morgue Overcrowding"

First of all, the law firms which litigate these cases are known to receive 30% of any "settlements". There go hundreds of millions of dollars that could have been used for R&D (Research & Development) at the pharmaceutical manufacturing level for new, life-bettering drugs; that could have motivated medication price-lowering at the pharmacy sales level.

And, what happens to these "settlements" of 70% of those multi-millions paid to each litigant state, city, town? It's claimed (who knows if this is actual) that these monies go to defray costs of hospital care, of "opioid epidemic" costs, of government police investigations, and yes they report, of "morgue overcrowding". Maybe if the DEA did its real job of interdicting illicits, arresting dealers, and remanding illicits users to detox, American morgues wouldn't be so full of dead drug addicts.

Walgreens and CVS dispute Florida's accusations of excess opioid distribution

More Evidence that Not Only the Feds are Fascistic, Now Florida is Vying for that Title

Attorney General Moody wants carte blanche power over Florida's PDMP, which would erode even more of patients' HIPAA rights – so information therein could be exposed during litigation. In that regard, watch out for Florida Senator Tom Lee who is eager to remove more of patients' rights to medical privacy in order to enrich Florida's coffers with filthy lucre, questionably gained through "settlements" some might believe are thinly-veiled coercions.

Florida Senator Against Pain Prescription Restrictions

Florida Senator Aaron Bean warned opiophobic Senator Tom Lee, **"Pharmacists are scared to death of your bill."**

Government "Shake-Down" of Pharmacies

Ocala, Florida Senator Dennis Baxley declared, "I have seen many an attorney-general across the country use the office to basically shake down large companies".

Chapter Sixteen

Plight of the Pain Care Physicians

Physicians Raided, Spied On, Hounded, Prosecuted, Imprisoned, Some Acquitted, Some Died Soon After

Even society's highly regarded professionals, the physicians among us who take excellent care of us, are daily victimized by a heedless, ill-informed, and intransigent autocracy based at HHS with its CDC, and at the DOJ with its DEA. Linked together in a seeming diabolical cabal, they've loosed such trepidation upon our fine doctors, across America, so that mounting numbers of MDs and other prescribing clinicians no longer will provide care for very sick and suffering pain patients. Thus, those federal autocrats' wrong-headed ideas about normal narcotic analgesic prescribing has produced a virulent coterie of federal and state anti-opioid zealots determined to destroy long-proven healthy, ethical medical care for Intractable Pain Patients. For those too sick to fight back, due to their life-limiting disabilities and never-ending pain, just managing to hold a job, barely able to be sociable, unable to live full lives.

And so, with the weaponization of the 2016 *CDC Guideline,* federal and state operatives, who never attended medical school, so are not supposed to dabble in writing even an aspirin prescription, now feel empowered to decide how many milligrams of a narcotic each particular pain patient should have, that these all should be the same dosage, despite hugely diverse diagnoses, levels of pain, aspects of disability and immobility. Such incredible hubris and meddling by nonmedical federal and state officials has resulted in pain doctors and professionals at pain clinics nationwide embarking on nonconsensual tapering, drastic *cold-turkeying*, under-dosing, and just plain turning pain patients away from care altogether. Malpracticing actions that have left pain patients in such poor health and insufferable conditions that they die suddenly, too young, from cardiac and other complications.

And there are even more unconscionable, unnecessary deaths due directly to these government interferers who have turned quality medical practice into the lowest level illness treatment analogous to medieval medical torture. Because, parallel to those government-engendered tragedies, are the rising suicide rates, around the nation, of untreated or under-treated pain patients whose suffering was too severe for them to remain earthbound. Both federal and state personnel who are participating in any part of this holocaust of thousands of suicides, therefore, ought to be charged with murder. Because, without their interference in normal, ethical medical care, all these patients would be alive today – and living some kind of a quality of life, not quite like people without daily pain, but participating in family life and work. And ALIVE!

A West Coast Inquisition: The Death Certificate Project of the Medical Board of California

This group targeted physicians who merely wrote the usual, normal prescriptions for their pain patients. However, pressured by fears of our nations runaway Department of Justice's ominous tactics, these overseers of medical practice in California all genuflect to the DOJ's threatening intimidations and commands. Just like the authorities on other State Medical Boards throughout our country.

This outrage Death Certificate Project occurred around the time of the drafting of the misguided 2016 *CDC Guideline* which "recommendations" eroded normal professional medical practice and stripped patients of their rights to have their sufferings diminished with the best medications known for pain alleviation – opiates and opioids! Indisputably!

Listen to this: 450 Medical Doctors have been thus attacked by this self-effacing California Medical Board which, genuflecting to the DOJ even more, implicated by referral to their healthcare boards a total of another 72 professionals: Nurse Practitioners, Physician Assistants, and Osteopaths. Cowardly California Medical Board! Instead of standing up for its upstanding professional physicians, capitulated to juris doctors who, I guess they suppose, studied medicine in law school!

Of the beleaguered 450 physicians, the board formally accused a mere 23 (frightening the rest of California's physicians overseen by the board) of "negligent prescribing". Which many California doctors are calling a Witch Hunt and an Inquisition. Even so, fear of these tactics, rumbling through the medical community, instigated by the DOJ's and DEA's relentlessly severe overreach has, thus, led California physicians, not yet on the "inquisition" radar to refuse narcotic prescriptions to patients they know medically deserve an opioid for their levels of pain.

Barbara McAneny, M.D., president of the American Medical Association and an Albuquerque, New Mexico oncologist, said the California board's witch hunt terrified her, that she knew other physicians felt the same way, and that they'd also be intimidated into not prescribing the opioid medications they knew their patients' conditions deserved. (See Dr. McAneny's full discussion of this in Section II PERIL, Chapter 10.)

California medical board officials treat MDs like they're in kindergarten. Gung-ho to change prescribing behaviors because blah, blah, blah from nonsensical DOJ pressures, they're sure to embarrass themselves with their dicta. Clueless, sitting at desks making proclamations, inventing problems and causes to comply with federal government know-nothings and even a State Attorney-General's goals to sue Pharma manufacturers, have set upon their ethically-practicing professionals, like the Donner Party cannibalizing its own.

Meanwhile, autocratically policing an honorable profession–all of whom know very well how to prescribe, what to prescribe, how much to prescribe, how often to prescribe, and for how long to prescribe a narcotic analgesic–what West Coast fools are these sitting there doing this to their own? Stop with the nonsense that MDs don't know prescribing. All physicians know prescribing for all kinds of medications, including for narcotic analgesics! They know! They've always known! I can't stomach the unconscionable disrespect these physicians and other clinicians are suffering from such emesis-producing, genuflecting by "Medical Boards" around the country. They're bowing so deeply to government tyranny that they're falling all over themselves like a failed circus act. For what? What's their payoff by complying with injustice?

Why wouldn't they challenge the DOJ overreach? Why is it a crime to abate your patient's pain? What is going on with professionals on these boards commiserating with lawyers, prosecutors, judges who have zero medical school credits and zero pharmaceutical knowledge? And yet such arrogance emboldens them to make laws impacting millions of pain patients and thousands of physicians, and to mount prosecutions against other health professionals such as nurses and pharmacists. What the...? Are we back in the Fifteenth Century with Castilian Dominican Friar Torquemada?

Physicians Received Threatening Letters from the California Medical Board It's widely known that less than 1% of patients treated with opioids ever graduate to addiction. This is true for patients on their prescription narcotics for years, even decades, due to lifelong afflictions. And those few who do were addicts prior to their pain diagnoses. All physicians avoid this complication by taking thorough medical histories and prescribing other therapies for known addicts. Albeit that opioids are best for certain kinds and severities of pain; in the case of addicts with a pain diagnosis, the physician has no other choice but to be creative by ordering physical therapies and/or other medications exclusive of opiates and opioids.

The California Board licenses 141,000 physicians. Just imagine the earthquake underfoot generated by the understandable shaking fears these intimidations of so many thousands of doctors are causing. Shame on California. Shame on all medical boards and medical organizations which don't stand up for their co-professionals, for the sacred Doctor-Patient relationship, for the right of every patient to not suffer to the best of our healthcare professions' abilities to engender healing and pain relief.

Let me repeat: Doctors prescribe medications for pain. Patients get instructions how to use these medications. If patients misuse them, where's the doctor's liability? What did he/she do wrong? And, addicts dying from street illicits...what has that to do with prescription medications? Nothing! Zero! Zilch! Nada! And, someone suiciding...what has that to do with physicians' prescriptions which are clearly discussed with patients and whose instructions are on the label of the vial containing the medication, along with extensive printed instructions coming from each pharmacist.

A key point: Many suicides by pain patients take place after the patient is left suffering from UNDER-DOSING or COLD-TURKEY-ING! Where is the "concern" of the medical boards around the country for these patients who are dying daily from the health ravages of intractable, untreated pain or, after despairing of ever again being relieved of pain, by suicide?

PHYSICIAN VICTIMS OF THE CALIFORNIA MEDICAL BOARD'S INQUISITION

San Francisco addiction specialist Dr. Ako Jacinto was threatened with a $1,000/day fine because a patient he'd long ago prescribed methadone for, without the doctor's knowledge took Benadryl (R) (diphenhydramine) along with it and died. In December 2018, Dr. Jacinto was still awaiting a hearing. These kinds of physician-intimidations impact the doctor's care of other patients, his family relationships, and his mental health. These have to stop STAT! This doctor did nothing wrong.

San Diego Dr. Paul Speckart reported that a number of his patients had received a letter from the California Medical Board demanding access to their medical records, questioning his patient care. Stunned, he said this upset his patients as well as him, severely, and disrupted his normal equanimity in his medical practice with all his other patients, because he feels it's not only about his medical license, it's also about the implication that he's a bad doctor.

More DOJ/DEA-Victimized Pain Physicians
Lesly Pompy, M.D., Michigan Pain Doctor Raided, Robbed of his Practice

Empowered by the crippling Guideline, the Drug Enforcement Administration (DEA) invades Pain Care Physicians' offices, and seizes patients' confidential medical charts. Dr. Lesly Pompy's unimaginable "capture" situation, in Michigan, by government intrusion on confidential patient care, and on the intricacies of focused medical practice in the complex specialty of the management of pain, is but one example of the looming threat spreading out across our nation, barging in on innocent doctors, scaring to death patients and nursing staff. And, ultimately neutering the ability of the medical profession to treat pain at all.

Dr. Pompy, who has done nothing wrong and has only used his medical knowledge to treat people in pain, ethically, has been so badly victimized that his is a horror story. However, his "capture" mirrors what hundreds of other clinicians have suffered at the hands of the dishonorable DEA and its DOJ overlords. Listen to this: A few years later, still awaiting adjudication of his case, and unable to practice his profession (remember, also, that the DOJ mandates the seizure of targeted physicians assets leaving them without money, effectively destroying what they've built over a lifetime), Dr. Pompy applied for a new job as an Emergency Medical Technician (EMT). Even this he awaits despite delay after delay. Seems to me the DEA and the DOJ are not really interested in protecting patients from specific medications. They're sadistically interested in destroying innocent physicians' livelihoods and lives. The latter I'll discuss in greater detail later in this chapter. It's important to note that some physicians, once acquitted die shortly thereafter. I consider these deaths murders by the Department of Justice with its tactics of stripping not-yet-prosecuted physicians of all their personal and professional assets, forcing medical boards to rescind their professional licenses, abandoning them in limbo as the oozingly slow judicial system steals their time, and without money, unable to afford an attorney.

Similar police state tactics are killing medical practices around the country. If it weren't so ominous, so destructive of normal medical care, and so unmitigatedly insensitive to pain patients' sufferings, these incursions would look like a grade D movie, even a Keystone Kops affair. But, there's nothing funny about these medical practice invasions generated by "permissions" implied in the 2016 *CDC Guideline*, which may as well have been titled *Mein Kampf*, and by the hubris and unchecked actions and antics of the DOJ and its DEA.

CALIFORNIA SCREAMING: MORE CALIFORNIA MEDICAL BOARD PERSECUTION

Corinne Vivian Basch, M.D., Another Doctor Persecuted, Fights Back The Medical Board of California, threatening to suspend Dr. Basch's Medical License, filed multiple charges against her specifying various applications of opioids and benzodiazepines (antianxiety meds), accusing her of "failure to taper" and other familiar charges applied incorrectly to physicians nationwide by DOJ prosecutors. Let me amend the latter to "applied viciously by DOJ persecutors!

Good for her: Dr. Basch is taking her case to court. In one report, Dr. Basch abhorred what many MDs now feel forced by DOJ physician-prosecutions to do: for example, lowering a morphine prescription of 340 mg/day to be cut overnight to merely 90MME. "That's appalling," she said. And all MDs would agree, highly dangerous to the patient.

Pain Patients Lose Each Time the DOJ and Rubber-Stamping State Medical Boards Attack Pain Doctors If the California Medical Board has its way, Dr. Basch's practice will close, stranding her 1400 patients who rely on her care and on their medicines. And this will leave an already medically-underserved community further doctorless.

In a Time of Insanity Caused by Government Overreach into American Healthcare, praise for Dr. Basch from a medical colleague (anonymous for this physician's protection from DOJ scrutiny): "You are admired for fighting this injustice. Your courage and integrity shine out in this era of insanity. As a pain doctor, I totally support your work."

A suddenly *cold-turkeyed* pain patient said, "This is appalling. Is my life in pain worth less than a street addict's life? Dr. Basch is doing professional and caring work. Shame on the Federal government and on California for interfering with her quality patient care."

Pain Patients as Well as Doctors Fear Federal and State Governments Here's what some were saying when they heard of Dr. Basch's plight:

> "I think they want all pain patients dead."
>
> "Did you DEA and DOJ attend medical school?"
>
> "Get out of the way between patients and their doctors."
>
> "Cease. Stop invading doctors' practices!"

More Supporters of Arcata, California's Dr. Basch

> "My doctor for 6 years. She is caring and dedicated."
>
> "Dr. Basch's pain care for me has been life-transforming. Chronic pain was horrific before."
>
> "Someone I knew was forced off her lifelong opioid. With severe withdrawal and plus return of severe pain, she collapsed and died. Our government is doing this to people."
>
> "I was reduced to 90MME. Now in constant pain. One size does not fit all. I applaud physicians like Dr. Basch, making a difference despite government and medical board intrusions."
>
> "How does the American government and Medical Boards do this? Doctors studied a long time in medical school. Doctors know their patients. Government knows zero about illness, pain, humans."

Mark Ibsen, M.D., of Helena, Montana wishes Dr. Basch good luck. "The only way to win is to fight back. The Board is not interested in the truth. Or outcomes, or safety. They are out to make an example of you. Don't let them." Also, "Lame, unscientific accusations. It's a witch hunt. Fight back, Dr. Basch."

According to Linda Cheek, M.D. of **doctorsofcourage.org**, the government's agenda against physicians is over a century old. Yet it is greatly magnified these days because of the media hype of misinformation creating massive opiophobia and unfounded popular hysteria blaming prescription narcotics for illicits addictions. Dr. Cheek calls, what the current onslaught by DOJ and DEA operatives has caused, "A Police State" and that "California is the worst in targeting and eliminating doctors."

"LEAVE NO DOCTOR UNSCATHED!"

?The Hidden Mantra of the DOJ and DEA?

Overall Toll of Physicians Victimized by the DOJ
Recent Physician Prosecutions Mirror Hundreds of Others Nationwide

1. **Frank D. Lazzerine, MD**, a 41-year-old Massillon, Ohio Family Practitioner, fell victim to the chicanery of the DOJ and DEA at his June 18, 2019 conviction. It's unnecessary to list the bogus charges. Simply, Dr. Lazzerine was thought to have been targeted by a competitor for his patients, Ohio's largest hospital chain, Mercy Medical Center, which may have alerted the DOJ with suspect accusations. In his practice, Dr. Lazzerine treated indigent pain patients – people other medical facilities ignored. In the beginning, in 2016, his office was raided. In 2018, Dr. Lazzerine was arrested and jailed for more than a year on $5,000 bond.

In jail, not earning income, with assets forfeiture-seized, physicians can't mount a defense.

Prosecutor Tampers with Local Jury Pool via a media Blitz of Untruths In Dr. Lazzerine's case, a local police officer and a

DOJ-planted "patient" lied in court, where illegally obtained "evidence" was unlawfully allowed. Finally, tainting public perception and prospective jurors with the Big Lie: Conflation of illicit street drug deaths with opioid prescribing for patients in pain, the prosecution made the public, and the subsequent jury, think they have some connection (which all physicians and scientists can attest they do not). Furthermore, outrageously, a bogus "expert," Theodore Paran, M.D. is called to wow the brainwashed jurors, even though he's only an internist with some concerns about addiction, but zero expertise in pain management medical care.

Thus, this young professional empath, a wonderful physician, languishes in prison. For what?

2. **Christopher R. Russo, MD**, a 50-year-old Birmingham, Michigan Pain Specialist, was targeted by DOJ/DEA miscreants, along with his five colleagues, in December of 2018. His practice was at The Pain Center in Warren, Michigan. After Medical School, Dr. Russo trained in a Pain Medicine Fellowship for two years, followed by subsequent training in Advanced Interventional Pain Management Techniques. His work had been focused on trigeminal disorders, vertebral compression fractures, spinal cord and occipital nerve stimulation, and radiofrequency ablation. He's also been concerned about chemical dependency and his records show his prescribing for patients has been squeaky clean.

   Unspeakably unfair, devised by the catch-22 world of DOJ plotters-against-clinicians, because of asset forfeiture during litigation pendancies, Dr. Russo, like all physicians so illegally-targeted, couldn't pay for a vigorous legal defense. Bogus charges - intimidations of Pain Center nursing staff into testifying against these pain specialists, with threats they too would go to prison if they didn't testify according to the prosecution's lies - are rampant. Not a conscience for truth exists in these DOJ craniums. These accuser-DOJ/DEA clones in our government, dressed up like sacrosanct citizens, are criminals and should be in prison themselves!

Inquisition Mania against empathic American doctors: Rumblings of 15th Century Torquemada.

As Mel Brooks would say, "You couldn't talk 'em outta anything!"

You'll notice, now, that this focus-on-physicians Witch-hunt has been going on even before the infamous Guideline of 2016, which only fanned the flames of this 15th Century-style auto-da-fe. In today's courtrooms against physicians, though, the "heretic" is not the hounded "defendant". It's the heretical government rogue malfeasors of the DOJ, the DEA, and the CDC who are responsible for all of America's misery regarding pain care in ER Acute, Postop, Dental and Intractable Pain. (Oh, by the way, when did these "juris doctors" obtain there medical degrees?)

The reader needs to research the outcomes of these cases I'm highlighting here. At this writing, I have no results about what has happened to Dr. Russo's case.

3. **Franck Fisher, M.D.**, a Shasta County, California General Practitioner, was charged in 1999 with murder and drug trafficking. Dr. Fisher lost his house, lost his medical practice, and was jailed for 5 months. When it was found that the deaths resulted from accidents and other health issues, he was released. But the human toll, the damage to spirit, finances, a sense of safety in a supposed just society were all shattered. In 2003, charges against Dr. Fisher were dropped, and he recovered his medical license. Then what? After 4 years in hell? Who should be in prison now?
4. **Eugene Evans, Jr. , M.D.**, of Northern New Jersey, was imprisoned for 5 years because he'd been a quality, compassionate physician and, saving troubled pain patients monthly trips to his office, he gave each patient 3 prescriptions, subsequent ones not to be filled before the

specified date of the end of the prior prescription. (Everyone knows that this is totally, medically, ethically correct. Nurses know this. Pharmacists know this. The second and third Rxs would not be filled until the prior ending dates had passed.) Nonetheless, Dr. Evans had been imprisoned because he'd pled guilty to the false charge of distributing Controlled Substances, to spare himself (as his public defender advised) the catch-22 "conspiracy" charge that would've sent him to jail for a quarter century. Note that most all doctors targeted by DOJ back-stabbing tactics have this ludicrous ominous bogus charge hanging over their heads which traps them in a No-Exit maze.

This ought to be illegal:

To be charged with "conspiracy," against which there is no legal defense. What's this catch-22 trap?

And the prosecution isn't mandated to explain the charge in each specific case. This abomination accounts for all the "guilty" pleas to untrue charges so innocent defendants can avoid severe sentences for the never-proven "conspiracy".

Conspiracies of perjury seem to be the order of the day for DOJ prosecutors, DEA operatives, and State Attorneys-General.

Reluctant witnesses for the prosecution are threatened with jail themselves if they don't march to the tune of the illegal vendetta against innocent doctors. The DOJ's cohorts in court are hell-bent on their greedy, money-grabbing via forced forfeitures of physicians' assets and other hidden-from-the-public perks they acquire with each case in which they destroy doctors.

5. **Joel Smithers, DO**, a 36-year-old Family Practitioner in Beckley, Virginia was invaded by a "guns-drawn" DEA squad at both his practice and his home, where also residing were his wife and 4 young children.

It appears the DEA targets doctors as criminals when pain patients come to them for treatment when they can't find pain care doctors in their home states. Americans! This DEA is way out of control!

Note too, the DEA's access to confidential HIPAA records also seems to empower them to intrude ever-deeper into patients' lives and into physicians' patient care. What the DEA is apparently doing with this confidential information is using numbers of prescriptions written to target doctors, and other prescribers, most likely to take a plea of guilty when faced with decades of imprisonment for that bogus non-sense "conspiracy".

"Conspiracy," is that elusive entity that legal sneaks have invented to victimize innocents because, somehow, this nonsensical aspect of the law permits "a charge for which there is no defense and about which the prosecution need not explain". What kind of insanity is that? But that's a story for another book, for an honorable juris doctor to write.

AMERICANS

MUST STOP

THE GESTAPO DOJ/DEA

Dr. Smithers, just like thousands of other DEA/DOJ beleaguered clinicians, is a victim of runaway government insanity. First the DOJ/DEA cabal taints the press and public with lies, conflating illicit drugs with normal prescription opioids ordered for pain. Then, instead of doing their jobs of illicit drug interdictions, dealer prosecutions and rehab remanding of known addicts, the DOJ/DEA ignores these imperatives and criminalizes normal pain-medicine prescribing – ruining doctors' lives, effectively murdering unmedicated pain sufferers to physical collapse and others to suicide.

From Dr. Smithers, they took his everything. Using that harshest of confiscations, meant for hardened criminals, our cold-turkey government agents used "civil forfeiture," robbing his family of all his assets so he could only have access to a public defender. At this writing, it's possible he'll be in jail for life, his wife spouseless, his very young children, fatherless.

6. **William Bauer, MD**, an Ohio Neurologist who has been caring for his patients in Sandusky, Erie and Huron Counties where he's been treating 1500 chronic pain patients...even as major pharmacy chains have been refusing to fill his legal prescriptions. This behavior on the part of giant drugstore chains risks his patients' health statuses, he worries. But, neither Ohio's Medical Board nor its Pharmacy Board would intercede while acknowledging he has all the licenses necessary to legally prescribe opioids.

   Dr. Bauer calls this *"drughibition"*. While demonizing prescription opioids, they're depriving pain patients of valid pain care. He says that smaller pharmacies cooperate with filling his scripts. It's the chain pharmacies which insurers intimidate, inhibiting them from filling opioid scripts that Dr. Bauer is fighting to change. We need more Dr. Bauers. Hopefully, the DOJ/DEA cabal won't target him, now that he's made his patient-centered focus determined and public.

Forced to Cut Opioid Prescribing by DEA GESTAPO, Two Top MDs Feel Awful that Several of their Patients Suicided

Neurologist, Stephen Nadeau, MD, was warned by a Gainesville, Florida hospital that all opioid prescribing must cease or he'd lose admitting privileges for his patients requiring hospitalization.

Mark Ibsen, MD of Helena, Montana was pressured by his state's medical board and by the DEA for the dosage levels he prescribed, knowing these ranges were needed by his patients in intractable pain. Apparently, a disgruntled, lying employee alerted the board which suspended his license. Then the DEA made 5 "visits," like storm-trooper spies pressuring him and threatening him with jail if he kept prescribing, in each case, each particular opioid and how much he knew his patients needed.

Soon thereafter, in both cases, several of both physicians' patients chose death by suicide in place of unbearable, unrelenting pain when these fine doctors were backed into a corner and threatened into stopping their pain-controlling medications by government rogues.

Hundreds of Healthcare Professionals Blast the Governments' Patient-Torture Tactics In their recent plea to the government officials at HHS/CDC, a group of healthcare professionals – doctors, nurses, pharmacists and other clinicians – decried that Intractable Pain Patients who'd been stable on long-term opioids were having their doses involuntarily reduced to untenably low, ineffective levels at the same time insurers were refusing coverage of alternative treatments or alternative medications which might help somewhat (though, admittedly never as well as their opioid that provided the most effective analgesia).

These clinicians further pointed out that the subsequent unconscionably-inflicted suffering sent some into the streets for illicits and propelled others to kill themselves. Still others end up languishing in hospitals as they deteriorated physically to ultimate premature deaths.

Pain Torture is a Human Rights Crime Not only is the denial of adequate pain treatment torture, nor is it simply unethical, but it also violates the Universal Declaration of Human Rights (UdHR) which explicitly says that refusing pain treatment is a kind of torture and is unacceptable. Our once great U.S.A. is a signatory country to this agreement.

Shame on America! Shame on the DOJ! Shame on State Attorneys-General! Shame on the DEA! Shame on prosecutors who ruin fine physicians' and other clinicians' lives!

The DOJ's Deadly Oppression of Pain Care causes Deaths: From health deterioration due to low MME doses, From suicides due to untreated pain

Our U.S. Attorney General must adamantly declare, "Government leaders victimizing physicians, and therefore the health of their patients, with unfounded prosecutions are criminals who should themselves be prosecuted."

Department of Justice Operatives Boast about their War Against Physicians

On April 17, 2019, the DOJ's public relations department was operating full force just like big bosses in business do. The whole purpose of this press release appears to have been a play for public kudos for their arrogant and questionable "accomplishment against America's physicians".

Listen to this title these hubris-ridden malfeasors cloak themselves in: **Appalachian Regional Prescription Opioid Strike Force (ARPO): Takedown Results Against 60 Individuals, including 53 Medical Professionals – ARPO Grows to 10 Districts including Western Virginia.** Colluders in this self-congratulatory militant attack on 31 physicians, 7 pharmacists, 8 nurse practitioners and other licensed professionals were basically for prescribing (isn't that what doctors do? normally?) and distributing (isn't that what pharmacists do normally?) HHS also boasts, in this press release, about stripping more than 2,000 health professionals and their associates of the right to participate in Medicare and Medicaid. Furthermore, the DEA boasts having issued 31 suspensions and forced 1,386 surrenders for so-called "Violations of the Controlled Substances Act".

Since December of 2018, Federal Agents plus 14 prosecutors had charged 60 defendants alleging what? That prescriptions for opioids were given to patients? Are they crazy? When will this insanity end?

Questionable HHS Secretary Azar Fuels DOJ Acrimony against MDs

The built-in lie: Alex Azar, JD, HHS Secretary, sounded sentimental toward illicits addicts while seeming to protect pain patients with this comment in this press release: "It is also vital that patients who need pain treatment do not see their care disrupted...why federal and local public health authorities have coordinated to ensure these needs are met in the wake of this enforcement operation."

It's a wonder Azar didn't choke on these lying words, because the whole world, at least in Canada and the U.S., as well as all over the

Twitterverse, knows that millions of pain patients have been subjected to suffering torture – death due to health-deteriorating consequences of lack of pain relief, and death by suicide due to unremitting, unbearable pain. The reader should note these vital facts when considering the sincerity and reliability of how Mr. Azar refers to the epidemic of untreated pain patients' sufferings. Azar is a former Eli Lilly executive giving him, at least past ties to Big Pharma. Has he broken all contacts with his Eli Lilly colleagues? Also, he's a lawyer. What does he know about practicing medicine?

Azar also oversees CDC activities. Aha! With his questionable credentials and possibly conflicting loyalties, he's head of this major Federal health agency, parent to the CDC, so he's also co-responsible for **the death document**, the CDC bombed the American medical world with in 2016, the infamously misguided *Guideline*.

Militant DOJ and State Government Lawyers have Blood on their Hands from Ever-Mounting Deaths of Under-treated Pain and from Suicides

The following legally-educated, not medically-educated, lawyers signed onto the boasting hubris of this outrageous press release. Be aware readers, you should know who your enemies are, who's out to get American clinicians, who doesn't care a whit about pain patient care. Also, as a citizen paying their salaries, you might wish to contact these officials:

- Attorney General Brian Benczkowski, Criminal Divison, Justice Dept.
- U.S. Attorney Robert M. Duncan, Jr., Eastern District, Kentucky
- U.S. Attorney Russel M. Colemen, Western District, Kentucky
- U.S. Attorney Benjamin C. Glassman, Southern District, Ohio
- U.S. Attorney William J. Powell, Northern District, West Virginia
- U.S. Attorney Michael B. Stuart, Southern District, West Virginia
- U.S. Attorney J. Douglas Overbey, Eastern District, Tennessee

- U.S. Attorney Don Cochran, Middle District, Tennessee
- U.S. Attorney D. Michael Dunavant, Western District, Tennessee
- U.S. Attorney Jay E. Town, Northern District, Alabama
- U.S. Attorney Thomas T. Cullen, Western District, Virginia
- Deputy Inspector General, Investigations Gary L. Cantrell, HHS (Office of the Inspector General-HHS-OIG)
- Assistant Administrator John J. Martin, DEA Diversion Control Division

GOOD NEWS, AS WE GO TO PRESS: Termination of "Adoptive Seizures"

On June 24, 2019, Citizens for Ethical Reforms in Government and Medicine (CERGM) reported something hopeful, that our American House of Representatives passed a bill terminating "adoptive seizures" by government law enforcers. Heretofore, seizures of personal and business assets for those merely "charged" with a crime were rife and federal and state policing entities would "share" the spoils. Everyone knew these were criminal, money-hungry behaviors due to broad federal powers gone wild among irresponsible, greedy officials.

However, some of these malfeasors may sample a taste of honesty because the Wahlberg Bill has passed, amending the prior overarching latitudes that the wrong people were benefiting from. This amendment prohibits the DOJ to perform adoptive seizures which, heretofore, circumvented state laws of forfeiture. As the CERGM article notes: "This will come as a blessing for many physicians who have been falsely accused by state medical boards of violation of the substance control act, placing a greater burden of proof on law enforcement" before taking such actions.

Thus, since doctors can now control their personal and work assets, they can more easily obtain quality legal help. And that will get them through the morass of DOJ chicanery to help them fight false allegations against them.

Police, Lawyers and Legislators Guilty of Criminalizing Quality Pain Care

Barging into normal American medical practices, DEA operatives are empowered by an unwritten carte-blanche to:

- do whatever they want to destroy physicians' and other clinicians' lives and livelihoods
- thoroughly rip normal narcotic analgesic prescribing away from doctors
- tear opioid therapies away from pain patients

These rogue police, operating with impunity under the direction of a dictatorial DEA and its parent DOJ may as well be Mafiosi, marking out their geographic territories, targeting honest, caring, ethical physicians, and other prescribing clinicians, on scurrilous, spurious charges in order to boast some kind of faux "solution" to an illicit street-drug "crisis" that has zero to do with narcotic analgesic prescribing for various painful conditions. These federal and state government assaults on millions of Americans in pain and on their physicians and pharmacists must stop STAT! Americans will no longer tolerate these police-state tactics. Rogue government leaders and their go-along-with henchmen and other operatives must be interrogated, publicly by Congress, and imprisoned when their misdeeds against citizen-patients and citizen-physicians are exposed.

The Hounds of Hell

According to Dr. Mark Ibsen of Helena, Montana (quoted earlier about Dr. Basch's plight in California), physicians nationwide are terrified by these DEA invasions. Pressures on clinicians, from clueless fools in undeserved, elevated roles in government (DOJ, DEA, HHS), have so heightened that doctors are running scared all over America and have no recourse but to abandon their pain patients to zero medical care. Is this America? Or have we descended into a netherworld of evil, the torture of innocent patients, the imprisonment of innocent physicians?

Since opioids are the best analgesics in most chronic pain conditions and, as well, for acute applications in Emergency Room care, postoperative care and dental care, Lynn Webster, MD, past president of the American Academy of Pain Medicine has pointed out that there is no other alternative, at this time, to this highly effective class of pharmaceuticals for these millions of suffering patients. Still, nearly 50% of physicians nationwide have ceased prescribing this best treatment for their patients' pain conditions, fearing the hounds of hell of the DOJ's DEA breathing down their fiery wrath on medical practices who dare to practice high quality pain care medicine. And yet another 68% reported sharply reducing their opioid prescribing for their pain patients, even those who really required higher doses.

Daniel Laird, MD, JD, a Nevada physician and medical malpractice attorney, is appalled by these evil happenings in our America. As a champion of quality care for pain patients with opioids when indicated, he reported having had a 6-month waiting list of pain patients, abandoned by other physicians, who'd been intimidated by this ongoing police state targeting paincare physicians. He's even been so inundated with abandoned pain patients that, feeling terrible about this, he's had to turn some away.

And, **J. Julian Grove, MD, of Phoenix, Arizona**, felt so affronted and pressured by this threatening missive from Walgreens – "You have issued prescriptions for opioids exceeding the CDC guideline" that he tweeted he's a pain specialist double-certified in anesthesiology, treating cancer patients and other complex pain conditions. He told his hoard of Twitter followers that this pharmacy onslaught was "insulting". And it is that. But Dr. Grove is too kind.

At the time of this writing, U.S. Attorney General Jay Pak, referring to 30 physicians targeted for being "outliers," clinicians who prescribed more opioids than others in Atlanta, had sent WARNING LETTERS to them about their "atypical prescribing". Although Pak pointed out that these same MDs hadn't actually been known to have done anything illegal, such letters and implied harshness of penalties are chilling to the freedom to practice medicine most ethically for each patient's best benefit.

These government nincompoops aim to cut down on opioid prescribing by forcing MDs to prescribe exactly alike for every patient in existence. Reminds me, again, of the invasive, intrusive letter I, and many other New Yorkers received from Consolidated Edison, which forced me to send them a strong retort and warning since they invaded my privacy and equanimity with this most ignorant missile (*sic*), essentially daring to affront me with, "You use more electricity than neighbors in your building". Idiots! Since I work at home and my neighbors work elsewhere...go figure. Suffice to say, they abruptly ended this abusive campaign dreamed up by a clueless someone (possibly a personality type like those invaders from the DEA).

Forcing medical practice and patient care into a one-size-fits-all cut-down in opioid dosages to 90MME and sometimes to merely 50MME is also a tyrannical imposition by untrained-in-medicine buffoons. Dangerous malfeasors because these kinds of forced practices put patients in danger of deteriorating health, early deaths and many suicides, turning buffoons into killers!

DOJ/DEA Unchecked Powers Kill Doctor's Lives and Livelihoods

According to one recent Fox News report about it, the DEA has the power to revoke the manufacture, distribution and dispensing of narcotics. Yearly, it brings 1500 new cases and arrests 2000 individuals. Also, about 800 clinicians each year are forced to surrender their DEA registrations which occurs when a DEA "investigation" is launched against them. Once underway, these questionable "investigations" include the seizure and forfeiture of medical records and personal assets often leading to physician bankruptcy. So, surrendering one's DEA registration is easier than fighting these DEA Goliath-powerful onslaughts.

Again, Mark Ibsen, MD of Montana, emphasized that, since they don't want to be imprisoned, physicians are pleading guilty to "whatever" lesser charges are invented by the DOJ/DEA malfeasors, because once they are targeted and their assets and medical records are seized, they're unable to earn a living or pay for a legal defense.

During the DEA's pressure on Dr. Ibsen, he'd referred his patients to Forest Tennant, MD, a renowned pain specialist and pain scientist. Whereupon DEA goons descended on Dr. Tennant's practice. Finally, this highly expert and beloved physician ceased practicing medicine in order to avoid these out-of-control government autocratic dangers, which deprived patients of a valuable physician, and deprived him of his cherished medical career.

Sadly too, but yet again, a pain patient suicide Once Dr. Tennant "retired" after the outrageous, vindictive rogue raid by the DEA, his pain patient, Jennifer Adams, a police officer, shot herself to death.

Physicians Fear, Pain Patients Suffer, Politicians Don't Care

This Los Angeles patient, with spinal stenosis and diabetic retinopathy, told me he tried getting a journalist to report that the federal government has deliberately confused the public by conflating illegal heroin and fentanyl with prescription pain medicines. His personal experience of being tapered way down to only 20% of his analgesic dosage, with no real pain relief, he attributes to the fact that, "My doctor and all the other doctors in California are afraid to prescribe narcotic medications because the government is breathing down their necks, ready any moment to imprison them."

A Chicago doctor emailed me, saying, "Doctors ought to be able to treat pain without fear of losing their cherished profession and livelihoods. We also have a right to the best for our families, our patients, and respect for our knowledge and expertise. We know how pain affects our patients, in different ways, in differing intensities. We know which drug and how much of it to prescribe. We know about the varying metabolic activities in differing patients which means some patients require higher opioid doses to acquire the best analgesia. It's essential that government bureaucrats remove themselves from the practice of medicine because their interference has condemned some patients to suffer endlessly, others to suicide." The government's restrictions to 90MME or even lower, down to 50MME, of narcotic medications for patients who've been having a relatively workable quality of life theretofore on higher doses, without addiction, is cruel punishment and exposes the idiocy of the government's one-size-fits-all dictum for narcotic dosing.

A Miami vendor suffering a painful, progressive condition, told me, "With my chronic pain, I wouldn't be able to work, buy insurance, enjoy my family without my hydrocodone. The government has no business telling our doctors what they can prescribe for us. My doctor is constantly afraid of being arrested for writing prescriptions to relieve pain." Finally, he said, "This is like some evil joke being played on the public and causing fear in all our doctors. When will it end?"

This grandmother in Queens, New York was mercilessly forced from 130MME to less than 90MME within two months. Where before these reductions she could care for her grandchildren (ages 3 years, 5 years, and 4 months), now she tells me, "I can no longer pick up the baby, I'm stuck in bed all day, no longer able to cook or do housework... politicians need to just let doctors take care of us, not the government. What about my quality of life? Why should I stay alive?"

A heart surgery patient in Atlanta, Georgia with a lifetime of suffering from Arnold-Chiari, Pseudomotor cerebri and Pituitary dysfunction, had worked as a teacher until she could no longer. In pain, on opioid medication and managing some quality of life, suddenly in 2016 (when the CDC Guideline was published), she was *cold-turkeyed* off her well-working narcotic throwing her health into chaos and soon thereafter requiring cardiac surgery. Reprehensively, she was blamed for being "a drug seeker". She reported that she's now in renal failure requiring dialysis, and, "I spend my days in bed with ice packs to my head. Please, may the laws change before any more of us get complications and die. I hope they free the doctors from fear of giving us our opioids for our pain."

One electrician in Portland, Oregon decries "doctors' practice of avoiding caring for pain patients. The way I was mishandled in that city... the cruel behaviors toward me despite my suffering. Oregon should be ashamed of the way it forces its doctors to mistreat pain patients." This man was in tears as he told me this on the phone, from another state to where he had to relocate in order to get opioid prescriptions.

Treated like a leper in Charlotte, North Carolina This spinal fusion patient's doctor refused to prescribe her usual opioid medication and told her he can't take care of her anymore. She emailed me, "I was forced to go to the streets to get whatever I could to manage my pain. Sometimes it doesn't really help, too weak. Other times it just knocks me out and I'm stuck in bed. Twice I had trouble breathing after one of those fentanyl things. I'm scared one day I won't wake up. But without my opioid pain relief, I may as well be dead."

A desperate musician denied pain medication sent me this note from Newark, New Jersey: "I sympathize with doctors being threatened by the DEA raids I heard about, but when my pain doctor told me he will no longer be prescribing for me and he's dismissing me from his care, I cried. As a man, I don't cry except at funerals. But, we'd had such a good relationship and my fentanyl patches controlled a lot of my pain. Now I'm lost. I think my doctor feels lost too."

One Oregonian Physician deplores the maltreatment of pain patients. I quote his email communication to me here: "I just examined a patient with a four-level back fusion, symptoms ten days ago, frontal plus dorsal incisions. He'd been prescribed only 7 days of a narcotic by his surgeon. Sobbing so deeply, he made my nurse cry, too. He'd had to drive all the way from Ohio to see me. As physicians, we should NEVER have to mistreat patients like this. SHAME on the American government for allowing the DOJ and DEA to cause all this suffering."

Patient-Doctor relationship sacrosanct for this Taos, New Mexico retiree who wrote me, "Treatment decisions about pain medicine belongs between patients and their doctors. Meddling politicians should be voted out of office."

This bedridden Real Estate Broker phoned me to insist, "What's needed is a Class Action Law Suit against the government agencies that are intimidating and imprisoning our doctors. It's criminal that in

America, unlike with our pets' veterinarians, human beings' doctors are prevented from helping relieve our pain."

A mother of 7 in pain in Detroit wrote me, "Because Vicodin had worked well after my Caesarian Section and for sciatica in the past, I'd asked my surgeon, after my recent operation, for it for pain. He looked at me like I was a leper and told me to manage on an OTC like ibuprofen. What suffering I went through. What happened to American doctors?"

A father of 3 in Milwaukee called me to sound off against "...the criminalization of physicians prescribing opioids for pain patients. Now I can't get any pain meds at all. My doctor seems to be trembling whenever I need a refill. What am I going to do if he stops helping me?"

This woman worried about her spouse wrote me a lengthy letter, "My husband has so much pain but he has a frightened doctor, too." Those blotchy spots on her stationary, were they from teardrops? She goes on, "I'm angry the government is attacking doctors for prescribing necessary medicines for their patients. I'm outraged the government has so much hidden power that even the news journalists don't report this problem accurately. My husband asked me to buy him a gun before his last vial of pills runs out because his doctor won't prescribe any more, he said."

This physician, an oncologist, reported to me that there are Catch-22 "roadblocks" when he tries his best to help his cancer patients. He told me that "our federal government has placed OxyContin in the cross-hairs of its focus". This, despite the fact that, used appropriately, it relieves much cancer suffering. Apparently, this doctor points out, OxyContin is difficult to prescribe because commercial insurers and Medicaid "...are practicing medicine by limiting its use...." The same is not true for long-acting morphine, which they "allow". However, this doctor says both OxyContin and morphine are good analgesics and it's up to the physician to choose which one is best based on various patients' allergies, swallowing abilities, intelligence, compliance capabilities, and so forth. "Both drugs are manufactured by the same pharmaceutical company, so this strangle-hold by outsiders is a mystery."

Yet another upset Physician, a Surgeon emails me that in 27 years as a physician he has evidence that different patients require different lengths of time of narcotic analgesic usage. Some require opiates for years, even decades, he said. Often such patients benefit from long-acting narcotics. Adamantly, this surgeon reports, "This current opiohysteria constraining us to prescribe a narcotic analgesic for only 3 days postoperatively is outrageous. Most patients require a week to 10 days of an opioid post-surgically. These politically-motivated restrictions are causing massive human suffering."

An angry middle-aged gardener called me to share, "I've been upset wondering why our pain doctors didn't get outraged when forced how to write their pain prescriptions, forced by a gang of know-nothings, lawyers and politicians."

Forced cut in his opioid medication by 50%, this former hockey athlete emailed me that, "I had to move from New York to California, where my new doctor immediately told me my opioid prescription would be cut in half. Having had three heart surgeries and the severe pain of my degenerative disc condition, I asked him about this drastic cut. He told me the government limits Primary Care Physicians and only surgeons can prescribe more. I'd been on hydrocodone successfully for over 15 years and was able to work at sport equipment sales. Now I can't work. My doctor needed to protect his career because of the federal government interference. When will this government-produced insecurity stop? We have to get rid of the politicians and lawyers in Congress and at the 'Justice' Department to stop this assault on patients with pain."

Finally, this patient feels abandoned by physicians and wrote to me: "A doctor needs to be the one to provide pain care, not a DEA agent looking at our private medical records. There's more to managing pain than just the medicine. Doses need to be matched to each patient differently. My doctor said that each patient's system handles opioids faster or slower. The government needs to get out of interfering in my doctor's care of his pain patients. How can our doctors keep working ethically in this atmosphere of prosecution when they're just doing the right thing for their pain patients? How did lawyers and congresspeople get to tell the medical profession how to practice medicine? I'm angry!"

For DEA/DOJ Promotions, Pay Raises and Other Perks, Physicians are Raided, Prosecuted, Ruined–Even Acquitted, Some MDs Died

According to Linda Cheek, MD, owner of **doctorsofcourage.org**, the DOJ and DEA are creating "Medical Political Prisoners". (She herself had been caught up in this outrageous maelstrom of injustice and been imprisoned for a time for nothing more than being an excellent physician.) Dr. Cheek contends that U.S. Attorneys get promotions, higher benefits and other perks when they pursue aggressive criminalization of physicians prescribing opioids. Also that physicians practicing independently (outside of a hospital conglomerate, say) are perceived by hospital executives as "competition" who are expendable and they find ways to taint these clinicians' reputations in complaints to the DOJ and DEA and, also, to State Medical Boards.

At **doctorsofcourage.org**, you'll find an extensive listing of prosecuted physicians, from every corner of America, running into the tens of hundreds. Most of these hundreds were strongly advised by their court-appointed counsel (assets seized, they couldn't afford their own defense attorneys) to plead to a lesser charge to avoid decades in prison on the spurious charge of "conspiracy" which has no defense and which the prosecution need not explicate in trial. Trapped, many pled as instructed and are wasting away emotionally, spiritually and unable to use their medical skills to help patients. What a tragedy. (DOJ and DEA persecuting scoundrels ought not to be able to sleep until these injustices are remedied.) Here is a representative example of those known to be acquitted, some suing the government in response.

And, then, IN MEMORIAM, with a deep moment of silence, I'll list the physicians and other clinicians who were deceased shortly after this attack on their lives and livelihoods by our DOJ-DEA cabal who illegally empower themselves to, in this manner, slaughter our medical empaths, pain care experts, for the crime of taking excellent, legal, and ethical care of suffering patients.

Please realize this adumbrated list comes from Dr. Cheek's work covering years of government invasions into doctors' and patients' lives. There are undoubtedly many other medical profession victims of our vicious government lawyers and police which have not yet been tabulated. Remember, though this is ongoing, rapidly widespread misery suffered by doctors and patients, somehow these facts have not penetrated the media enough to generate bold anti-DOJ and anti-DEA outcries to have them cease and desist.

Following are the Acquittals

2015 George Azapios, MD Carmel, Indiana	**Charges Dropped SUING CITY**
2015 Luella Bangura, MD Carmel, Indiana	**Charges Dropped SUING CITY**
2015 Aaron Borengasser Physician Assistant Little Rock, Arkansas	**Acquitted**
2015 Roland Brutus, MD Winter Park, Florida	**Case Dismissed, Police Misconduct**
2011 Cesar Deleon, MD Lake Worth, Florida	**Acquitted 2015, 4 years later**
2015 Roland Chalifoux, DO, McMechen, West Virginia	**Acquitted 2017, 2 years later**
2005 Frank Fisher, MD location unknown	**Vindicated**
2011 Jerry B. Hankins, MD Brmingham, Alabama	**Charges Dropped**
2003 Cecil Knox, MD Roanoke, Virginia	**Acquitted 2003**
2014 Larry Ley, MD Carmel, Indiana	**Acquitted 2016, 2 years later**
2018 Gary Alan Moore, MD Hixson, Tennessee	**Acquitted 2019, 1 year later**

2016 Joseph Oesterling, MD Saginaw, Michigan	**Acquitted 2017, 1 year later**
2011 Lisa Pliner, RN Boston, Massachusetts	**Acquitted 2015, 4 years later**
2010 Debra Roggrow, MD Fort Myers, Florida	**Acquitted 2012, 2 years later**
2013 Alan J. Salerian, MD Washington, D.C.	**Charges Dropped**
2016 Richard Snellgrove, MD Fairhope, Alabama	**Acquitted 2018, 2 years later**
2016 John K. Sturman, Jr., MD Anderson, Indiana	**Acquitted 2018, 2 years later**
2015 Ronald Vierk, MD Carmel, Indiana	**Charges Dropped, SUING CITY**
2013 Marilyn Wagoner, MD Kokomo, Indiana	**Charges Dismissed**
2011 Joseph Zolot, MD Boston, Massachusetts	**Acquitted 2015, 4 years later**

IN MEMORIAM
DOCTORS AND OTHER CLINICIANS WHO DIED UNDER DURESS, STRESS, AND STRIPPED OF ASSETS TO DEFEND THEMSELVES

Sept. 2015 Sukhveen Kaur Ajrawat, MD Potomac, Maryland
DIED February 2016, 5 months later

Feb. 2009 Bernard Baso, MD Los Angeles, California
DIED June 2009, 4 months later

Feb. 2015 Jay Cho, MD Mechanicsburg, Pennsylvania
DIED November 2015, 9 months later

Mar. 2016 Michael Cossi, MD Fort Wayne, Indiana
DIED August 2018, 2 years later

Aug. 2014	Vincent Cozzarelli, PharmD Bellevile, New Jersey
	DIED April 2015, 8 months later
2018	Michael Cozzi, MD Fort Wayne, Indiana
	DIED August 2018, same year as charged
2011	Victor Georgescu, MD Wheelersburg, Ohio
	DIED August 2012 SUICIDE
Nov. 2016	David Goldfield, Pharm D Medford Lakes, New Jersey
	DIED December 27, 2018, 2 years later
Mar. 2015	David L. Jones, Nurse Practitioner Portales, New Mexico
	DIED May 13, 2016, 14 months later
Plea Jan. 2017	Kevin B. Lake, DO New Albany, Ohio
	DIED June 2017, 5 months later
Mar. 2015	Cynthia Masso (unknown credential) Philadelphia, Pennsylvania
	DIED June 2015, 3 months later
Aug. 2004	Ronald Allen McIver, DO Hodges, South Carolina
	DIED September 2011, 7 years later
Mar. 2012	Richard Minicozzi, MD Philadelphia, Pennsylvania
	DIED June 28, 2015, 3 years later
Plea 2002	Benjamin Moore, MD Winston Salem, North Carolina
	SUICIDE (date?)
April 2016	Ronald Myers, MD Roland, Oklahoma
	DIED September 2018, 2 years later
Raided 2017	Nikhil Nihalani, MD Jacksonville, Florida
	DIED June 2017, the same year
Oct. 2015	Alfred Ramirez, MD Orange City, New York
	DIED October 2016, 1 year later, in home confinement

June 2016	Sandeep Sherlekar, MD Germantown, Maryland
	DIED September 2016, 3 months later
June 2016	Charles R. Szyman, MD Manitowoc, Wisconsin
	Acquitted November 2017
	DIED February 2018, 3 months after acquittal
Plea June 2016	Nicola Tauraco, MD Frederick, Maryland
	DIED August2016, 2 months after forced plea
Plea Feb. 2014	Tomasito Virey, MD Bronx, New York
	SUICIDE February 2014
June 2013	Norman Werther, MD Fort Washington, Pennsylvania
	Sentenced to 25 years, DIED October 2015
Dec. 2003	Freddie J. Williams, MD Panama City, Florida
	Life Sentence in 2004
	DIED OF CANCER in 2006 at Age 56

PANDEMONIUM

Physicians Raided, Spied-on, Hounded, Prosecuted, Imprisoned, Some Acquitted, Some Die Soon After

Ominous Results of DOJ Overreach: Crippling Doctors from Accurate Opioid Prescribing

On May 15, 2019, the American Academy of Family Physicians (AAFP) **https://www.aafp.org/** published "Frontline Physicians Call on Politicians to End Political Interference in the Delivery of Evidenced Based Medicine," a document backed equally by the:

~ American Academy of Pediatrics (AAP)

~ American College of Physicians (ACP)

~ American Osteopathic Association (AOA)

~ American Psychiatric Association (APA)

~ American College of Obstetricians and Gynecologists (ACOG)

It is a strong, mince-no-words response to the harsh, medically-unconscionable constraints by the Department of Justice (DOJ) and the Drug Enforcement Agency (DEA) that have trapped physicians in catch-22 situations such as, "I know my Sickle Cell Disease patient will benefit from an opioid for this severe, life-long genetic condition, but the DEA just phoned, warning me about my doses of the narcotic I prescribed for him."

Finally, fed up, and with their deep Hippocratic Oath consciences fiery hot, three years after the badly misguided 2016 *CDC Guideline* generated such draconian behaviors by these government judicial and policing agencies, physicians in diverse specialties, from childbirth doctors to mental health clinicians, have gone public with their fears for the well-being and very lives of American Intractable Pain Patients.

All six medical organizations abhor what the federal HHS/CDC and DOJ/DEA have been inflicting on American Pain Patients by infecting state politicians with misinformation and mass hysteria that prescription opioids for pain are related to illicit drug deaths. Having spread this erroneous opiophobia, these feds, without cautioning against medical negligence in pain care, have allowed by proxy, an onslaught against prescription narcotic analgesia and against any physician who dares to carefully individualize dosages, sometimes high for rapid metabolizers.

The clarion call from organizations representing a total of over half a million American physicians, state unequivocally: "Our organizations are firmly opposed to efforts in state legislatures across the United States that inappropriately interfere with the patient-physician relationship, unnecessarily regulate the evidence-based practice of medicine and, in some cases, even criminalize physicians who deliver safe, legal, and necessary medical care."

Furthermore, this public document goes on: "The insertion of politics between patients and their physicians undermines the foundation of trust this relationship is built on and inhibits the delivery of safe, timely, and comprehensive care. Outside interference endangers our patients' health by limiting, and sometimes altogether eliminating, access to medically accurate information and to the full range of health care."

"Physicians should never face imprisonment or other penalties for providing necessary care. Politically-motivated laws force physicians to decide between their patients and facing criminal proceedings. Physicians must be able to practice medicine that is informed by their years of medical education, training, experience, and the available evidence, freely and without threat of criminal punishment." (Signed by all the signatories to this demand).

Chapter Seventeen

Veterans in Pain, Suiciding at Alarming Rates due to VA Opiohysteria

The United States Department of Veterans Affairs at **va.gov** is a cabinet-level federal agency which was created to provide almost comprehensive healthcare services to military veterans at VA medical centers. Formally, it's the Veterans Health Administration, often called the Veterans Administration (VA). By 2014, it had 377,805 employees.

The VA Motto: "To care for him who shall have borne the battle and for his widow, and his orphan." Ironic when so much wrong has been done to newer and older veterans by the VA itself.

American *OMERTA*: The VA Code of Silence on its Medical Neglect and Denial of Rx Opioids to Our Wounded and Sick Warriors

According to a 2014 article in *Newsweek*, 60% of veterans who fought in the Middle East and 50% of older veterans suffer chronic pain. Nonetheless, these statistics didn't halt tragic actions by the VA that continue to negatively impact the health of those who served, leaving them in excruciating pain without surcease, condemning many to suicide. The VA decided to institute mandated opioid cold-turkeying even though such wresting from well-working narcotic analgesia is known to be dangerously unsafe for patients on opioid therapy for pain. At the time of this *Newsweek* report, in Arizona alone, veteran suicides were 53.6 per 100,000 of our brave warriors.

One Marine veteran, Robert Rose, has been fighting the VA's negligent, uncaring system of abrupt and dangerous opioid treatment disruption. Where, when on his narcotic medication for intractable pain, he was able to work at skilled wood-crafting and play with his grandchildren, he's now wheelchair-bound due to lack of his narcotic medication for his military service acquired spinal, knee and neck injuries. Additionally, as a diabetic, his health is at further risk. Now bedbound at times and wheelchair-confined at others, lack of exercise puts his health at further risk. This valiant soldier is now pushed, by sadistic VA fiat to vent angrily at this feelingless assault on veterans' health and well-being.

Reportedly the VA is infested with do-nothing lackeys forced to adhere to low-level expectations unworthy of our valiant soldiers. A code of silence, internally at the VA, is said to be rife. This involves production of misinformation, delays, and intimidations of whistle blowers. None of the latter feel safe, in this *omerta* environment, to expose any criminal or medically unethical actions they are, as insiders, fully aware of. Afraid of losing their pensions, and their assured government jobs, VA operatives are too intimidated to intercede in individual cases, or to report to the public via the press the intolerable conditions the VA is forcing our military survivors to endure.

VA Facilities Routinely Delay Medical Care or Deny Healthcare Altogether VA-related suicides abound, incidents consequent to drastic restrictions in what was once normal narcotic prescribing for our veterans suffering chronic pain. In 2014, an indifferent VA led veteran Kevin Keller, at age 52, to shoot himself to death rather than live with his unending pain. Which, no matter how hard he'd tried to get the VA to help him, the VA's callous indifference forced him to take this only way out. This, and many other such veteran tragedies, are iatrogenic, directly resulting from harsh new VA policies that ignore critical and safe medical practices. Due to these stringent restrictions, veterans suffering proven chronic pain are enduring severe harm because they're not receiving the pain relief levels they require and deserve.

Weeping VA Physicians Feel Helpless against VA Anti-Opioid Rules The VA pain pendulum swings between pain-unmedicated veterans feeling forced to use illicit street drugs, and suicide by those without any pain relief whatsoever. That's because far too many VA facilities have been pressuring VA physicians to drastically cut, and way too swiftly, opioid dosages or to cold-turkey veterans' narcotic analgesics altogether. Sadly, some VA nurses reported witnessing any number of VA physicians shedding tears about being forced to deny opioid pain care absent the mandatory safeguards of gradually tapering opioid dosages and the provision of added supportive medical and psychological care.

Intimidations of Ethical VA Clinicians Abound at VA Facilities Patient-focused, committed, empathic physicians and other healthcare professionals, working at VA hospitals and its other facilities, experience ongoing intimidations and demotions when they dare to step outside unethical VA barriers by providing quality patient care for our deserving veterans. Cover-ups, pressures of job-loss, and a general air of suffocation – of tightening the invisible noose around the necks of clinicians desperately trying to do the right thing for America's valiant soldiers – prevail. This has got to stop. Our veterans deserve supreme quality medical care. Physicians and other clinicians treating them deserve the highest levels of support and encouragement from VA management staff. Americans feel in our hearts that veterans deserve timely diagnoses and treatments – not long pain-filled delays. And we know they deserve to be rendered as pain-free as possible with the best prescription analgesic for each one's level of pain.

Therefore, veterans suffering various pain-producing conditions must receive, starting now, the highest quality pain management with prescription opioids selected specifically for what's ailing each ill warrior, at varied dosage levels depending on each individual's degrees of pain and each's metabolism of specific narcotic compounds. Remember, this is imperative, physicians who treat pain are the ones to decide what each veteran needs to dampen the suffering. Not some bureaucrat, sitting at a desk, far away from a veteran's illness and life circumstances. Not some congressional legislation roadblocking high quality pain care. That's why we call them "Doctors". Because they know how to take care of patients in pain. You VA bureaucrats and administrators mismanaging the healthcare of our valiant ones should be ashamed. And some of you, who are depriving veterans of their medically-justified opioids should be terminated from your jobs. Americans abhor heartless people in power oppressing others. Moreso, Americans are wounded by such maltreatment, even torture, of our bravest souls.

Some Examples of VA Callousness toward Veterans in Pain A number of mistreated, under-treated, untreated and otherwise severely mishandled veterans with chronic illnesses and pain are being left to fend for themselves due to ever-increasing stringencies restricting quality opioid treatment by VA fiat. Despairing opioid-deprived veterans with intractable pain resort to suicide. This is because many are being abandoned or abruptly cold-turkeyed without supportive medical measures to help them transition to less suffering without their effective narcotic analgesic. Here are but a few examples of this forced suffering:

A Navy Veteran writes me, "Pain patients are being tapered down or completely cut off from their pain meds. It's happenings all over the country."

A retired Air Force doctor emails me, "Once the VA restricted opioid prescribing, my pain doctor cut my medication in half and this was done so fast that my withdrawal symptoms were terrible. As I am a doctor too, he confided in me he felt intimidated by the medically-ignorant directive."

An Army nurse amputee told me, "The Veterans Administration needs to be reminded that we veterans are human and have a right to request and receive pain relief. My VA doctor is so intimidated by VA pressure about prescribing opioids that he cut my opioid down by 50% and wanted to force me off it altogether. With this low dose, I may as well be on nothing. Before, I could work in the hospital library. Now I'm home in bed without a job."

This Army Medic Veteran emailed me, "With my herniated discs and a spinal fusion and lots of pain, my VA hospital viewed me as a 'drug addict,' wouldn't take my pain seriously. Even after additional spinal surgeries, leaving me bedridden, the VA would not prescribe opioid medication for my nonstop pain. I have to jump through hoops, gather huge amounts of records each time my primary care MD sees me. He's very kind and helpful but hampered by VA interference and by faulty interpretations of my PDMP medical records. It seems the DEA police are creeping into VA paincare decisions."

A Marine Veteran wrote me, "I've contacted politicians about these harsh VA restrictions which forced a VA doctor to suddenly lower my really good pain control narcotic to 70MME. Totally ineffective. He may as well have prescribed WATER. I called state officials and my governor. No response. I contacted local newspapers but their journalists are convinced it's bad doctors to blame for drug addicts dying so they won't investigate my story. I used to work full time, enjoyed my family and some social life. Without effective pain medicine, I've lost my job and spend 90% of my time in bed. Is this what I fought for my country for me to come home to?"

This ex-Infantryman, with PTSD and an amputated right arm plus an amputated left leg, told me, "My cluster headaches were mostly relieved by a small dose of opioid plus a small dose of Valium. Suddenly, in 2014, the VA forced my doctor to cut my meds off cold turkey. The headaches came back. I don't ever expect to be fully pain-free, but I think I deserve the right painkiller at the right dose to help me live somehow."

A Navy Veteran with a Parkinsonian-type progressive neurologic condition, emailed me, "I couldn't sleep and deteriorated. We helped keep

America free but no one cares about us. They view us, veterans with pain, as addicts. Relentless pain caused many of my buddies to kill themselves. I'm on the verge of making such plans. Depriving us of the best medicines – the opioids – that subdue our pain is cruel. We fought in faraway lands to keep Americans safe. As humans, do we not deserve humane care?"

VETERANS' FRIENDS, FAMILIES, AND OTHER CONCERNED AMERICANS CONTACTED ME

Brain Pain: "My husband served for five years and came home without part of his face. Doesn't he deserve pain medicine for brain pain?"

A Nightmare: "What a nightmare that an American agency that's supposed to help our returning wounded soldiers turns their backs on them, let's them suffer."

Shameful: "We take better care of our pet animals than we do of our veterans. For shame."

Diabetic Neglect: "The staff at our VA hospital are smooth talkers but do nothing to help. Appointments are long-delayed. Even physicians ignored my Navy brother's ketoacidosis crisis. He had to go to an Emergency Department elsewhere and was hospitalized for his diabetes. The VA is still not treating his pain."

Double-Amputee Neglect: "My double-amputee sister, an army veteran, was told she's an addict and was reduced to only 90MME of her opioid, which doesn't take care of 90% of her nerve pain in her thigh areas. Why is the VA torturing veterans who sacrificed so much for all of us?"

Pain Ignored: "As an old army veteran, I trusted my America when my pain became too strong for aspirin. Why can't the VA see we have a right to be comfortable like every other citizen? I got a form letter back from a congressman I wrote to: 'Thank you for your letter.' That's it? This is how we soldiers are being ignored while hurting very badly."

An Army Veteran Physician who is also a Pain Patient emailed me: 'What right has the VA to mistreat us veterans in pain? As an army major, I did my job, risked my life to run into fields of fire to help my men. Now, when I need my opioid to relieve chronic war-related-injury pain, the VA abandons me. What kind of country have we become?"

A Navy SEAL called me to say, "My quality of life is gone. They stopped my pain medicine just like that. Cold turkey. Like they didn't care about the withdrawal suffering or the pain returning. It's not a Veterans Administration. It's a Veterans' Nightmare. And, daily I read about another suicide by a veteran whose pain drug had been stopped by the VA."

SOME VETERANS ARE FORCED INTO EXILE, TO OTHER COUNTRIES WHERE PAIN IS PROPERLY TREATED

Shaming and Blaming Real Pain Patients: This valiant American soldier, abandoned by a VA hospital, went into exile to get dependable pain care. "I've left Amerika," this pain-filled American veteran spells out, because the VA staff kept calling him an addict, shamed him, had him "running in circles", then stopped his pain medication altogether. "My pain was so severe, I sent myself into exile, far from my own country. Here, doctors treat my pain quickly with a shot and will prescribe whatever I need to control my pain." Sadly, this veteran felt impelled to warn bureaucrats, politicians, and Veterans Administration regulators: "May your turn for agony arrive and may you suffer it, too, without an opioid."

Rigid VA Autocrats Prescribe Death to Veterans in Pain:

Veteran Suicides Caused by VA Refusals of Medically-Safe Opioid Care

There will be many more veteran suicides before the VA malpracticing physicians stand up to the VA and fight for the right to treat their pain patients with the opioid appropriate for their specific conditions. One American veteran told me, in that regard, "We are veteran women and men without a country. It's okay to the VA that we're committing suicide day after day because they can't feel our pain."

Daring Physician Advocates Legal Recourse for Veterans in Pain

Daniel Laird, MD, JD is a Las Vegas physician who treats pain conditions. He is also a valiant advocate for fully adequate opioid dosages for patients with unremitting pain, as well as for other acute, moderate, postop, cancer and other hospice pain needs. All pain deserving to be treated effectively, he asserts. Also an attorney, Dr. Laird handles medical malpractice, personal injury and related medicolegal cases. You can contact him at **LairdLaw.com** Dr. Laird takes cases on a contingency basis, meaning that only with an outcome in the litigant's favor, will a percentage accrue to his law firm.

I hope, some way, veterans in pain and all wronged pain patients will mount countless Class Action law suits against malfeasing individuals, and against government entities and the autocrats who run them, in order to halt the anti-opioid holocaust against American Veterans as well as against all the other 50 million Americans who are victims of ill-treated or untreated pain.

Section V

PAIN MARTYRS POST MORTEM

Chapter Eighteen

In Memoriam: Suicides due to Untreated Pain

This chapter is a memorial for all the unnecessary life-endings by suicide–of patients in unbearable, untreated pain–that are happening daily all over America since the 2016 *CDC Guideline* emboldened DOJ prosecutors and DEA police to wrest the practice of pain care medicine away from physicians, to leave pain patients unmedicated and desperate.

At the close of this section, is a dirge I wrote to honor these avant-garde heroes and heroines whose ultimate sacrifices are empowering the fight for the rights of patients in pain to receive their legal prescription opioids. My **DIRGE FOR PAIN WARRIORS** is followed by a simple obituary of precious lost lives from around the nation. It is but a very small sampling of the great numbers, nationally, of the list of the lost.

According to a Human Rights Watch (**www.hrw.org)** report of December 18, 2018, once the 2016 *CDC Guideline* had been erroneously turned into law, millions of chronic pain patients in America, on what some may consider "high doses" of narcotic analgesics (patients on "high doses" metabolize opioids at different rates than those on lower doses), have been struggling to access paincare physicians. Thus they've been abandoned to zero pain relief altogether.

Because many MDs, intimidated by the nefarious autocratic actions of the DOJ and DEA, have simply "retired" or shut down their pain care clinics.

Those "retirings" and pain practice closings are no coincidence. They've been going on nationwide for three years because clinicians are deathly afraid of DEA raids and are, fearfully, intimidated by DOJ prosecutory entrapments. Entrapments such as the catch-22 charge of "conspiracy," which carries a sentence of at least 25 years in prison, that DOJ prosecutors hang over the heads of capriciously-charged physicians and other clinicians (nurses, pharmacists, nurse practitioners and physician assistants) if they don't plead guilty to a lesser charge. That scurrilous coercion, even though the lesser charge has no basis in reality. And, if the doctor won't plead to the lesser bogus charge, the DOJ prosecutor need not explain to the judge what the "conspiracy" charge entails in each specific case. In this pain-filled world of deep injustices, add this one: there is no defense to the charge of "conspiracy". Go figure. What lame-brain *juris doctor* allowed this catch-22 concept to sail into legal acceptance? With this kind of Keystone-Kop law – "conspiracy without proof" – this is not justice and the accuser-agency should be renamed the DOI, Department of Injustice.

Thus, the majority of healthcare professionals, mostly MDs, targeted by the DOJ, will spend time in jail or on house arrest, without having done anything wrong. Too, they will also lose their professional licenses, and by DOJ gestapo-style seizures, will forfeit all their personal and professional assets, and their patients' medical charts.

With this kind of scenario hanging over the heads of all government-targeted physicians, it's no wonder thousands of other doctors are closing up bona fide pain-treating practices and never ever prescribing any medications for pain relief again and retiring from medicine altogether. In this climate, American physicians are feeling they've a target painted on the backs of their white medical coats. The scene is set for physicians, with stethoscopes around their necks and shackles around their wrists, led away by federal fools.

What tragedies the DOJ-DEA cabal is visiting on innocent doctors and their patients. (See Chapter 16, "Plight of the Paincare Physicians," for unjust imprisonments and DOCTOR DEATHS within a few months of DOJ-DEA incursions into their lives and professions.) No wonder patients can't find pain-treating clinicians. Human Rights Watch is very concerned that pain patients are suffering as a direct result of these illegal actions by DOJ operatives who seem to have been awarded *carte blanche* to implement Hitlerian tactics, to answer to no one, to destroy doctors' lives with the added fall-out being the destruction of pain patients' lives.

The purported "guideline" that triggered clinician trepidation, instead of supporting ethical narcotic prescribing, has caused great physical, mental and social anguish to chronic pain patients – which has also crept into all other medical areas where pain is encountered, e.g., acute ER pain, postoperative pain, and dental pain. Now excruciating pain is "acceptable," as MDs and RNs turn their backs on suffering patients. An outrage. A crime.

On the coattails of this misguided missive, the DOJ and DEA persecutions and prosecutions of physicians have so infected the Hippocratic practice of medicine that doctors are abandoning patients in pain altogether, too often ending in pain patient deaths. For, while many struggle with sudden, rapid tapering or *cold-turkeying*, off their trusty pain medications, some dying suddenly due to the physically-deteriorating effects on heart and brain of under-treated or untreated pain, others living in pain-beyond-unbearable opt for SUICIDE. This chapter is a Memorial for all of them.

DIRGE FOR PAIN WARRIORS (R.I.P.)
by Helen Borel

There are no tears.
Just anger mixed
with grief and sadness.
Rest sweetly out of misery.

And no more fears
of crushing insane pain;
O how they miss their families,
Yet suffer not again.

And no more cares
That Doctors turn deaf ears,
and ER Nurses jeer,
Because you hurt so bad
for many years.

Still no one hears
Your loud but silent cry.
O why, O why must others die
Before our country cares?

AMERICAN GENOCIDE: They Now Live Where Nothing Can Hurt Them Anymore*

Suicide Dates are listed

Jennifer Adams	41	Montana	April 2018
Dawn Anderson	52	Indiana	March 2019
Debra Bales	52	California	January 2018
Jesse Schmaltz Baroda	31	US Marine Corps	October 2017
Kellie Bernson	59	Colorado	December 2017
Donald Beyer	47	Idaho	May 2016

Robert Breault	52	New Hampshire	May 2018
Lee Cole	38	US Army	April 2018
Paul Fitzpatrick	56		October 2018
Robert Charles Foster	65	Veteran	October 2018
Katherine Goddard	52	Civilian	June 2017
Doug Hale	53	Vermont	October 2016
Daniel P. Hartsgrove	62	Civilian	May 2017
Rory G. Hosking	50	US Army	February 2019
Carla Howard	?	Tennessee	March 2019
Charles Richard Ingram III	51	US Navy	March 2016
Sonja Mae Jonsson	42	Oregon	August 2016
Sarah Kershaw	49	New York	February 2016
Allison Kimberly	30	Colorado	June 2017
Phillip Kuykendall	63	North Carolina	December 2016
Sherri Little	53	California	July 2016
Robert Markel	56		June 2016
Bob Mason	67	Montana	January 2016
Mercedes McGuire	25	Indiana	August 2017
Travis "Patt" Patterson	26	US Army [Combat Iraq/Afghanistan]	January 2017
Denny Peck	58	Washington State	September 2016
Marsha Reid	59	Texas	November 2016
Jessica Simpson	28	Civilian	July 2017
Brian Spece	54	US Marine Corps	May 2017
Ryan Trunzo	26	Iraq Veteran (Massachusetts)	Suicide Date ?
Zack Williams	35	US Army, Iraq Veteran	Suicide Date ?

Note: **This obituary of pain patient suicides is only a minuscule microcosm of the actual scope of such needless deaths occurring nationwide. When will politicians and legislators rescind the Department of Justice and Drug Enforcement Administration carte blanche that inhumanly prevents appropriate opioid prescribing? A medical decision that must only be made, on a case by case individual basis, and only between a physician, or other prescribing clinician, and each patient in pain.*

Section VI

PERPETRATORS: A Confederacy of Ignorance and Greed

Chapter Nineteen

Prescriptions for Disaster

The terrible mishandling of pain care issues by CDC functionaries is very sad, even inexplicable, considering all the exemplary work the CDC does handling the complexities of epidemics and pandemics involving infectious diseases and toxic threats. Thus, it baffles knowledgeable healthcare professionals that the CDC continues to downplay, even ignore, the mass suffering its unfortunate "recommendations" continue to inflict on patients in pain all over America.

Worse, our CDC, America's agency to conquer epidemics, is completely blind and deaf to the epidemic of premature deaths and suicides of pain patients all over this country–including veterans suiciding daily–whose untreated, unrelenting pain is triggering these sad demises.

How Suspect Motives Negatively Impact Pain Patients

Let me review a few key facts before continuing this discussion about the CDC's mishandling of this national crisis of untreated pain and the suicides that have resulted therefrom. (Seemingly disparate discussions in this book have turned out to be so intricately intertwined that it has to boggle a reader's mind to grasp all of them as elements of the same story. I empathize with you, dear reader, because even I, the researcher and writer of *American AGONY*, have been struggling to make sense of the facts I've uncovered. And to present them in some kind of cohesive whole.)

To sum up about pain itself: **Pain** is a physical sensation due to injury or disease. When it occurs suddenly, or postoperatively, it's **Acute Pain** and lasts for a short time, minutes, hours, up to a few months. When it continues for over 3 months to about 6 months, even after healing, it's **Chronic Pain**, which sometimes lasts lifelong. Excruciating, unrelenting, intolerable pain is called **Chronic Intractable Pain** (its patients are usually referred to as **Intractable Pain Patients–IPPs**) which causes the patient to be bedridden, housebound and wheelchair-bound, and can lead to premature death if not treated accurately with the prescription opioid that the individual has been successfully medically-managed on.

Chronic Untreated Pain leads to immobility, sleep troubles, depression, physical malfunctioning, job loss, absent social relationships, being housebound, being bedridden, being wheelchair-dependent, and unable to do most everything for oneself. Even one of these often makes the sufferer feel hopeless. Hopelessness can produce dire consequences, like suicides.

About 100 Million Americans Suffer Chronic Pain

These numbers should make it evident that this is an epidemic...an epidemic of pain untreated, followed by companion epidemics of (1) premature deaths due to the physiologic effects of untreated pain and (2) suicides due to unbearable, untreated pain. In these cases, why is the CDC doing nothing to prevent these untimely, distressing deaths occurring in epidemic proportions? **IPPs comprise 20% of the 100 millions in pain**. The ignorance about, mishandling of, and ignoring of this pain epidemic–also an epidemic of untreated pain–starts with the bumbling bunglers at the CDC, which has also turned its back on The Pain Patient Suicide Epidemic. What's up, Docs? Doctors at the CDC? Your prevention tactics are needed STAT!

Untimely Early Deaths due to Under-Treated and Untreated Pain

One result of many opioid-medication discontinuances or drastic dosage reductions is untimely, early deaths due to the physiologic complications of untreated pain. These include those pain patients whose normal

MMEs (morphine milligram equivalents) of their usual opioid dosages have been tapered so low that they wouldn't relieve the pain of a flea. Some to only 90MME, others to a laughable 50MME.

Another is the widely-known epidemic of pain patient suicides, including those of our Valiant Veterans–whose suicides continue to be wrongly publicized in the press as due to PTSD–due to lifelong, unrelenting, unbearable pain. These have got to stop, STAT! Immediately! Which means the DOJ, the DEA, many state and federal legislators, and organized anti-prescription-opioid proponents need to be exposed for their true agendas–government overreach, hidden perks for some government functionaries, and singular examples of pure greed. (You'll learn more about these latter in the following chapters in this section.)

A Tsunami of Misinformation Disseminated by Our Government

The CDC's opioid-specific monitoring, from 2011 onward, and the dissemination of its purported data to all Americans via outrageous, unscrupulous publicity techniques–enlisting clueless journalists and vast print and broadcast media sources–created a tsunami of misinformation, engulfing our country in a national hysteria, still raging, the likes of which has not been seen since the McCarthy hearings that ruined so many lives before fellow congresspeople admitted to themselves that Joe McCarthy was operating with a few less marbles than they themselves, who initially supported his insanity. And, analogous too, to America's Salem Witch Hunts and Trials in the 1600s.

IPPs, as a result, became targets of the sorely misinformed media, which further fueled, and is still so doing, the untruths about the misconstrued "epidemic". IPPs soon were being turned away from care by their longtime pain management physicians. At the same time, doctors who were still prescribing narcotic analgesics for their pain patients were stunned when pharmacies began refusing to fill these legal, medically-accurate opioid prescriptions. Soon IPPs began growing desperate for relief and the restoration of a semblance of normalcy, of what little quality of life their narcotic medications had provided them. Whereupon, health insurers added more grief to IPPs by refusing to pay their contracted portions for patients' prescription narcotic medications.

In this atmosphere, fueled by intrusive and abusive actions of federal government functionaries, most severely in this last decade–you've already read, and there's more in Chapter 22, about what the DEA and the DOJ have been, and are still doing, to physicians and the great harm these unleashed activities have caused to pain patients–IPPs began being tortured by involuntary tapering by their own longtime doctors, of their well-working prescription opioids, some even by sudden *cold-turkeying.*

Despite these immoral, nonmedical actions against IPPs, the statistics of deaths due to illicit drugs continued to rise. And, this mortality rate was known by HHS and CDC officials to be attributable to street drug use of adulterated fentanyl and fentanylized heroin, each often mixed with anxiolytics and/or alcohol. Which didn't stop the CDC from deliberately conflating normal IPPs use of prescribed narcotic analgesics with drug addicts' use of tainted illicits.

CDC principals also have been confusing the American public by claiming that normally prescribed opioids can't be differentiated from heroin. These CDC confabulations, thus, energized DEA operatives to invade legitimate, ethical physicians' offices, to mislabel suffering IPPs as addicts, to deprive postsurgical pain patients, acute ER pain patients, and dental pain patients of even their medically-correct short-term narcotic analgesic prescriptions. Despicably, the DOJ empowered the DEA to relentlessly label IPPs as "drug seekers". Thus, not only have IPPs been deprived of their legitimate pain medications, and continue to be so maltreated and vilified, they're forced to suffer the humiliation of being labeled "junkies". And all other patients with conditions, diseases and injuries that generate acute pain, short-term pain, or somewhat longer periods of pain, are abandoned without medically-indicated opioid treatment at all.

Medication Refugees have emerged from this federal government manufactured crisis. For, many IPPs are forced from their home states to travel, sometimes hundreds of miles, sometimes to relocate–from a lifetime of family and familiar environs–just to find a physician to treat their pain and a pharmacist who will fill their medically legal narcotic prescriptions.

Suicides: Their Final Analgesic

Finally, IPPs were, and are still, doomed to never-ending suffering. And they're committing suicide as their final analgesic. This is iatrogenic. It's a medical crime against innocent pain patients whose conditions, by valid statistics, have zero to do with addiction. Whose use of narcotic analgesics is medically justified, previously permitting them a semblance of normalcy. And it's criminal to equate their normal use of prescription opioids for pain control with drug addicts' deaths by tainted illicits.

Suicides by these patients can be directly attributed to the myopic CDC functionaries who approved its misguided 2016 *Guideline*. And to the gestapo actions of the DEA whose unchecked marauding of physicians' practices have been leaving patients without their long-time doctors, with no one to prescribe their pain medicines. Finally, also to the prosecutory zeal of conscienceless DOJ prosecutors who, I'm sure, are itching to indict the Perdue Chicken. I say the latter because, these DOJ weasels have been tricking innocent doctors into a catch-22 of pleadings to lesser, though bogus charges, to avoid the nebulous "conspiracy" charge which the dirty dealing DOJ lawyers don't have to explain but carries a sentence of at least 25 years.

These ruthless, reprehensible government strongarm tactics are bullying our nation with disinformation and are bullying clinicians in all specialties from ever prescribing anything stronger than water for pain. Medical abandonment of patients in pain is the disgusting result of these government fools who should all be in jail for practicing medicine without a scintilla of knowledge thereof. And, any physicians who are employees of the CDC, the DEA, the DOJ, or of HHS should be ashamed of not resigning in protest of the torture being inflicted on pain-sufferers by the agencies we pay to do the right thing for all Americans. The horrific results of all this government outright lying, subterfuge, spying on patients' records, destroying medical careers, mandating flea-sized doses of MMEs that won't even help a flea, are catastrophic. They include the destruction of professional medical, professional nursing and professional pharmacy practice at the highest levels of skill and empathy. Shoddy healthcare is now the norm by the incompetent dictates of these government miscreants. And, the ultimate, destruction of pain patients' lives by government viciousness propelling them to suicide.

Suicide is the horrific last resort of under-treated and untreated pain for patients–whose opioid medications controlled their pain for years, often decades. Now, with unrelenting physical suffering, they can no longer work, no longer get out of bed or are stuck in a wheelchair, are unable to participate socially or with family members. Trapped like this, suffering physically, severely, they see only one way out. Death.

Such deaths should be laid at the feet of the foolish functionaries who are perpetuating this American Holocaust–HHS, CDC, DOJ, DEA. As well as, at those state and local legislative authorities who are also impeding autonomous medical care for pain patients. Medical care should not be compromised by mini-brained government interference.

Brain Changes Worsen the Suffering of Unrelieved Pain

It's important to note the effects on the brain and the body's nociceptors (pain-sensing nerves) and on the quality of life of patients enduring under-treated or untreated pain. Long-term mismanaged pain control by under-dosages, or zero opioids altogether, produces severe brain changes. Damage happens to cerebral and spinal neurons and throws neurochemicals out of balance. It's a kind of poisoning of the Central Nervous System (CNS), which is the whole brain plus the spinal cord. IPPs so mistreated may also be suffering daily lives worse than anyone can imagine because they're robbed of any real quality of life due to pain, immobility, loneliness and so they prefer suicide.

Still, despite these awful facts, it's the rare IPP who'd resort to illicit street drugs to supplement their too-low-dose prescription opioids.

Opioid Classifications Recognized by the CDC and Illicit Drugs Threatening Addicts' Lives

Illegal–heroin

Natural–codeine, morphine sulfate

Semi-synthetic Opioids–oxycodone, hydrocodone

Synthetic–methadone, fentanyl, tramadol

The Carfentanil Threat and Misreported Mortalities by the CDC

About six years ago (2013), the American illicit market of fentanyl exploded with Chinese imports via Mexico. Soon thereafter, the synthetic carfentanil–an extremely more powerful fentanyl analog–found its U.S. market online. The CDC, then, deliberately misreported mortalities due to these illicits as prescription-opioid-related deaths. This, despite the report, by Gladden, et al. that almost every death attributed to fentanyl was not that by diversion of prescription fentanyl, but was due to illegal street-bought and internet-purchased fentanyl.

Erroneous Reporting of Illicit Drug Deaths: CDC Skews Statistics

Turns out, according to the DEA itself in a 2015 "threat assessment report," that morphine appeared to be the culprit in numerous overdose deaths when heroin was the actual culprit. This because of the heroin metabolite that swiftly morphs into morphine and is, then, detected on toxicologic examination post mortem as 6-monoacetylMORPHINE. Thus, severe "mistakes" have been made classifying heroin deaths as due to prescription morphine. Worse, such mis-categorizations, of vital statistics like these by CDC officials, have further fueled the government- promoted fiction and national terror that has been misplaced onto medically-appropriate narcotics and have sorely harmed millions of pain-sufferers who badly need their legal prescription opioids for their therapeutic benefits.

Could these manipulated, fake "statistics" be deliberately publicized to bolster the lie that prescription opioids cause drug abuse deaths?

Who Loses in this Opiohysteria Fiasco?

1. **Intractable Pain Patients** whose pain medication needs have zero to do with addiction since less than 1% of patients on prescription opioids become addicted to them
2. **Relatives, Friends and Co-Workers** of IPPs who are no longer able to connect with the sickly housebound, bedridden, pain-racked patient
3. **Former Employers** who've relied on the knowledge, skills and profits once generated from their educated, talented and experienced employees, now side-lined by untreated pain and various levels of immobility
4. **Families Mourning** their pain-crushed loved ones who've suicided
5. **Our Economy**, we taxpayers, Medicare and Medicaid must absorb many of the costs of the burdensome care of untreated, bedridden, pain-crippled patients
6. **Drug Addicts**, where the focus on illicit drugs really belongs.

What's being visited on American pain patients by our government agencies and certain individuals (some clueless, some just plain greedy) is criminal. As mentioned earlier, key players in this sweeping, deathly agenda, an actual cabal against Hippocratically beneficent treatment of pain, are Health and Human Services (HHS), the Centers for Disease Control and Prevention (CDC), the Department of Justice (DOJ), the Drug Enforcement Administration (DEA), various State Attorneys-General, many politicians, legislators at various levels of federal and state power, and private organizations bent on their narrow agendas that are blind to the sufferings, wasting-away deaths, and suicides of patients in severe unbearable pain.

As an R.N., and as a veteran medical science and prescription pharmaceuticals writer (in "Medicine Avenue" advertising agencies in New York City), and now as a practicing psychotherapist, I am very wounded by the unconscionable idiocy and cruelty of our government agencies' actions, many of these entities headed by nonmedical desk-warmers who have zero knowledge of anatomy, physiology, neurology, nociceptors, pain-causing diseases, injuries, the Central Nervous System (brain and spinal cord), and zilch about pharmacology, pharmaceuticals, or the intricacies of pain management. One example heads HHS, Alex Azar, JD, a lawyer and former Eli Lilly executive. This is a man who has inside familiarity with how Big Pharma does its Research & Development, how drug manufacturers acquire FDA approvals for their pharmaceuticals, and the intricacies of how they market their medicines.

A Possible Diabolical Scenario

Then, consider this possible thought-process by a cadre of some self-aggrandizing insiders: Do everything you can to kill the prescribing of average-cost narcotic analgesics - e.g., morphine sulfate, Demerol® (meperidine HCl), Dilaudid® (hydromorphone), codeine, and Percodan® (oxycodone HCl + aspirin), which manage the intractable pain of millions of patients throughout the nation, and you open the door for the medical market to be flooded with more expensive opioid analogs, including copycat analgesic products by eager generics manufacturers.

And, bear in mind the Suboxone bonanza. A stratospherically lucrative morphine product (see Chapter Twenty, "The Suboxone Hoax"), Suboxone permits wide-scale use of a legal morphine purportedly to detox and reverse drug addiction to illicit opioids.

A Nurse's Perspective on Pain and its Treatment

As an R.N., I've taken care of hundreds of patients with various acute and chronic illnesses that subjected them to varied kinds and degrees of pain. I've administered oral narcotics as well as injectable narcotics.

I've seen, over the many lives I've tended to, the benefits of taking care of pain.

Known definitely is that when (1) acute pain is controlled, illnesses and surgical wounds heal faster, and (2) when chronic pain is quelled, patients' qualities of life improve dramatically. The pain-afflicted can often work and partake in life with family and friends. Not languish, housebound, bedridden, hopeless, suicidal.

Relentless Pressure against Prescription Opioids, Except for the Morphine Product, Suboxone®

In the last decade, a crescendo of prohibitions, fueled by government agency leaders and certain private interests, has been building up against American patients in pain. Increasingly denied, by ever-escalating proscriptions of federal and state interlopers, their appropriate, legal narcotic analgesic dosages, they continue to be harshly victimized. That because of the uneducated or unscrupulous functionaries at the alphabet agencies mentioned earlier.

Thus, those clueless operatives have been and continue to be bolstered by anti-opioid pressures about prescription narcotic analgesics from leaders and board members of Physicians for Responsible Opioid Prescribing (PROP) - as though, in their hubris, PROP's members can't admit that all physicians went to medical school to take excellent care of patients, to relieve their sufferings, and certainly know how to "responsibly" prescribe a whole litany of medications, including morphine and its analogs.

The conceit that only those few PROP members have the secret to pain relief - that opioids are deleterious medicines; that other physicians are very low in intelligence, responsibility, ethics, pharmaco-chemistry knowledge, experience in treating various painful conditions, and in prescribing dosages and timings of narcotic analgesics for patients in pain - is hubris beyond hubris. It's blind arrogance.

Furthermore, it shrinks patients' rights to rely on their own physicians for Hippocratic care. It frightens all the rest of America's physicians, who are not members of the PROP club, into not providing pain care of any kind, and certainly not opioids - just what's been happening all over America for years, especially since the advent of the 2016 *CDC Guideline* heavily influenced by "advisors" connected to PROP.

This mindset, furthermore, has served to embolden our federal and state government leaders to ignore constitutional protections of citizens, to invade doctors' practices, to haul away patients' confidential medical records, to confiscate physicians' assets, to persecute, prosecute and imprison innocent clinicians - all to be sure that suffering pain patients are denied medically-appropriate legal prescription narcotic analgesia for their painful conditions.

For shame! Today, millions upon millions of Americans in pain are being involuntarily tapered or abruptly *cold-turkeyed* off their well-working prescription narcotic regimens because of the out-of-thin-air invention of opiohysteria whipped up by thick-headed, conscienceless government dimwits, and by private entities and individuals dead (*sic*) set on promoting their painful and lethal agenda. (In the following chapters in this section, you'll learn the details.)

Further muddying the facts has been and continues to befuddle those with research-based contrary data, is the ongoing deliberate conflation of drug addicts' overdose deaths (many of whom could've been revived with naloxone) with normal prescription treatment of patients in pain. Due to which, pain patient suicides continue as I write this.

Chapter Twenty

The Suboxone Hoax

Suboxone® (buprenorphine/naloxone), long-promoted as this salubrious, anti-addiction formulation for the Medication Assisted Treatment (MAT) of drug addiction, is only now beginning to be recognized, paradoxically, as an addiction threat itself. And many healthcare professionals, today, even view Suboxone's widespread effusive promotion and mandatory prescription for addicts as instigating and perpetuating addiction to it's morphine component, buprenorphine. How, then, did medical professionals arrive at this conflation - addicting addicts to a legal opioid to, eerily, replace illicit drugs? And, who, or what entities, beside Indivior and its parent corporation Reckitt Benckiser, stand to benefit from the largesse of $uboxone ale?

At this writing in 2019, Suboxone® (buprenorphine/naloxone), manufactured by Reckitt Benckiser subsidiary, Indivior, has been sold and prescribed for 17 years, purportedly for the treatment of drug addicts during detox in rehab and, subsequently for maintenance of a "clean and sober" existence for them. I understand that some of these patients, later, no longer require the Suboxone at all. However, from my research, it appears that, due to the morphine component, the buprenorphine (called "bupe" on the streets, to where it's often been diverted), many of these so-designated "detoxed" patients appear to have to remain on Suboxone for life.

In 2016, eligible Suboxone-prescribing physicians, who were limited by law to treat up to 100 addicts, became eligible to increase these census limits to 275 such patients by the federal government. Also, at that time, via the 21st Century Cures Act, a billion dollars was allocated to treat drug addicts. And, many of those billions have gone to purchase Suboxone, purportedly for "addiction treatment."

However, an unforeseen (but expectable by neurochemistry-knowledgeable physicians) denouement followed this widespread "treatment". Addicts were able to divert it to be sold and used on the street. This is one of the many questionable outcomes, that are definitely not therapeutic, that buprenorphine (a morphine) alone, or in its combinations with the narcotic antagonist, naloxone, has visited on America. (Note: Other buprenorphine/naloxone combinations are also on the market.)

So far, too, I've found no studies which demonstrate that the morphine buprenorphine has been successful in getting addicts off it, itself. Some drug addicts appear to need to remain on it for life. Others seem to revert back to their prior drug abuse.

My own evidence, of but one strange case, is that of one of my psychotherapy patients, who was working with me on his social, employment, and family issues related to his alcoholism. He was also a patient at an addictions clinic where he was prescribed Suboxone. Nevertheless, he reported to me that, even while on Suboxone regularly, he continued to drink alcohol, as much as was his usual habit, while ingesting this so-called "curer of addictions".

Pain Patients, Falsely Labelled "Addicts," Forced Off their Opioid Analgesics, Forced onto Suboxone

With this history of Suboxone's failure to cure addictions, the ignorant enforcers of opioid abstinence still pressured physicians to label all their pain patients as addicts. A wrong diagnosis nonetheless upping the censuses for Suboxone prescribers, upping shady motivation$ to classify as many pain patients as possible in this "addict" category to enrich Suboxone prescriber$ (of which there are hundreds nationwide), to magnify addiction levels beyond reality, to justify in the fabled minds of most

State Attorneys-General bogus lawsuits vs. nearly every drug company on the face of the earth which manufactures a narcotic analgesic.

Cruel Stupidity is Forcing Pain Patients to "Detox" on Ineffective Suboxone, Instead of Being Treated for Pain

The devastating nationwide onslaught by nonmedical government interferers into crucial pain care has falsely classified pain patients as addicts. Thereby, forcing many into "treatment" with this laughable Suboxone detox regimen. First of all, it appears not to be working so well in the lives of illicits addicts. More importantly, a morphine (buprenorphine) modified by a narcotic antagonist (naloxone) is unlikely to quell severe, intractable pain since the naloxone counters any analgesia the buprenorphine might provide. (Remember, Suboxone detoxing is meant to eliminate "cravings" by addicts for their illicits of choice. Pain patients do not have cravings. Pain patients have pain. So this whole fictionally-derived protocol is a hoax that is severely harming pain patients everywhere in America.

Nonetheless, these biochemical truths have had zero effect on the current government functionaries' forced protocols on suffering pain patients. Reminds me of the Danny Kaye film, THE INSPECTOR GENERAL, about fawning government lackeys, and of the early twentieth century Keystone Kops, idiotically clueless about reality, too stupid to see the obvious.

U.S. Government Magicians and Other Anti-Opioid Tricksters Against Narcotic Analgesics for Pain Patients are now on shaky ground – willingly blind to the evidence that Suboxone itself is an addicting opioid! What remains to be sorted out is who in federal and state government agencies, who in academia acquiring opioid research grants, which "nonprofit" organizations, and which individuals have been benefitting from this lucrative largesse – in addition to Suboxone's manufacturer.

Importantly, too, even the state Prescription Drug Monitoring Programs (PDMPs) have a disclaimer instructing doctors and pharmacists to not count the morphine, buprenorphine (and its naloxone-added combination drugs) in their opioid totals. Instructed like so: "Buprenorphine products have no agreed upon morphine equivalency and as partial opioid agonists, are not expected to be associated with overdose risk in the same dose dependent manner as doses for full agonist opioids." That, government sanctioned hooey despite everyone's awareness that drug addicts are overdosing on bupe, as the diverted Suboxone component is referred to on the street.

Some Facts about Suboxone's Manufacturer

In April of 2019, DOJ prosecutors charged that Indivior – the Reckitt Benckiser subsidiary which manufactures Suboxone – misled the medical community and U.S. government healthcare programs by convincing them that the sublingual (under-the-tongue) film formulation of this drug was safer than similar competitive buprenorphine products and had less abuse potential.

Meanwhile and significantly, for quite some time, federal agency leaders and their operatives at the CDC, DOJ and DEA, have been stubbornly scrambling to make normal medical prescribing for opiates and opioids a crime, to make prescribers criminals, to magically transform pain patients into addicts. Bumbling, but too often like a herd of cattle thundering blindly toward unknown destinations, they unethically, decided to blame the rising rate of illicit drug deaths, known to be due to adulterated fentanyl, fentanylized heroin, plus assorted additives like alcohol and the benzodiazepines on medically-appropriate opioid pharmaceuticals.

And, so determined were they to criminalize legal prescription narcotics that they gave themselves permission to hound and beleaguer physician-prescribers, to demoralize, intimidate and dehumanize patients in pain, to proscribe any pain relief at all for nearly every American. The latter is not an exaggeration since, as I've mentioned earlier, this opioid war against the long-term, sometimes lifelong, medically-appropriate use of opioid drugs for Intractable Pain Patients (IPPs) has metastasized to every single pain category you can imagine. This fact would be a joke if it weren't so cruel, dangerous, and deadly.

Orthopedist: "You just had a knee replacement? Take two Tylenol and call me in the morning."

ER Doctor: "Your finger just got sliced off in your blender? Take two aspirin and get over it."

Dentist: "Your tooth extraction site is pulsating with pain? Rinse your mouth out with some saline."

Oncology MD: "Dying of cancer? Sorry, the DEA won't let me prescribe the opioid analgesic you're entitled to."

The Diversion Aspersion

The fictions abounding in federal circles, still, are that patients in pain on legally-prescribed, medically-accurate opioid analgesic dosages have been and are, somehow, having their medications diverted to the street. And that most drug addictions should be blamed on legitimately-prescribed narcotics for pain. The parallel fiction, that federal conspiracy theorists have been feeding to the naïve radio, television and newspaper media - scaring the public to death - is that hundreds and hundreds of American physicians all over our nation have been mis-prescribing and over-prescribing opioid analgesics. This fake "fact" has been bolstered by the raw stupidity of untruth upon untruth disseminated throughout the medical community by the irresponsible 2016 *CDC Guideline* "recommendations". And by the further (would you believe?) brashness of the DEA police mandating limitations on the MMEs (morphine milligram equivalents) physicians are allowed to prescribe for their variously-afflicted patients in pain. Dear reader: So the DEA police also have medical degrees?

Settled are these true facts: 1) Less than 1% of patients prescribed an opioid for pain ever become addicts; and most of those were addicts prior to their pain diagnoses. So that kills confabulations and nonsense about pain patients getting addicted. 2) Millions of pain patients don't go to seedy parts of their cities to sell their opioids to addicts. Clueless government propagandists can't think clearly: Patient has severe pain. Patient consumes opioid medication to alleviate pain. Patient wouldn't part with a milligram of morphine or other narcotic analgesic. They need theirs to daily cope with a life never totally free of excruciating suffering. That government notion is just plain stupid. Which doesn't stop brainless persons in power from spreading this rumor.

Magical Unrealism of Government Tricksters and Private Profiteers

With all that, and recognizing, finally, the Suboxone hoax and the probability that it's not the reverser of addictions, to this day still so touted, Suboxone is still promoted as a Medication Assisted Treatment (MAT) for addicts. Unfortunately, it's also falsely promoted as an analgesic for pain patients forced off their well-working prescription opioids and deliberately mislabeled "addicts". As mentioned earlier, the buprenorphine in the Suboxone formulation is cut by its naloxone component, thereby nullifying any potential analgesic properties the buprenorphine might, I say might, provide.

Our Same Government Chastises Suboxone to the Tune of Billion$

Thereafter, thus, in July 2019, Justice Department prosecutors won a judgment of $1.4 billion from Indivior's parent company, Reckitt Benckiser Group Plc. That because Reckitt Benckiser chose to settle rather than waste money and distractions on lengthy court proceedings. That is said to be the largest settlement of an opioid case in American legal history.

Unfortunately, none of the major news outlets have reported this turnabout for Suboxone. The mainstream media is turning a blind eye to the obvious. This absence of publicity about Suboxone's troubles, plus all the disinformation abounding about pain patients, their physicians, and the manufactured-out-of-whole-cloth story that prescription opioids have any relation to drug addicts' deaths from illicts has plunged America into a death spiral of formerly well-medicated pain patients whose failing health due to untreated pain is killing them, or whose hopelessly unbearable pain is plunging them to kill themselves.

Government Shenanigans with Suboxone: A Final Display of the Arrogance of Unchecked Power

Bearing in mind the billions our United States just won from Reckitt Benckiser, its once partner in escorting Suboxone into the American medication market, note these facts: Seventeen years ago, we Americans, via our government functionaries, ushered Suboxone, a product of British pharmaceutical science, into the U.S. by spending $54 million on American scientific testing and another $22 million on Suboxone clinical trials to slickly slip Suboxone into the American pharmacopeia for treating addicts. In addition to that "treatment," now being questioned by medical experts, our government clowns have now turned our protégé corporation, Reckitt Benckiser, into our adversary. Go figure.

Million$ Still being Earned on Suboxone, Questionable for its Purported Indication

Despite all these doings, Reckitt Benckiser still expects revenues between $670 million to $720 million, the net expectation being between $80 million to $130 million this year.

Wealth earned on Suboxone prescribing has been a veritable bonanza for its independent clinician prescribers and for addiction treatment businesses around the country. One confidante referred to the opiohysteria fiasco and faux Suboxone "cures" as egregious and greedy entanglements in the promotion of and profiteering from the addictions-treatment industry by some politicians and journalists. It's a business. A big business. And another anonymous insider reports to me that some congresspeople suddenly have lucrative employment at 12-Step corporations, referring to "most rehabilitation centers" as "crony patronage systems". In that regard, this person referred to four famous addiction treatment businesses.

Addiction$ Businesse$ Reap Billion$

About three years ago, the Substance Abuse and Mental Health Administration (SAMHSA) anticipated that the addiction detox and rehabilitation

The Games Government Plays at the Expense of Pain Sufferers

These kinds of behind-the-scenes shenanigans, these conflicting goings-on during the last 17 years must be exposed. To sum up, our America has been:

1. Shepherding a foreign country's (Britain's) anticipated blockbuster drug, purportedly as a detox agent, into our country, into the soaring American profits Suboxone continues to generate for addiction treatment businesses;
2. Bolstering those activities using American taxpayer dollars of $54 million for laboratory testing and $22 million for clinical tests;
3. Doing so, though increasingly aware of accumulating clinical evidence demonstrating Suboxone's buprenorphine component is, itself, addictive;
4. Promoting Suboxone's use, to this day, despite its ineffectiveness for its indicated purpose
5. Approving, via the Food and Drug Administration (FDA), its continued marketing for detox purposes, in spite of that questionable efficacy;
6. Turning around and suing Suboxone's manufacturer – which American money propped up in the first place – and winning the handsome sum, in July 2019, of $1.4 billions.

A hefty profit from our country's initial investment in a product that continues to disappoint therapeutically; that at least the scientific and medical communities always knew it couldn't do what's been claimed it could.

America, once their conniving partner, then their enemy, but still selling their sued pharmaceutical.

Hanky-panky. Cranky Yankee!

industry of $35 billion annually would reach $42 billion by 2018, which it exceeded. Could that "excess" be because of the false labeling of millions of pain patients as "addicts" and remanding them to Suboxone-prescribing facilities and Suboxone-prescribing doctors? Where, by the way, their pain was not relieved.

Money Motive$

Since 2004, the early advocates for Suboxone, including members and associates of Physicians for Responsible Opioid Prescribing (PROP), have been propping up this product as a miracle medicine to reverse drug addiction. That, even though it, itself, is a morphine substance. By some convoluted persuasions, such buprenorphine proponents have indoctrinated thousands of doctors and addiction treatment facilities throughout our country to make Suboxone the cornerstone of the treatment of drug addiction, particularly of opioid addictions. (It's "anti-addiction" applications, however, have spread to Suboxone prescriptions for alcoholics and other substance abusers.)

As mentioned earlier, once opiohysteria hit the newspapers and the public outcry screamed louder, a windfall possibility was emerging in certain money-salivating minds. It appeared that the drug addict market for the Suboxone "cure" was saturated. But doctors with permits to prescribe it had government-limited quotas for how many addicts they could treat with this agent. Ergo, these Suboxone advocates now had to harvest a new crop of "addicts" to apply their questionable Suboxone protocol to. Voilá - bamboozle the public that addict deaths are due to prescription narcotics. Abruptly cut off supplies of medicinal opioids to pharmacies. Harass, raid, and jail pain management physicians. Force doctors to label their pain patients as "addicts". Coerce such nonaddict patients to endure "Suboxone detox". Oh, by the way, the federal government, in the wake of the opiohysteria its functionaries created, then increased the patient quotas for Suboxone-prescribing doctors by at least 100%.

Now that the rest of us know what its early and ongoing proponents have always known about the Suboxone hoax, we should all expect a revelation, sometime soon it is hoped, about the true chemistry of buprenorphine and its workings in the brain. Whereupon, it will be abandoned for its purported "benefits" as we look to the horizon for some new magical chemical or device, to replace it. And to generate new wealth for certain individuals and groups eager to profit from other people's pain.

Chapter Twenty-One

Hidden Agendas of Anti-Opioid Proponent$

Apparently, the ardent proponents of Suboxone as curative for drug addiction are still advocating for its use in that illness despite their admitted awareness of the contrary. That it's a potent opioid, that its use is also addictive. Further known by prescribers of Suboxone and so-called "anti-opioid proponents" is that the drug was, and is still, being diverted by addicts for illicit use of its morphine component, buprenorphine (bupe, in street lingo).

In fact, in it's case against Reckitt Benckiser, DOJ prosecutors accused the company of promoting Suboxone to doctors for uses "unsafe, ineffective... medically unnecessary and often diverted" for illicit uses. Nonetheless, Health and Human Services (HHS) leaders and members of Physicians for Responsible Opioid Prescribing (PROP) ignored this growing health threat to addicts, especially those outside the safety net of the healthcare system.

Money Motive$ Exposed

On the pretense that it was ever necessary to instruct well-trained American physicians on the minute but widely-known details of narcotic analgesic therapies – well-known by both doctors and nurses for at least a century – a group sprung up publicizing its hubris that its few members alone possess the key to the knowledge and integrity of how to use

– really how Not to use – morphine and its semi-synthetic and synthetic analogs "responsibly".

The edict of this organization is moronic and insulting to the entire medical profession who are empathic, knowledgeable opioid prescribers. And, as well, insulting to RNs whose knowledge and expertise permits us to administer these drugs to hospital patients and in acute settings, such as Emergency Rooms, in close collaboration with each physician-prescriber.

Nevertheless, these facts have never pricked the consciences of persons associated with PROP. The outlandishness of what's implicit in this group's self-designation seems to escape over the, supposedly intelligent, heads of its leader and its members.

Purportedly, PROP came into being for the "noble" reason of limiting opiate and opioid prescribing based on the bold-faced erroneous dictum that such medications are across-the-board "dangerous" and that patients in pain have many other pain-control options which have less worrisome side effects. Strange, because the "side effects" of many of these "options" often turn out to be their ineffectiveness against pain. Such misfires have included Yoga, spinal implants, physiotherapy, meditation, psychotherapy and assorted other pain-patient intrusions that have never proven anywhere near as effective and successful as opioid medications against pain, if at all. So much for "alternatives to opioids for pain therapy".

Importantly, we should quickly avoid advising wonderful-for-milder-pain acetylsalicylic acid (Aspirin) for serious pain. Also, we should never promote all the other NSAIDs (nonsteroidal anti-inflammatory drugs), and certainly not acetaminophen (Tylenol) for dire, intractable pain. They just don't do the job that morphine and its derivatives do so well. And, believe me, the leader of PROP and the chief proponent of its purported anti-opioid agenda, Dr. Andrew Kolodny, is well aware of these widely known pharmaceutical facts.

It's imperative, therefore, that the public be made aware of some aspects of Dr. Kolodny's ardent campaign against quality pain control in

America. As well as to sort out a possible hidden agenda – a *PROPagenda* – that has zero to do, at all, either with the well-being of pain patients or the recovery of drug addicts!

Because, in the guise of "saving" pain patients from the "horrors" of addiction – bearing in mind, again, that less than 1% of patients prescribed opioids ever become addicted – under the reckless rubric that "all opioids are harmful," millions of patients suffering excruciating pain are made to endure virulent rapid tapering that thrusts many into severely declining health, eradicated life quality, and early death from debilities arising from untreated pain. Others, suddenly *cold-turkeyed*, with no alternatives but to suffer hopelessly, choose suicide. Suicides which continue daily as I write this.

Thus, the scourge of untreated pain is blood on the hands of those appearing so eager, and seeming so medically sincere, to rip well-working prescription narcotic analgesics from their healing roles in the lives of patients unfortunate enough to suffer diseases, inherited conditions, or injuries whose inflictions of severe pain are destined to never cease.

Many proponents against therapeutic opioid prescribing – at various dosage levels depending upon each individual patient's rates of metabolizing narcotics (not the idiotic limitations of only 90MME [morphine milligram equivalents] or even as low as 50MME mandated by medically-naive government operatives) – are making such crucial decisions from an addictions expertise perspective, not from a pain specialist's perspective. The leader of such thinking is psychiatrist Andrew Kolodny. And some other PROP members are psychiatrists, too. I don't think Dr. Freud would have approved of these shrinks' unempathic attitudes against therapeutic opioid interventions for patients in dire pain.

Add to that anti-opioid mindset, the fact that disproportionate numbers of PROP members were heavily consulted about, contributed to, and inflicted their skewed views on the incipient misguidances in the doomed 2016 *CDC Guideline*. It is baffling, unfathomable, that admitted specialists in addiction care like Dr. Kolodny, who was once Chief Medical Officer of the addiction treatment consortium, Phoenix House (appointed in 2013), would inflict irrelevant views on vital issues related to the care and comfort of an entirely separate patient population, those with all kinds and levels of pain.

It further boggles mental clarity that admitted specialists in addiction care were even invited to contribute to meetings at the CDC dealing with that entirely different area of medicine – the evaluation and treatment of pain. Yet (see Chapter Seven) about the infamous 2016 *CDC Guideline*, there they were, advising away, way out of their league.

Patients in All Pain Categories are *PROPagenda* Victims, Too

In this regard, it's imperative to remind healthcare professionals in particular, and all Americans in general, that this fumbling, amateurish, unprofessional behavior against Intractable Pain Patients (IPPs) has had a horrible trickle-down effect on the time-honored medical treatment of all kinds and levels of pain. Apparently, no one, suffering any pain conditions whatsoever, will ever again be allowed anything but aspirin or other NSAIDs, all equally ineffective against severe acute, chronic or cancer pain. And, forget about that visit to your dentist to have that root canal done. The Drug Enforcement Administration (DEA) has tied the prescribing hands of your dentist, too.

The destruction of chronic pain management, via the PROPagenda has now infected every kind of pain in existence that normally warrants a narcotic prescription. These include postsurgical pain, dental pain, migraine pain, acute wound pain in the ER, and carcinogenic pain. What's more, due to PROP's coercive influence on the CDC's "recommendations", the DOJ's DEA co-opted to itself coercive tactics to strike the fear of prosecution and imprisonment into the hearts of pain care physicians. And they succeeded. (See Chapter Sixteen).

Follow the TestiMONEY

One self-appointed disseminator of opiophobic hysteria – who, strangely is a proponent of the failed morphine, buprenorphine, the key ingredient in the Suboxone Medication Assisted Treatment (MAT) regimen – is Dr. Kolodny, again a psychiatrist whose background is in public health and addictions medicine which do not qualify him to lead a war against opioid treatments for pain. He does not treat pain patients, so his claimed expertise and knowledge of the neuroanatomy and neurochemistry of pain and of the wide variety of painful disorders extant is suspect.

Nevertheless, he purports to be an expert in these complex fields, publicizes himself as such, and just, at the rate of $725 an hour, earned $500,000 in Oklahoma vs. Johnson & Johnson, in July 2019, as an "expert" witness for the Oklahoma Attorney General's case. (It's important to note that many, even most A-Gs' cases against Big Pharma are considered bogus and are settled by the drug companies just so the nonsense can end and they can get back to their R&D (Research & Development) activities to create new and better analgesics and life-saving drugs.

Imperatively, you the reader should be aghast at the potential that 49 other states may pay for Dr. Kolodny's "expertise" at such fees in cases vs., not only Johnson & Johnson, but every other Pharma company on the planet which manufactures a narcotic analgesic. For all we know, certain American litigants may go after extraterrestrial pharmaceutical companies. Next, too, The Perdue Chicken!

For, as I write this, over 1500 municipal, country and state cases – against pharmaceutical manufacturers of opioids for pain – are consolidated in an Ohio court for adjudication in October 2019. What a splendiferous opportunity for government profiteer$.

Finally, it's very important too, for grant-awarders and donors to look into the activities at Brandeis University, with which Dr. Kolodny is associated. Does this university's activities, research, affiliations have any bearing on how millions of American pain patients are now being medically abandoned and suiciding?

Chapter Twenty-Two

THE WRONG ARMS OF THE LAW: State Attorneys-General, the DEA and the DOJ

The overreach of government lawyers, police, and prosecutors into the lives of patients in pain, which has been going on for years and is still happening, has gone from distressing to death-promoting. Too many, almost all, of these autocrats have been blithely abusing their unrestricted powers. Which abusers include many State prosecutors who've gone overboard in their zeal to bring down an entire industry - Prescription Medicine Manufacturing - vital to 21st Century health and survival. Which include Big Pharma corporations that have developed and manufacture opioid medications commonly used for over a century to treat various levels of pain.

With these omnipresent State vendettas ongoing, the CDC then bumbled its way into normal opioid prescribing for pain, weaponizing its misguided 2016 *Guideline* by ripping from physicians their legal rights to prescribe appropriate narcotic analgesics for their patients in pain. This missile then emboldened the Department of Justice (DOJ) to empower its Drug Enforcement Administration (DEA) agents to embark on storm trooper actions that do not belong in the United States of America.

In subsequent segments of this chapter, I'll discuss questionable, possibly criminal, actions of the DEA and the DOJ that will make your head spin. "Renegades" is the best word I can think of at the moment, for you to keep in mind. because these government-created rogue police and prosecutors are feared by physicians nationwide, by other prescribing clinicians, by pharmacists, and by fifty millions of Americans in pain whose legal narcotic medications are being denied to them, force-tapered, cold-turkeyed; whose lives are ruined thereby, many suiciding.

State Attorneys-General: Wrong Indictments by Injudicious Lawyers

For starters, let's look at what the anti-Pharma State Attorneys-General are doing to harm, not only pain-sufferers and the makers of essential medicines, but all American citizens who ever require any kind of prescription medication for any and all diseases, inherited disabilities, injuries, and surgeries.

Prosecutorial overreach of State Attorneys-General against manufacturers of legal opioids harms pain patients and, ultimately, all patients. Unconscionably, as you've been witnessing in all the distressing facts throughout this book, this legal fenagling is ongoing, seemingly neverending. And these stories of how various government functionaries have inserted themselves into our personal, confidential healthcare lives, causing untold added suffering along with untreated miseries, are only magnified via the blatant attacks by State prosecutors on the very corporations which exist to keep us well, to cure many diseases, to palliate others, to relieve pain.

Along with the private vested interests mentioned in earlier chapters - the organization PROP, the Suboxone bonanza enjoyed by the addictions treatment industry, for examples - when State Attorneys-General sue makers of vital medicines on such a huge scale, as I'll describe below, they're planting the seeds for the constriction of an industry that does vital research to produce pain-relieving and life-saving medications for all of us.

A strange catch-22 in these anti-Pharma-company state litigations is that - when Dr. Kolodny (see Chapter 21, Hiddent Agenda$ of Anti-Opioid Proponent$) is the testifying "expert," who, remember, earns $750 an hour for his trial preparations and on-the-stand opinions - everything he says may well fly in the face of the anti-opioid stance he and his

PROP organization stand for. That's because he's pro-Suboxone for the MAT (Medicine Assisted Treatment) of addicts, despite what everyone, by now, knows about its buprenorphine component being truly, also, an addictive morphine. (See Chapter 20, "The Suboxone Hoax".) There he sits, on the witness stand, scurrilously expounding on the horrors of prescription opiates and opioids, assisting the current prosecutor he's working with in faulting Big Pharma makers of morphine and its derivatives while, hypocritically, ardently, effusively supporting Suboxone, "the legal morphine" for the treatment of addictions. A treatment which everyone now knows is suspect and, at best, must be a lifetime millstone for addicts using it, now, in place of the illicit narcotic they originally used and supposedly detoxed from.

Why Many State Attorneys-General are Blameworthy for Pain Patient's Sufferings

Patients suffering various increments of pain have been for years, and continue to be, victimized by State prosecutory actions that extend well beyond legitimate boundaries of society's concern for lawful behaviors and a healthy citizenry. It seems, with the shot-gun deploying of the 2016 *CDC Guideline* missile (see Chapter 7, Critique of the Guideline), everyone and his cousin with a J.D. degree has jumped on the taint-the-opioid bandwagon to incorrectly demonize narcotic medications, to demoralize opioid-medicated patients in pain, to detain and imprison opioid-prescribing physicians, to further inflict chaos, added suffering, and even death onto innocent pain patients' lives.

Thus, while the DEA and the DOJ (see discussions below) are reveling in their *carte blanche* tactics, unbridled and unchecked by any other government agency or congressional entity, treating pain patients and their physicians like criminals in a netherworld of their own autocratic concoction, an unsettling number of American states have also given *carte blanche* to their Attorneys-General to prosecute, at will, any and all companies which dare to manufacture prescription opioid medications. To reiterate: These prosecutors earned their MD degrees in Law School?

What's particularly important about this troublesome arm of the law to Americans in agony is that these State prosecutors inflict heavy impingements on flourishing Pharma manufacturers and distributors which could, someday, shrink the development and supply, not only of more and even safer opioids, but of many other vital medications as well. The constant litigation these A-Gs inflict on Pharma corporations would seem comical if these constrictive actions didn't wound so many millions of patients in America and worldwide. Seriously, though, it's like these state prosecutors intend to put these medicine makers out of business.

What's in it for the Plaintiff A-Gs?

When state A-Gs decide to sue a pharmaceutical company, beside the winnings or conceded settlements to the state of 70% of millions or more – litigating firms take 30% – these lawyers and their staffs know very well that there are implicit perks that accompany such bounty. Promotions? Raised salaries? Increased employee benefits? Bonuses? They know what's expected of them in these cases. They are also not so naive as to think they won't be rewarded for helping their state strip a pharmaceutical corporation of some of its working capital.

Supposedly, too, that 70% goes to the plaintiff state's coffers to defray costs of the "opioid crisis" of illnesses and deaths due to illicit drugs said to be burdening that state's healthcare system. In that regard, it'd be interesting if auditors could look at these monies' dispersals to determine exactly what they are actually being used for. And to ferret out any potential misuse of, or diversion of, this wealth.

Why don't we just de-legitimize all pharmaceutical manufacturers – and be done with this obvious State thievery of monies that could be earmarked for Research and Development of new and better prescription pharmaceuticals? What a waste of resources, both state taxpayers' funds and drug company funds. What rampant displays of greed. Especially greed built on the deliberate conflation of two distinct patient groups – (1) drug addicts and (2) patients in physical pain.

The winnings from these wink-wink, nod-nod trials, strangely enough, are meant to be spent on drug addicts – supposed "victims" of legally-prescribed opioids, a fiction daily infused by irresponsible journalists into the public consciousness. And, even though the latter is totally false – because we all know by now that less than 1% of patients prescribed opioid medications ever go on to addiction – that fact hasn't stopped these sorry prosecutors from inflicting their erroneous accusations on Pharma companies anyway.

Meanwhile, parallel to these windfalls and false focus solely on drug addicts in these A-Gs' states, patients in pain are being summarily denied their narcotic analgesics altogether. Nonetheless, our legal system permits these incursions into the normal workings of the pharmaceutical industry with alacrity. So doing, these state lawyers have set up – and continue to do so as I write this – two distinct patient groups as adversarial, pain patients and drug addicts, when these two have zero to do with each other's illnesses. Zero!

Attorneys-General Victimize Big Pharma, Contribute to Pain Patient Abandonment

Expecting Americans to believe the opio-fiction – equating drug addicts seeking "highs" and dying on overdoses of illicits as having even a nano-relationship to pain patients simply experiencing pain relief from their prescription opioids – many State A-Gs have discovered a goldmine in casting pharmaceutical companies all over the planet as villains who "flood" American communities with painkillers for their own nefarious enrichment. Yet, it's the A-Gs, the states for which they prosecute and their litigation firms that eye the gold-filled cornucopia in their intimidations of Big Pharma. Bear in mind that the treasures these A-Gs are salivating for are monies the targeted pharma companies could've used for Research & Development (R&D) of new curative, life-saving, and pain-relieving drugs. Instead, federal and state government hanky-panky and pressureful legal maneuvering often forces drug manufacturers to summarily "settle" these bogus cases so they can get back to their very important medicine manufacturing.

Behind the Scenes, these Wrong Arms of the Law have been Laughing at All of Us

State A-Gs, with a greedy eye, focus on every Pharma manufacturer which happens to market an opiate – morphine – or opioids, the latter being semi-synthetic or synthetic analogs of morphine. They laugh behind our backs as they drum up elaborate charges all the while knowing that most drug companies will "settle" rather than waste their teams of lawyers' time and corporate funds to defend such ludicrous but pressureful cases. Truly sad, because those million$ and billion$ could have gone to the development of new and better drugs for the sick and suffering.

A-G Meddlers in Medical Affairs

Various State A-Gs apparently studied medicine in law school. I guess a J.D. automatically confers knowledge of anatomy, physiology, neurology, pharmacology, Central Nervous System (brain and spinal cord) pain circuits, neurochemistry, nociceptors, the clotting cascade which relates to pain, etc., etc. And, of course, the intricacies of various modes of patient care.

The Greedy Eyes of Plaintiffs: More than 1500 Class Action Lawsuits vs. Big Pharma by State A-Gs and many Municipal and County Prosecutors

Speaking of windfalls, I know for sure, with these A-G onslaughts, their J.D. degrees apparently didn't confer empathy on these money-motivated lawyers. Worse yet, according to a report made to me in April of 2019, most A-Gs are financially motivated to vilify prescription opioids because they are plaintiffs in over 1500 class action law suits against Pharma manufacturers, expecting to win billion$ from makers of opioid medications – via municipal, county and state judicial systems.

In fact, for the mere sum of $270 million, Oklahoma Attorney General, Mike Hunter, recently settled that state's suit against Purdue Pharma. It's important to bear in mind that most, if not all, such suits are "settled" by the pharma corporation to be relieved of the time-wasting, exorbitant legal expenses and to get back to work doing what they do best – researching, developing and manufacturing life-saving and pain-relieving medications for the sick and dying. Thanks a lot, Mike. That $270 million could have gone, instead, to Purdue Pharma's R&D division to bring new miracle medicines to market to help us all.

Top Profits for the Litigating Law Firm vs. Hundreds of Drug Companies

One law firm, Simmons, Hardy, Conroy, stands to enjoy Big Pharma "settled" spoils. Because, as the litigating firm, it is suing multiple opioid manufacturers on behalf of those municipal, county and state governments, earning a third of the "settlements". These legal maneuvers, blinding the common sense of journalists reporting them, and so infecting the national consciousness, are a smokescreen hiding the gross ineptitude of government lawyers.

The true victims of this institutionalized opiohysteria, the real losers and convenient targets are patients in pain, opioid-prescribing physicians, opioid-dispensing pharmacists, AND narcotic analgesic manufacturers.

A-Gs Collude with Kolodny, the PROP "expert"

Andrew Kolodny,MD, is these A-Gs' other "partner" in these attacks on pharmaceutical manufacturers. Remember, he's trained in psychiatry (See Chapter 21, about Dr. Kolodny's role in opiophobia and his organization PROP) yet he appears to pop up everywhere, advertising an "opioid epidemic" which he wrongly attributes to prescription narcotic analgesics. Yes, his once association with Phoenix House as its Medical Director assures his knowledge about addictions, as well as other mental illnesses. However, his resume does not show any immersion in the highly specialized field of pain management which usually relies on the intricate expertise of anesthesiologists, neurologists and other clinicians who've taken in-depth pain physiology and analgesic pharmacochemistry trainings. Nonetheless, when it comes to his agenda, and those of various state A-Gs, he has been cleared as an "expert" in these aggressive litigations against pharmaceutical manufacturers of opioid medications.

Paradoxically, this proponent of "the legal morphine" buprenorphine, in July of 2019, at the rate of $725 per hour, earned $500,000 for his testimony in Oklahoma vs. Johnson & Johnson. It's important to note that J&J's subsidiary, Janssen, manufactures among its many products, the pharmaceutical Duragesic® (fentanyl transdermal), a legal opioid with specific patient instructions on its use, and which has zero relationship to the adulterated fentanyl from which drug addicts are dying.

Enlightened Judge Dismisses North Dakota vs. Purdue Pharma

In May of 2018, on the momentum of the opiohysteria epidemic, North Dakota Attorney General Wayne Stenchjem sued major narcotics manufacturer Purdue Pharma Inc., claiming its opioid products played a causative role in illicit drug deaths. Instructively, the week of July 23, 2019, this suit was dismissed by a wise judge. That, even though many American states, via their state A-Gs, have been chomping at the bit to reap the spoils of burgeoning law suits – against Purdue Pharma and other legitimate pharmaceutical manufacturers – and are still doing so.

In this Grand Forks County, North Dakota case, A-G Stenchjem sought huge sums of money from Purdue. The charges: That "aggressive marketing" to increase its opioid sales somehow led to the purported "epidemic". The crime: Marketing opioids to treat chronic pain.

The stupidity of such chief lawyers of our American states, so ignorant of what drugs are for, what marketing of all products – clothes, cars, toys, food, jewelry, insulin, antibiotics – entails, is glaring. This affliction of marketing ignorance among high-powered lawyers is illustrated by the overzealous resort to these epidemics of lawsuits they're inflicting on innocent manufacturers of life-saving and pain-relieving drugs. At this writing in August, 2019, almost every one of our 50 states is suing various pharmaceutical manufacturers. Add to those bogus actions, some 2,000 counties, cities and Native American tribes that have joined in the fray to divvy up the envied spoils.

Fortuitously, in addition to the North Dakota case being dismissed, so too have some municipalities cases been dropped. And Purdue Pharma also reached "nuisance" settlements with Kentucky in 2015 and with

Oklahoma in March of 2019. What a waste of clean money that could've been used for Purdue Pharma's Research & Development (R&D) of new life-saving and pain-relieving pharmaceuticals!

Why Judge James Hill Wisely Dismissed North Dakota vs. Purdue Pharma Inc.

Over Attorney General Stenchjem's objections, then, Judge James Hill of the Burleigh County District Court, dismissed his case against Purdue Pharma Inc. as "oversimplifying" a public health problem by suing one company. At which time, Judge Hill instructed that, having abided by Food and Drug Administration (FDA) product labeling regulations, Purdue Pharma's marketing behaviors were legitimate. Furthermore, he pointed out that, though the state's assertions were known to the FDA for years, and which the FDA carefully studied, it nonetheless required no warnings nor drug labeling changes by Purdue.

Outrageous Prosecutorial Targeting of Opioid Manufacturers

Not to relax about these prosecutorial incursions, dear reader, because in Cleveland, Ohio in October 2019, one judge has been designated to adjudicate the consolidated group of nearly 1,500 lawsuits against manufacturers of opioids. Anyone who doesn't see the ridiculousness, and waste of drug corporation resources and drain on government funds, in this misapplication of legal processes is clearly ignorant of business practices, of sales objectives, of profits goals, of advertising and of marketing – not to mention, in the pharmaceuticals industry, the humane analgesic goals of opioid products.

Thus, the various state governments' manufactured charges versus all these bona fide pharmaceutical companies' salubrious objectives are as stupid as if they were applied to manufacturers of other products we humans purchase and consume.

Recalling North Dakota vs. Purdue Pharma, the charges further eroded credulity when they went from outright wrong to utter cluelessness as Attorney General Stenchjem claimed that, once their narcotic products were sold, Purdue didn't control their distribution, didn't control their manner of pharmacy dispensings, didn't control their prescribings. Duh! Physicians prescribe! Pharmacists with PhGs dispense! Distribution quantities are according to what's needed by patients in pain in each community.

Most, if not all, these state prosecutions (I'm inclined to call them "persecutions") by myopic attorneys-general are bogus – founded on the shifting winds of opportunism (for greed and fame) and of marketing ignorance. As the straightforward wisdom of Judge James Hill instructed and emphasized:

1. All prescription drugs are approved, overseen, marketed and advertised under extraordinarily tight parameters and scrutiny by the FDA.
2. The FDA removes any drug from the market that shows dangerous side effects.
3. The FDA monitors all medical journal advertising of drugs and mandates changes when deemed necessary. The same stringent actions apply to public advertising of any drug.
4. Conversations, emails, conferences, meetings, and sales talks about drug products are normal business occurrences – the same kinds of discussions about growing any business providing products or services. What? You're not allowed to talk about how to grow your business, product benefits, new medical indications for an existing drug?
5. The marketing of opioids for patients in pain is not a crime against addicts. Addicts voluntarily use illicit adulterated fentanyl, fentanylized heroin, at times with ethanol and anxiolytics. Overdoses of these can kill. None of which has any relationship to analgesia for pain, MMEs prescribed, or numbers of prescriptions.

Drug Enforcement Administration (DEA): Wrong Policing by Lawless Agents

In this section, I'll report to you about the blatant abuses of the DEA federal police, unelected, who write their own regulations which, magically are transmuted into "law" which, then, further increases these renegade powers. Such autocratic activities against innocent citizens then devolve into renegade actions – DEA agents, like gestapo, take it upon themselves to close down doctors' practices, to get staff fired from their jobs, to confiscate patients' confidential medical records, to arrest innocent physicians, to seize all personal and professional assets from these physicians. These rogues have no one to answer to – not any congressional oversight – while good doctors flounder, pain care is shut down, pain patients flounder, and the DEA couldn't care less. Apparently, Congress is wearing blinders or couldn't care less about this run-amok agency. Here, legislators, is an outrageous abuse of power by renegade DEA operatives given unlimited *carte blanche* to harm patients, doctors, pharmacists and anyone in the healthcare population, who dares to act normally in any of their capacities both healthcare workers and people receiving their care. Why is this?

How has the DEA, along with its overseer the DOJ, eluded exposure of its questionable, I believe criminal, and blatantly dangerous incursions into our liberties and our healthcare system all these years? Even before the incredulous "misguideline" document from the CDC in 2016?

Who is responsible for giving these unregulated "regulators" such dangerous power? Who is to blame for allowing them to barge into the field of medicine and totally disrupt a once compassionate, death-defying, suffering-allaying system? Much of the DEA's "regulations" and actions are unconstitutional. So how come the DEA is getting away with these inhuman, illegal incursions?

Lawmakers have an urgent obligation to interrogate, publicly, this lawless group; to disband it immediately, and to create in its place a licit entity whose sole duties will be to focus on imported illicit drugs (from

China, Mexico, the Internet), drug kingpins, drug dealers, and drug addicts of illicits. The latter being remanded to Medical Assisted Treatment (MAT) at a detox facility (Caution: See Chapter 20, "The Suboxone Hoax"). The former being prosecuted and imprisoned.

Those are you duties. DEA! Those drug purveyors are your criminals, DOJ! Yes those, instead of all the innocent physicians and other blameless clinicians this rogue DEA, via its DOJ prosecutors, have harshly, maliciously imprisoned (see Chapter 16 for the deaths and suicides of too many of these innocent doctors).

Draconian DEA

Note too, the DEA invented an even more intrusive division in 2013 which is called "Diversion". An entity whose functionaries came up with an even more ridiculous construct, the 20% Rule, which resulted in the decree that no American pharmacy could sell Controlled Substances (which are usually prescription narcotic analgesics) exceeding 19% of their businesses. Otherwise they'd be unable to access those drugs for their dispensing inventory for 90 days.

Turns out this has been an unrealistic, arbitrary restriction of Controlled Substances and has weighed heavily over the professional obligations pharmacists have toward their prescribing doctors and sick patients.

In this modern era, well beyond the years from 1776 all the way to 2013, local drug stores have carried only what their communities' inhabitants needed. Unfortunately, even in this lunar-travel-capability era with its ever-expanding digital-world opportunities, tiny micro-mentalities exist who only know how to invent constrictions. Such mini-minds inhibit responsibility-challenged DEA leaders and their operatives who adhere, blindly, to their religion of abuse of power and abuse of their fellow citizens. They also operate under the delusion that they are qualified to practice medicine, so they proceed – clumsily, dangerously – to make medical care and medication dosage decisions that are alarming and deadly to patients.

Congress and Other National Leaders, Please End these DEA Abuses

These "diversion" religionists must be immediately diverted from their illicit and unconstitutional goals of:

1. Practicing medicine
2. Interfering in patient care
3. Spying on physicians and other clinicians
4. Threatening physicians and other clinicians
5. Preventing sufficient opioids from being supplied to all pharmacies nationwide
6. Dictating less than physician-determined opioid dosages for various patients
7. Accessing confidential medical files (even carting them away in gestapo-style raids) out of doctors' offices, arrogantly, in front of frightened patients and staff
8. Accessing confidential medical records via the ominous Prescription Drug Monitoring Program (PDMP) set up in most states. The PDMPs of many states are now "open books" to these DEA spies. By what legitimate authority has this loose-cannon cadre, this autocratic government-shielded entity, awarded itself these naked intrusions into American patients' medical privacy rights?

Is this an America we want? Is this ideal, Hippocratically curative American healthcare? Does any American really want this unelected, out-of-control cadre of medical know-nothings to be in charge of the highly specialized scientific application of narcotic analgesic care of pain-suffering self, family and friends?

How long will our Congress and all levels of government – federal, state, county, municipal – look the other way while Intractable Pain

Patients (IPPs) and other patients in pain suffer and choose suicide? How long, you who are empowered to reverse all this misery, will you do nothing while fine, empathic physicians, and other clinicians and pharmacists are raided, assets seized, and imprisoned on dubious charges?

Operatives of the DEA are Human Rights Violators

Permitting the DEA to continue to exist in its current arrogant structure, blatant anti-citizen restrictions, and criminal interferences in medical practice and pain patient care is unfathomably irresponsible.

To American legislators, politicians, governors, mayors, attorneys-general – if ever there were a time to act, an urgency like that of Pearl Harbor (1941), a toll of suffering like that of 911 (2001), a merciless mortality rate like that of the Bubonic Plague (1347-1351) – this is the time for you to summon your courage and take up the challenge of shutting down the DEA, including its "diversion" division. You can't cure a malignant entity with tiny little admonishments here and there. You need to dismantle it altogether. (Think of its existence like that of a Stachybotrys mold infestation where a whole house must be demolished or anyone who lives there will become catastrophically ill and die prematurely from its effects.)

Then start a new entity that focuses on illicit chemical imports and their offshoots, dealers and addicts using street drugs. This means hands off pain patients' prescriptions, their physicians and their pharmacists. And, by the way, Storm Troopers have no place in America. Ergo, they have zero qualifications to ration pharmaceuticals, in various therapeutic categories, from being supplied to pharmacies–which must be available for dispensing promptly for suffering patients who need them. This edict must apply to all classes of drugs, including all medicines and pharmaceuticals the DEA has heretofore "scheduled".

Note: Some cough medicines may contain a narcotic chemical known to control a dry, hacking cough. We don't need clueless government DEA gendarmes – who can't know that a neverending cough could lead to respiratory distress which could lead to a grave situation for such patients – to dictate cough medicine dosages or cough medicine inventory limits for pharmacies.

Criminal DEA Agents Prosecuted: More Reasons to Dissolve the DEA

Here is just a small sampling of criminal behaviors by DEA agents – selling illicit drugs, stealing huge sums of money, threatening bodily harm to arrestees, falsifying official records, and commiting perjury.

It seems the effects of wrongful detention of innocent physicians, seizures of MDs' professional and personal assets, threatening and coercing doctors over medical issues the DEA had no business in in the first place, have so infected DEA operatives that these inhuman behaviors criminalized some of them. I'm reporting here something that's difficult to stomach – the blatant criminal behaviors of some DEA agents – trafficking in the very illicit drugs they are duty-bound to interdict, stealing huge sums of money supposedly seized for legal government sequestering.

According to an October 2017 report about certain DEA rogue agents, four of them were facing federal charges for conspiracy and corruption. Their crimes included perjury, misidentifying suspects in drug crime cases, and recording lies in DEA documentation. Such reprehensible behaviors that caused at least one wrongful two-year jailing of an innocent person. These are the known accused: Once Task Force Officers Johnny Domingue, Rodney Gemar and Karl Newman of the New Orleans division of the DEA. And Special Agent Chad Scott with the DEA since 1997.

That 2017 indictment accused Gemar, Scott and Newman of "seizing" property and cash from their arrestees and keeping these spoils for themselves. (It's important to remind the reader of the DEA's widespread wanton seizures of all assets of wrongly targeted physicians who treat pain patients – spoils which are earmarked for the DEA/DOJ to keep.) Strangely, the DEA making its own "laws" for itself as it goes along, unchecked by law-abiding others, did not call those criminal actions "theft," as they should have! The DEA simply called these "embezzlements". Too, this thievery continued for at least seven years according to the government's own records.

Special Agent Scott slickly accepted a federal defendant's bribe of $10,000. He also tampered with a defendant's testimony by coercion and perjured himself in this case. And DEA Task Force Officer Newman was arrested in 2016 because, after his seizure of thousands of dollars worth of oxycodone and cocaine, he sold these at a significant profit for himself instead of turning them in the official way. Outlandishly, in his "seizure," he was said to have used threats of violence and injury to the drug dealer, all while brandishing his gun. At the time, Newman pled guilty to "conspiracy to convert property" and to using a gun in a violent crime.

This snippet from the criminal actions of DEA renegades just hints at the wild permissiveness and corruption this out-of-control government entity has awarded itself. And it is only a tiny picture of the wanton behaviors DEA agents have inflicted on innocent physicians all across America. And on innocent other prescribing clinicians and on innocent dispensing pharmacists and innocent owners of businesses honestly taking ethical care of patients in pain.

These DEA employees were easily corrupted by the unchecked arrogance of this corrupt federal entity that needs to be disbanded at once to clean out all the rot and corruption, all the dirty permissions DEA leaders have awarded themselves. See Section VII for ways to create positive government entities and a new agency which will be empowered to solely oversee issues related to illicit drugs. Hands off the practice of medicine. Hands off opioid prescriptions for the care of all kinds of pain. The Doctor is in. The DEA is out! But, until this change can occur, it's imperative to pay attention to the DEA overreach that has not let up as I write this.

Threatening Phone Calls by DEA Agents to Prescribing Physicians

Congress and all legislators nationwide and every politically active and influential American also need to put an immediate stop to DEA operatives' threatening phone calls they've bombarded innocent physicians with. Intimidating them. Threatening doctors with ominous "warnings" about "dosage amounts" they are prescribing as being excessive.

When were physicians instructed in medical school that they'd be answering idiotic questions about substantively complex medical decisions to law school and police academy graduates? If the tragedies – the suicidal inflictions on pain patients and the prosecutorial inflictions on skilled and blameless physicians – that ensue from the actions of these lawless "lawmen" weren't so dire and deadly, these DEA behaviors would be comedic.

Imagine a satire wherein a bumbling, know-nothing DEA agent is telephone-admonishing a professor of neurology and anesthesiology (of which I've mentioned more than a few in this book), who's been a pain management clinician for decades and has saved the lives of thousands of chronic pain patients (many of whom might have suicided without their analgesic opioid medication). You can see the idiocy of such a story plot, right? The horrible truth, though, is that these implied-threat "warning calls" are happening even as you read this.

State Boards of Medicine Must Protect their Credentialed Physicians and Stop Bowing and Cow-towing to Phony DEA Charges

It's exceedingly imperative that all 50 states' Boards of Medicine (as well as the respective professional boards of NPs, PAs, DOs, and PhGs) rebel against DEA interference in medical practice, in the physician-patient relationship, and in all other professional-prescriber-patient relationships. State Boards should not genuflect, as they've been shamefully doing against their co-professionals, to manufactured DEA accusations. I demand this because my research shows that most doctors invaded by DEA gestapo tactics and then cleared have not been initially bolstered by their boards. Instead, across the country, Medical Boards have folded like disposable stethoscopes in the wrathful path of DEA dead-wrong accusations. (California is particularly egregious against its credentialed physicians.) Unjustly, they've summarily rescinded MDs' hard-earned licenses and chastised them unapologetically, helping rogue DEA operatives destroy fine physicians' lives and livelihoods.

Many medical organizations (see Chapter 10) are finally speaking up against the misguided 2016 *CDC Guideline*, against mini-dose MMEs that don't control pain for IPPs, against prosecution of physicians who've done nothing but prescribe, appropriately, the opioid medication in the individualized dosages each individual patient's condition and metabolism requires.

It's time for all Americans and our American government leaders to interrogate DEA and DOJ trouble-makers. Time to disband the DEA. Time to create a patient-friendly, physician-friendly, constitutional-rights-friendly entity which should be empowered to solely target criminals. That means their sole focus and responsibilities will be on interdiction of illicit drug imports, on arresting dealers of illicit drugs, and on directing drug addicts to detox facilities. Period. Those are their only jobs. Nor shall they ever again come near medical practices nor interfere with normal prescription opioids for patients in pain. Never!

The American Inquisition by the DOJ: Wrong Prosecutions and Imprisonments

A great pain care specialist, Forest Tennant,MD (See all about him in Chapter 12 and how the U.S. Injustice system killed his life's work.) maintains that claims that pain is etiologically psychological are "ploys" to distract the unknowledgeable from the neurologic truth about pain, from the medically-justified use of prescription opiates and opioids to target and ameliorate pain. I say the latter because in chronic, intractable cases, pain is never completely obliterated. Instead, it's ameliorated, alleviated enough so the afflicted can get out of bed, out of the house, go to work, live a modicum of a normal life.

(Acute pain, of course, like a toothache, a postsurgical wound, and other non-chronic pain conditions, can respond pain-free for up to four hours starting at about fifteen minutes after the patient swallows or is injected with an opioid. Then, if the acute pain persists after four hours, another intramuscular (in the hospital) injection or pill of an opioid drug can be administered again. This is standard pain care in hospital settings...and, in pill-form, for patients at home.)

But, for chronic pain patients at home, their physicians develop individual opioid doses and dosage-timing regimens depending on many individual factors differing from patient to patient. These include the type of pain, the disease or injury causing it, the locations of the pain, the intensity level of the pain, the individual patient response to varied dosage protocols of different opioids, the knowledge that some patients (and doctors can only discover who these are as they monitor each pain patient's responses to specific dosages and ingestion-timing protocols), metabolize opioids at rates requiring higher doses than others with seemingly similar pain levels. This fact alone accounts for justified high-dose prescribing in such patients.

Unjust DOJ Invasions

Unfortunately, such correct medical care has been turned into a crime by clueless DOJ/DEA raiders/inquisitors/prosecutors. And, if their rogue actions weren't so ominous, their attacks on, and imprisonments of, innocent physicians could be attributed to the Jacques Clouseau kind of fictional bumbling like the defective detective of French cinema. That's because these renegades haven't bothered to educate themselves about the medical facts just enumerated which all doctors, nurses and other clinicians are profoundly aware of.

The DOJ's Conspiracy to Frame Innocent Physicians

It's understandable that DOJ prosecutors wouldn't know such detailed medical facts any more than MDs have a clue about some obscure legal practices that, for instance, have been imprisoning innocent physicians for decades – outrageously adjudicating long sentences on the catch-22 charge of "conspiracy". A "crime" accusation which DOJ prosecutors have no obligation to explain to the judge. A looming threat to clinicians caught in the web of prosecutorial falsehoods.

For, if a DOJ-targeted physician refuses to plead guilty to DOJ-manufactured "lesser" charges (whatever these Inquisitors might taint them with, whatever they might fabricate but which carry less than the 25 years in prison for "conspiracy"), off they go, wrongfully convicted. Off to the latter years of their lives in prison! For what? I say for DOJ ignorance, overreach, out-of-control institutionalized stupidity. For lack of intricate medical knowledge. Lack of intricate pharmaceutical chemistry knowledge. A lack of human caring for other Americans, who happen to be painfully ill. And lack of conscience about their destructions of empathic physicians who are ethically following their Hippocratic obligations to FIRST DO NO HARM.

One of the ancient Ten Commandments is: "Thou shalt not bear false witness against thy neighbor." In this regard both the DEA and the DOJ are themselves breaking Divine law. Because of their, for years, ongoing specious fabrications against honest, caring, correctly-prescribing physicians and other professionals, the DEA/DOJ cabal has swept up, in its steel-lockjaw net, far too many honest medical professionals who have either died shortly after these unjust accusations or have suicided. Other wrongly-convicted professionals are sequestered away where they can no longer do any good for their patients or their families...a goal which Suboxone advocates, PROP, and lawsuit-hungry States suing every opioid manufacturer in the universe must be gleefully applauding.

As you've been reading above, about DEA police flagrantly flaunting their renegade actions against presumed-innocent physician-targets – ignoring civil rights, human rights, and truth itself – the DEA mirrors its parent, the Department of Justice. A DOJ *Reichstag* that, with *carte blanche*, bumbling wildly out of control, ignorantly singles out prescription opioids, the doctors who prescribe them, and the painfully ill patients who need them to survive.

Answering to no one, DOJ inquisitors have been given free rein to intimidate, falsely accuse, and trap opioid-prescribing clinicians in catch-22 traps that assure their Inquisition tactics never fail to indict blameless medical and other professionals providing empathic pain care to long-suffering patients. As a result, the DOJ has created this American holocaust – the daily torture of millions and millions of Americans cold-turkeyed off their well-working opioid regimens or involuntarily tapered to such low MMEs (morphine milligram equivalents) of their opioid analgesic that it wouldn't relieve the pain of a gnat. Then, those who can no longer withstand this government-sanctioned torture, have been daily, all around the nation, committing suicide.

This is an epidemic of suicides, these untreated pain-patient life-endings, which the DOJ's companion agency, the CDC with its skewed focus on prescription opioids, has managed to irresponsibly avoid. A suicide epidemic ignored by the CDC. Strangely so, since the CDC's mandate is to investigate and end epidemics.

Ominous Operations of the DOJ are Killing Pain Patient Care

The DOJ – overseen by the U.S. Attorney General, at this writing he is Jeff Sessions – is supposed to enforce U.S. law, ensure public safety, and lead the nation in preventing crime and assuring impartial adjudication of cases. (It's important to note, here, that the DEA, an arm of the DOJ is simply tasked with fighting illicit drug importations and dealer distributions. Nonetheless, as you've read about the DEA's gestapo-like actions above, the DEA's rogue incursions have far exceeded this entity's *raison d'etre*, yet are sanctioned by the DOJ's blind-eye inertia toward the DEA's outrageous invasions of patients' and physicians' rights.

DOJ Autocrats against Opioid Pain Relief: Physicians Deliberately Targeted, Pain Patients Deliberately Abandoned

Recently, U.S. Attorney General Sessions boasted about yet another "task force" targeting opioid prescribers. He seems gleeful in aiming to imprison clinicians. To bolster this goal, DOJ manipulations have morphed from announcing an "opioid epidemic" to calling it a "prescription opioid epidemic," thereby diverting public and media attention from the DOJ-DEA cadre's failure to control illicit drug trafficking.

The DOJ Plays Doctor by Dictating Medical Narcotic Prescribing

So these law school graduates know the intricacies of medical practice? Have studied pain patient disparities in metabolizing opioid dosages? Have learned the pharmacologic facts about various opioid formulations? Intimately know all the diseases, inherited conditions, injuries and surgeries that require the strengths of opioid narcotics? Have immersed themselves in neurology, brain anatomy and physiology, neurochemistry, anesthesiology and pain perception variations and intensities? Not!

Despite its operatives ignorance of those vital facts, U.S. Attorney General Sessions has funded, with yours and my tax dollars, twelve Assistant U.S. Attorneys who've been directed to initiate prosecutions related to prescription opioids. (In that regard, bear in mind that it's still a fact that less than 1% of patients prescribed opioid medications ever go on to addiction. Thus, Sessions' focus thereon is bogus, a waste of public monies, a diversion from what the DOJ-DEA are paid to do about illicit street drugs.)

Even though these newly-appointed U.S. Attorneys, and their DEA counterparts, didn't study in-depth medical subjects in law school, or any for that matter, they still are empowered by DOJ *carte blanche* arrogance to make opioid dosage decisions. The effects of which they haven't a clue. About how to do this therapeutically, with precision dosages and timings, they're at a loss. So, too, the pain patient is at a horrific loss.

These medically-naive JDs are now empowered to dictate medication dosages to pain management specialists and other prescribing clinicians. And. stupidly, the DOJ autocracy has decided that there's such a thing as "a normal opioid dose" beyond which "norm" clinicians should tremble in anticipation of severe DOJ consequences. (See Chapter 16 for a large sample of professionals imprisoned, some dead, due to this ignorant prosecutorial zeal.)

DOJ: Intrusive, Abusive, Inexcusable, Unjust

Because of the varied medical conditions producing pain (See Chapter 1), because of varying human genetics and metabolic idiosyncracies, because of various physical challenges like jobs and family responsibilities, and because of a variety of mobility constraints, these government lawyers' simplistic one-dosage-size-fits-all, mandated by DOJ mini-minds, would be laughable if it weren't so dangerous. Dangerous to patients who are prevented from receiving prescription opioid medications in dosages arrived at by a clinician who intimately knows each individual patient's needs. Dangerous to physicians and other pain practice principals who the DOJ is, thereby, setting up for ominous prosecutions and imprisonments.

It's a roundup of innocents to cause our nation to focus away from what the DOJ and its DEA should be focusing on – illicit drug interdiction, dealer apprehension and imprisonment, and remanding known addicts to detox facilities. And, while they're at it – these wrongly-focused, anti-doctor zealots – shouldn't the DOJ, so publicly hysterical about all the overdose deaths, be prosecuting those dealers for murder? Isn't the distribution of adulterated fentanyl, fentanylized heroin and other impure and questionably-dosed illicits the same as poisoning? Mass poisonings? Last time I heard, purposeful poisoning is considered murder! Shouldn't those issues be the prime focus of DEA police and DOJ prosecutors?

Note, however, despite these exigencies, how Sessions managed to deflect the nation's attention from what the DOJ should be focused on to this militant, anti-medical, anti-pain-patient, anti-pharmacy directive: "Our DOJ prosecutors, working with the FBI, the DEA, the HHS and our state and local partners will help us target and prosecute these doctors, pharmacists and medical providers who are furthering this epidemic."

What "epidemic," Jeff? Oh, you mean the one of drug addicts dying of illicits they were never prescribed? The epidemic of illicits your DOJ and DEA are failing to quell? Miserably failing!

When will you DOJ lawyers honestly admit that you're aware that less than 1% of patients prescribed opioids ever go on to addiction? When will you DOJ prosecutors evidence the truth that prescription opioids for patients in pain have no relationship to overdose deaths of addicts choosing to use illicit substances? When? The time is NOW. STAT!

Physicians have a DOJ Target on their Backs

If the DOJ doesn't cease this witch-hunt against physicians and other prescribing clinicians soon, there won't be a doctor in America from whom any patient can expect empathic pain care with appropriate opioid medications.

These designated DOJ prosecutors are not going to report back to Jeff Sessions that they can't find any dastardly doctor defendants. To keep their jobs, they have to dig up medical professionals to charge, no matter the "crime" being suspiciously false, in order to justify the fiction for which they've been hired in the first place. All American doctors who prescribe any drug for pain, may as well wear a sign saying, "I treat pain. Target me!"

Despicable Fall-Out from this DOJ Inquisition

In addition to - as noted throughout *American AGONY* – the DOJ/DEA stranglehold on legal prescription narcotics resulting in ongoing pain patient suicides throughout the country, millions of other patients, still braving severe pain, are forced to resort to impure street illicits. A paradox considering the existence of nontoxic, highly therapeutic, dependably pure and consistently manufactured Big Pharma opioids. The latter demonized and mischaracterized by nonmedical, brain-constricted government functionaries.

Thus, we're back in the streets. The streets of illicits which the DEA can't seem to handle at all – otherwise, why the soaring illicit drug deaths? The time is NOW to rein in the bursting-at-the-seams powers of the runaway DOJ. Time to set limits. Time for them to extirpate that crackpot "conspiracy" hoax inflicted on innocents, trapping innocent physician-defendants in a DOJ net of deceit.

Finally, when will the DOJ and the DEA get it? When will these policing and prosecutorial entities realize they should not be in the business of spying on patients, their records, their doctors' prescribings?

When will these government clowns get it that ONLY LESS THAN 1% of patients prescribed a narcotic analgesic ever proceed to addiction? And that that percentage can be offered alternative (though not as analgesically-effective as opioids) treatments for their pain conditions.

May I say, dear reader, at this point, I must so describe these government employees as I do because I am so very angry at the suicides and sufferings millions of Americans have been, and are still enduring, because of the ongoing, unconscionable DOJ prosecutions and DOJ-sanctioned DEA actions. These must stop immediately to save lives, to save those right this minute planning to kill themselves because hoards of misguided government functionaries are blocking normal opioid prescribing.

Section VII

SOLUTIONS: Putting Physicians Back in Charge of Opioid Prescribing with Zero DOJ and DEA Interference

Chapter Twenty-three

Heroines and Heroes, Professionals and Patients: Passionate Proponents for Pain Patients' Rights to their Opioid Medications

In addition to honoring pain care advocates in general, this chapter serves as an Honor Roll of medical and other healthcare professionals who are standing up to the medical microcephalics (e.g., DOJ and DEA operatives) who have caused so much added pain to already suffering Intractable Pain Patients. They deserve infinite accolades. For some have already fallen victim to the autocratic cruelties of the DEA and the DOJ – Raids, Seizures of all assets, Prosecutions. Others are speaking out boldly, despite DOJ/DEA clouds looming, ever-present over their heads, their medical careers, threatening their pain patients very dependence on their practices remaining open.

Pain Treatment Advocacy Heroes and Heroines: Professionals

Josh Bloom, PhD @JoshBloomACSH
Dr. Bloom is Director of Chemical and Pharmaceutical Science at the American Council on Science and Health. At his site, you'll find delicious, no-holds-barred detonations against opiohysterics and opio-liars like self-enriching Dr. Kolodny, who Dr. Bloom excoriates and confronts with irrefutable truths about pain and pain management. Here's a June 12, 2019 article to get you revved up – ACSH "Loonies, Lawyers & Activists" https://www.acsh.org/profile/josh-bloom/articles

Linda Cheek, MD @LindaCheekMD after bogus charges and some years in prison, Dr. Cheek keeps speaking out loudly against the nazi-like current onslaughts wounding the medical care of pain patients. And about the gross injustices inflicted on innocent physicians and other clinicians. (See Chapter Sixteen to grasp the enormity of the egregious actions with which our DOJ is still invading the lives and medical practices of innocent professional doctors.) In response, Dr. Cheek started the organization, DOCTORS OF COURAGE. Keep up-to-date with its ongoing work to help save our innocent medical professionals here-> https://doctorsofcourage.org/

Mark Ibsen, MD of Helena, Montana @MarkIbsenMD Dr. Ibsen has been the owner of Urgent Care Medical Practice. Despite official harassment and interruption in his empathic work for patients in pain, Dr. Ibsen fights on. https://doctorsofcourage.org/mark-ibsen-md/

Stefan G. Kertesz, MD, MSc @StefanKertesz Dr. Kertesz is a Physician at the Birmingham Veterans Affairs Medical Center and Professor, University of Alabama Birmingham School of Medicine. In this article: "No More 'Shortcuts' in Prescribing Opioids for Chronic Pain: Millions of Americans Need Nuanced Care," co-authored by Kate Nicholson, JD (see below) you will find his passionate advocacy for his pain patients. https://www.statnews.com/2019/04/26/no-shortcuts-prescribing-opioids-chronic-pain/

Thomas F. Kline, MD, PhD @ThomasKlineMD With 42 years of providing Primary Medical Care, having been the Chief of Hospital in Home Service at Harvard Medical School, Dr. Kline is a Raleigh, North Carolina physician who is very outspoken about the rights of pain-suffering patients and about the centuries of excellence of opium and its modern analogs for treating pain. Visit his website thomasklinemd.com And also get stirred up by his passionate pro-pain-patient talks here (Excellent youtube videos) passionately advocating for pain patients' rights.https://www.youtube.com/playlist?list=PLqz4lJbZaER7Szi0znDO5PNJx7q6UAZdK

Daniel Laird, MD, JD @DanLairdMD Dr. Laird cares for pain patients in his Medical Practice. And he's doubly helpful to pain patients as a Physician/Attorney who is a passionate proponent for the best interests of and medical requirements for patients in pain.

Dr. Laird decries the Suboxone® (buprenorphine/naloxone) cornucopia created by default like so: Declares as does Andrew Kolodny, MD, who I consider to be a nonexpert in pain management does, that all patients on prescription opioids are addicts (or, in the language police phrase, Opioid Use Disorder patients) and, voila', you have a whole new stream of millions of pain patients you can now subject to Suboxone against their will. Which represents a windfall for the likes of Suboxone clinics and solo Suboxone prescribers. Seems, this morphine is difficult to "detox" from once it itself has detoxed the real addict from his/her original heroin or fentanyl.

Suboxone "treatments" represent a gold-mine for its proponents despite the lack of substantial statistics about how and if it works to benefit detoxing real addicts. Despite the lack of proof that a morphine combined with an opioid antagonist (naloxone) produces life-long or long-term abstinence from addictive illicits for known addicts; nonetheless, even though it also has not been shown to relieve pain, far too many pain patients are being *cold-turkeyed* off their well-working opioid analgesics only to be forced to take Suboxone and frustratingly experience zero analgesia.

Also, Dr. Laird recently tweeted that Veterans in Chronic Pain who've been forced to taper off their pain meds by a VA employee have recourse: You can file a claim. Get form SF-95 at www.gsa.gov/forms-library/claim-damage-injury-or-death

Wonderful too, Dr. Laird just opened his own law firm in Las Vegas, Nevada. https://www.lairdlaw.com/ Personal Injury . Medical Malpractice.etc.

R. Lamartiniere, MD @rlamartini Baton Rouge, Louisiana Dr. Lamartiniere has been virtually crucified for being a fine physician to suffering patients in pain. See this article https://www.theadvocate.com/baton_rouge/news/crime_police/article_f5d023aa-982f-5682-85a6-fb06e8b61f43.html

Despite what he's been put through, and is still being menaced by, Dr. Lamartiniere won't back down from continuing to be a fine physician deeply concerned for his patients. I know he was recently hospitalized for an illness. I wouldn't be surprised if it also was complicated by all the horrible autocratic government and medical board stress imposed on this fine doctor. Nevertheless, he continues to speak out about the injustice of targeting patient-centered doctors; and about the awful burden these sieges and prosecutions place on Hippocratic-Oath adhering physicians.

Richard A. "Red" Lawhern, PhD @lawhern1 Dr. Lawhern is Director of Research and a Board member of the Alliance for the Treatment of Intractable Pain (ATIP). He's a staunch Pain Patient Advocate and a Passionate Proponent for suffering patients everywhere. Plus he's a Healthcare Writer, with 70 published papers to his credit.

According to one of Dr. Lawhern's tweets: "DEA may be operating what amounts to a bounty hunter system, awarding cash bonuses to drug diversion investigators based on the fines paid by doctors who they investigate. Profoundly unethical!" www.lawhern.org

He goes on in a follow-up tweet: "I invite physicians...to join the Alliance for the Treatment of Intractable Pain as knowledgeable advocates on behalf of patients denied effective treatment. He may be reached at lawhern@hotmail.com

Sean Mackey, MD, PhD @DrSeanMackey Dr. Mackey is Redlich Professor, Chief, Division of Pain Medicine, Stanford University and Director, Stanford Systems Neuroscience and Pain Laboratory, Department of Anesthesiology, Perioperative and Pain Medicine Neurosciences and Neurology Stanford University School of Medicine This in-depth pdf explains what's wrong with what's been happening to pain patients and what to do to ameliorate the terrible nationwide suffering caused by government autocrats. https://drseanmackey.com/s/Oregon-HERC-3122019.pdf

Stephen E. Nadeau, MD @StephenNadeau9 Associate Chief of Staff for Research, Malcom Randall VA Memorial Center, Gainesville, Florida; Professor of Neurology, University of Florida College of Medicine, Gainesville. Check out Dr. Nadeau's Patient-Centered Opioid Prescribing here: https://www.practicalpainmanagement.com/resources/news-and-research/alliance-offers-patient-centered-opioid-prescribing-recommendations

Kate M. Nicholson, JD @speakingabtpain Attorney Nicholson is Co-Chair of the Chronic Pain/Opioids Task Force for the National Centers on Independent Living and a civil rights attorney formerly with the U.S. Department of Justice. https://www.nicholsonherrick.com/our-team

Ted Noel, MD Retired Anesthesiologist @vidzette #PainPatientsVote #dontpunishpain And, see Dr.Noel's refutation of a 60 Minutes television program attacking quality medical practice opiate prescribing. https://www.americanthinker.com/articles/2019/03/the_emotherem_opiate_problem.html

Pharmacist Steve @Pharmaciststeve This pharmacist is gung-ho for the rights of pain patients to their opioid medications. And his website is a blast of fun but seriously taking on the establishment of know-nothings about narcotic analgesics. Pictorially, imaginatively rich, Steve, PhG, never met an intruder into the world of analgesic prescriptions that he didn't rake over the coals for their stupidity and cruelty against patients in pain. http://www.pharmaciststeve.com steve@steveariens.com 502-938-2414

Michael Schatman, PhD @headdock Dr. Schatman, a Clinical Psychologist, has devoted 32 years to the multidisciplinary management of chronic pain. He's on the faculty of Tufts University School of Medicine's Department of Public Health & Community Medicine. He's also Director of Research & Network Development, Boston Pain Care, Waltham, Massachusetts. On the subject of chronic pain management, Dr. Schatman has published 100 professional journal papers and he has been, for five years, the Journal of Pain Research's Editor-in-Chief.

Dr. Schatman is very passionate about this subject of the treatment of pain patients and, in my interactions with him, he has always presented a caring demeanor about what pain patients need and the exigencies of what the science demonstrates.

Presentations of Specialists in Pain Care Issues Including Dr. Schatman provided this comprehensive article: "Time for Pain Practitioners to Take Back Pain Prescribing" https://www.practicalpainmanagement.com/meeting-summary/time-pain-practitioners-take-back-pain-prescribing

Heroines and Heroes: Pain Patients and Pain Care Advocates at Twitter

This following segment lists as many pain care activists as I could identify at this writing from around our country. Most are in great pain and most, nearly all, have either been forcibly cut off their normal prescription narcotic analgesics or have been forcibly tapered to doses that wouldn't touch the pain of a flea. That ridiculous 90MME (morphine milligram equivalents) that the misguided 2016 *CDC Guideline* inflicted on prescribing clinicians as *de rigueur* treatment for all chronic pain patients, despite the scientific fact that different people metabolize ingested chemicals differently. Meaning that some pain patients require higher doses of their narcotic medicines to experience the analgesic effect that others will experience at lower doses. It's about individuation. Humans are not clones. Not automatons. But the cold turkeys at the CDC, seated at their tax-payer-financed desk jobs, even those with medical degrees but far removed from hands-on patient care, couldn't care less about the devastation they've wrought on millions of pain-sufferers.

Here is a small sampling of pain-suffering patients and advocates for a return to the sanity of normal medical care and normal opioid prescribing for pain patients including legal protections for all American patients to prevent DEA and DOJ interference in everyone's medical care. And with immunity against asset seizure and prosecution of pain-treating physicians. No more prosecuting imaginary, nonexistent crimes and catch-22 "conspiracies" against perfectly innocent clinicians.

We must thank the heroines and heroes, listed here. Most are pain patients, others are caring healthcare professionals, yet others are both in healthcare and in pain – plus the 50 million pain patients, yet to be tabulated – for their advocacy work and their pro-patient efforts on social media. For, in spite of terrible suffering, those pain patients who haven't suicided, are bravely struggling to live while fighting the cruel federal and state systems forcing their physicians to withhold their opioids. All these advocates, working for this anti-torture cause, are destined to reach a critical mass of loudness, the volume of which will reach voting booths all over America to summarily oust officials, legislators, governors and other politicians who've allowed these years of unrelenting physical torture to afflict millions.

Thank you, our American heroines and heroes on behalf of all patients in pain and their doctors in prison. American medical care must return to Hippocratic ethics. And these are the advocates who will make sure this comes true.

Adam C Lake MD	@ACLakeMD
Advocatefight	@chattyknana
Alex Smith	@CommentaryNow
Allison Wallis	@allylovespono
Amanda	@AmandaLatronica
Amara	@AmaraAdvocate
Amy Partridge	@Amy_I_Partridge

Andrea Anderson	@aander1987
Andrew Koster	@northender480
Andrew in Pain	@AndrewHohentha2
angela dawn sparling	@SparlingAngela
Angie Glaser	@CMLifeblog
Anne Fuqua, RN	@PainPtFightBack
Anne Jones	@Ineatgirl
Arianne Grand	@ravensspirit68
Arizona C50	@ArizonaC50
Audrey29	@Bisby2610
Audrey Lynn	@AudreyL44703843
Aunt Tritsy	@AuntTritsy
Barbara	@barbkaplitz
BEACHES1953	@beaches1953
Becky Brandt, RN	@bbhomebody
Beth Darnall, PhD	@BethDarnall
Bill Murphy	@MisterBMurphy1
BLR	@beachnut826
Boone	@DanBoon63784314
Brett	@brettkktterb
Brett Golightly	@golightly_brett
BrettNPain	@Prescot65779543
browndotflop	@browndotflop
Burning Nights CRPS	@BNightsCRPS
Candis	@Candis21403757

Carole Proffitt	@carole_profitt
Carla Howard	@WHoward1373
Carol Adams	@WarriorCarol
Carreen Sagar-Cannon	@CareenSusan
Casualty of CDC	@Talkeetna101
CatoHealth	@CateHealth
Chad Kollas MD	@chadDKollas
Charlene	@Cbedford0315
CAW 360 NETWORK	@CAW360
Caye	@Caye95148494
Cheryl Isanogle	@cherylIsanogle
Chris Gresham	@ChrisGresham12
Chris Reno	@ChrisRenos
ChristchronicpainDAD	@ChronicPainDad
Christine Garland	@kristnah
Chronically_tough	@HeatherKraus14
Chronic Pain	@acmcrn
Chronic pain advocate	@Iamchronicpain
chronic pain advocate	@painadvocateAR
Chronic pain fighter	@Ninjaofchronicp
Chronic Pain India	@chronicpainind
Chronic Pain is Our Reality	@ChronicPainR1
ChronicPainSucks	@ChronicSucks
Chronic Pain Warrior	@JohannaMagers
CIAAG	@ciaagofficial

Claudia Merandi	@CMerandi
Collena Ramsay	@RamsayCollena
CPNerve Center	@Cpnervecenter
CRPS Awareness	@CRPS_Awareness
Cyndi Garland	@garland_cyndi
David W Cole	@DavidWCole1
Dawn	@PainOmbudsman
Daxx Khan	@DaxxKahn
Debra WINTERROTH	@DebraWinterroth
Dee	@Deenst
Dee Giles	@DEEGILES0410
Dee Snutts	@DeeSnutts6
Diana Martins-Welch, MD	@MartinsWelchMD
Doctor Elle	@McKnightmdEllen
Don Nelson	@Donnelsonguy
Doc	@RidemDoc
Doesn't Sleep	@Dsntslp
Dr. Ginevra Liptan	@drliptan
Dr. Linda Bluestein, M.D.	@BluesteinLinda
DrMargaretAranda	@MediBasket
Dr.Melissa Geraghty, PsyD.	@MindfulDrG
Dr Patrice Harris	@PatriceHarrisMD
Dr Pompy Trial Files	@ForPompy
Dr. Wayne Phimister	@WaynePhimister
Earl D Barnes	@EarlDBarnes2

Ellyn Ingalls	@ellynarizona
Enough	@Enough212
facesofpainproject	@facesofpainproj
Fantasia Funkypie	@FantasiaFunky6
Fibro Sloth	@FibroSloth
Fight4paindoctors	@Fight4paindoc11
FightingwithFibro	@FightingwithF
FightingWithFibro	@fibro_with
Fight The Flame 5k	@FightTheFlame5k
FredSavage187	@FredSavage187
Gail Bigard	@BigardGail
Geek Keeper	@GhostinGeek
GermaLo	@germaine7676
Give Pain A Voice	@GivePainAVoice
Grammy	@dm_mahmurphy
Green Man	@shutterbug_in
HilaryKimMorden	@HilaryKimMorden
Holly Kai	@HollyKai2
Inga Dawson	@DawsonInga
J.A.G.	@puppyluvr312
Jamie Peterson	@jamie5577jamie
Janasue	@garjansue
Jane Stanley	@JaneStanley64
Janell	@Enchantress0125
janet zurecki	@downtowin

Janice	@JSG_54
Jason Jensen	@03_jensen
Jeanne	@kaake_rn
Jeff Slavinsky	@JeffSlavinsky
Jen Webb	@jen_the_Spidey
JennWade6	@Wade6Jenn
Jennifer Hah MD	@JenniferHahMD
Jennifer Ham Credico	@CredicoHam
Jennifer Wade	@jennife90117914
Jess	@QueenCitysless
Jillian Marie	@jellyannjiggs
Jim	@jim22890024
Jessica Minerd-Massey	@MasseyMinerd
Jinxthejinx	@Jinxthejjinx
J. Julian Grove	@JulianGroveMD
Jmkillingnyc	@jmkillingnyc
Jo	@Jo74596327
Joe Newman	@JoeAllenNewman
john	@John69nj
Jonathan Mayer, PhD	@jmayer0716
Jonelle Elgaway	@JonelleElgaway
Joseph Falzone, MD	@JosephFalzone3
J Sandherr	@Delta33_1976
Julie Shaw	@Julie44shaw
Julie walters	@Juliewalters60

Justice For Vets	@Justice4Vets
JustSayin'	@stupor2016
Kari	@K_MooreTweets
Kathy	@KathyN115
Katie Martucci PhD	@DrKatieMartucci
Kcdee	@Tami_KCD
Katamac	@Katamac1967
Kate	@MaritimerKate
Kathleen Aiella	@kathleenaie
Kathleen Sneed Skorpenske	@skorpenske
Kelly-Anne Bryan, RN	@KellyAnneBryan1
Kelly Lawler	@Irishbrat1966
Kevin MacDonald	@Kevinmfilms
kim I	@OutofTouchwPeop
Kim Miller	@KimmeeKMiller
Koa Still I Rise	@Chronicallykoa
Lance	@Lance65057698
Lauren Deluca, CPCU	@CIAAG_Lauren
Laura Spoonie	@LauraSpoonie
Lavishly Hers	@LavishlyHers
Leah	@LMovieLowdown
lee h. alderman	@reversechapter
leela lumos	@LeelaLumos
Lelena	@LelenaPeacock
Leslie Pease	@LesliePease1

Leslie Wren Vandever	@RheumaBlog_Wren
Lexilady	@Lexiladylv
Linda Richardson	@stopcppain
Lisa Davis Budzinski	@lisabudzinski
Lisa Yriberry Reist	@lisamreist
Lori A.	@SheepHeadLori
Lori fibrogal	@LFrioult
Loura	@Loura_Stories
Lupus Video Channel	@LupusChannel
MakeThisLookAwesome	@MakeThisLookAwe
MamaBear	@esteckler2
Margaret Aranda, MD	@ChronicLifeDiet
Marilyn M	@masonis_marilyn
Marla Morton	@mommak36
Marty	@PainPlayhouse
Mary Cremer	@cremer_mary
Mass Confuzion	@mass_confuzion
Maxx Lamb	@maxx_lamb
MelodiusBeek	@BeekMelodious
Mera	@WriterMera
Merri	@mlvanbrit
Michelle Caccamisi	@NurseMichelle50
Miami Lincoln	@CLincoln65
Michelle Wagner Talley	@cshel0607
Misha	@Ms_HotMess_

moaningmyrtle	@MyCatDidThat
Moderndaygypsy	@jeanneshowalte2
MoogiemonsterC	@MoogieMonsters
Mrs. C.	@CarolynColson
MyCaringFriends	@mycaringfriends
Myositis Support	@MyositisSupport
My Sisters Keeper	@SistersLove_2
Mystical Moon	@mysticmoonmaid
Nica Alban	@AlbanNika
Nick Carlin	@NickCarlin6
Nicole In Pain	@NicoleInPain
Number 11	@CahngStrong
nunya	@nunsjya
PAC	@PACRiseUp
Painer	@painer_n
Painfully Disabled	@karlarabel
PAINS Project	@PAINSProject
Pain Warrior	@marias_pain
PainWarriorsUnite-Tamara Stewart	@fightpaindaily
Pain Warriors Unite - War on Pain	@War_On_Pain
PainWeek2018	@PainWeek2018
Pam	@djsjrb
Pam Winterhalter	@PamWinterhalte2
Pandora Summerz	@sleeprmustawake
Patients Surviving with Chronic Pain	@CPPCommunity3

People in Pain Unite	@Ppl_InPainUnite
Peppermint Patti	@Angelsgal02
peter grinspoon (MD)	@Peter_Grinspoon
Peter Morley	@morethanmySLE
P. Hillman	@PHillman20
Pinkster C	@PinksterC_87
Princess, The Tower	@ApainPrincess
P. Tudsbury	@hlpngHands
Rachel Beals	@RBeals1976
Reese Tyrell	@ReeseSTyrell
Rev Ree	@magichoney12
Rhonda Favero	@FaveroRhonda
ricky kelly	@rickyke15718874
RN advocating	@RNadvocating
@RoaringInPain	@roaringinpain
Robert D. Rose, Jr.	@RobertDRoseJr1
RogerDis	@dis_roger
SadDays4Us	@UsDays4
Sally Parker-Nash	@SallyParker1661K
Sandosays	@sandosays
Sandra Newman	@Bris516
SerenityNow	@Serenit77890794
shareourpainMS	@shareourpainMS
Sheila Purcell	@kypaincare
Shelley	@Shelley_bean60

Sheri (LupusDiva)(osaxy)	@osaxy
she's in pain	@BodyEstranged
SMH (Veteran)	@InPAINpatient
Sonya	@sonya_lala_
Spike Under Fire CRPS	@SpikeUnderFire
Starvin Larry	@StarvinLarry
Stop Bad Doctors	@StopBadDoctors
Support Fibromyalgia	@teamfibro
SuzH16	@tampastamper12
SydneyInPain	@SydneyInPain
Tami Morse	@morse_tami
Ted Thompson	@tedt0308
Terri	@Terri27903773
Terri Lewis, PhD	@tal7291
Terry	@Terry31722579
Tess Gomez	@Tessgomez6
The Fugly Frog	@TheFuglyFrog
The Hummingbird	@HummingBird3027
TheMyalgiaFibroWarriorUK	@AmzFibro
The Sarge (Veteran)	@TheSarge11
@ThisHasToStopNow	@OurPainIsReal
todd	@ourpainsreal
Together We Heal AZ	@az_together
TonyF	@TonyTtonyff
Trazy	@TrazyPain

Truth Crusader	@ClarisseTru
2punk4u	@Havasunburn1My
Use_our_voices	@TheGrateKate
veronica	@Veronica417752363
Vicki Teixeira	@VickiTeixeira
Vivian The Truth About Opioids	@Vopioids
V. Thornley, M.D.	@VThornley
WALTER W BALDREE	@baldree_w
Wendy Sinclair	@Wendysinclairme
WonderWoman	@Imgrocks20653
Zyp Czyk	@ZypCzyk

Chapter Twenty-Four

ACTIONS TO RELIEVE AMERICAN AGONY

Part I THE VICTIMS: Pain Patients, Physicians, Veterans in Pain, Families of Suiciders, Pharmaceutical Manufacturers

Before I go into the specific actions patients in pain, physicians, military veterans, families of pain patients, and even pharmaceutical manufacturers must take to protect your rights– all directly affected victims of the out-of-control unapologetic Department of Justice (DOJ) and its Drug Enforcement Administration (DEA) – it's imperative that all Americans be aware, even though you may not yet be a patient in dire, unbearable, untreated pain, that it's very likely at some time in your life you're going to suffer some type of pain that will require medical care and the appropriate analgesic effects of a prescription opioid.

In some of you, this will be cancer pain. In others, it will be pain following a surgical procedure. Still others will suffer the pain of a sudden accident or a developing disease. And most of you will, sooner or later, experience the pain of a dental operation.

Action Essentials: Freedom for Prescription Opioid Relief

First demand HIPAA (Health Insurance Portability and Accountability Act) privacies and PDMP (Prescription Drug Monitoring Program) privacies be adhered to by nonessential others. Which means such access should only be available to patients and their physicians. Period! No exceptions.

What pain patients can do – until the DOJ and its DEA can be halted from their intransigent intrusions into the medical practice of paincare and their disruption of the doctor-patient relationship, with their uneducated bad "advice" about prescription opioid medications – is to consider the following actions and implement those ones most facile for you considering your pain levels, mobility issues and your finances.

Refuse certain elective surgeries if you can't be assured in writing, from your surgeon, that you'll receive the appropriate opioid normally prescribed after such operations. Don't be bamboozled into accepting the nonsense that Tylenol® (acetaminophen) or Aspirin (acetylsalicylic acid) are sufficient for such sufferings.

Consider law suits, individual if you can afford such, or class actions where legal fees come out of your winnings. Class actions, if many are mounted, or one covering millions, even thousands, of pain patients will have powerful effects on the press reporting on opioid-related issues; will help turn the tide of public opinion toward the benefit of patients suffering without their usual opioid medications; will put federal and state agencies, hospitals and other medical facilities, and all prescribing clinicians on notice that pain patients are not going to relent until normal opioid prescribing is restored all over our nation. Until government victimizers get out of the practice of medicine and and cease restricting the legal distribution of prescription opioids. (Class Action lawsuits and litigations against federal government and state government agencies and/or their employees are discussed toward the close of this segment, Part I.)

Sue Emergency Room physicians and their hospitals for negligence and medical malpractice. You are entitled to quality, standard-of-care treatment. But, if you present in the ER with an injury or illness that would've normally deserved an opioid analgesic and you were left to suffer instead – for example, Sickle Cell Crisis needs morphine, ditto nephrolithiasis, kidney stones moving through your ureter, and other painful conditions doctors are well aware are not candidates for less than opioid-strength analgesia – this is medical malpractice. Remember, not only the individual physician who did not prescribe the indicated opioid for you, but also her/his hospital is liable due to the concept known as *Respondeat Superior*, an employer is responsible for all employees' actions. It's possible that, in this federally-induced climate of tremulous fear of opioids, among the legions of medical practitioners and medical facilities, a growing nationwide barrage of lawsuits could get these frightened folks' attention so that they, too, resist DOJ, DEA and state government functionaries' overreach. Maybe, then, pain patients will have their opioids restored. Maybe then our nation can return to sanity in medical practice.

The same principle can be applied to Intensive Care Units (ICUs), clinics, pain care centers, dental facilities, freestanding emergency centers, and so forth. (Again, see later in this Part I for specifics about law suits and class actions.

There's also a PETITION in this Section VII for you to use at your discretion. It highlights demands for change toward fulfilling your rights to your usual prescription opioid medications at your usual dosage levels and their usual, for you, time intervals. You may decide to use it as is, or alter it to suit your specific, or your organization's specific needs. It's meant to nudge politicians and legislators to budge out of their lethargy or enmity about prescription opioid analgesia and take action on behalf of patients in pain STAT! That, in medical-speak, means immediately! No time to waste, People are dying from under-treated pain. People, including our valiant veterans, are suiciding nationwide because of unbearable untreated pain. **Demand your rights to your opioid medications**.

Your rights to financial government benefits as long as this anti-opioid malignancy infests American medical practice due to DOJ, DEA, VA and other government entities. As long as they force on you unnecessary urinalyses, extra doctor visits, extra blood tests, nonconsentual tapering, cold-turkeying, and forced surgical implants and spinal injections. As long as they cruelly label you a "drug seeker" and force you to get "detoxed" (when you're not an addict} with Suboxone, "the legal morphine". At times forcing you to take Suboxone as an analgesic, a failure in this regard because its morphine component, buprenorphine, is muted by its naloxone component Duh! Therefore, **demand reimbursement for extra transportation, for a caregiver** to help dress you and get you out of your bedridden state into a wheelchair to attend the unneeded office visits. **Demand remimbursement for all unnecessary lab tests you are being subjected to**.

Meet with other pain patients in the clinic or practice and contact a lawyer to mount a class action suit against these inhumane practices. (See below about Class Actions.)

Do not pay for any unnecessary visits and tests. You have plenty of medical evidence – x-rays, CAT and PET scans, healthcare records and records of your hospitalizations, as well as photos of any pain illness that can be visibly viewed. These can be shown to a judge by your attorney defending you against unnecessary doctor clinic or office visits.

Point out to any officious ancillary doctor's office staff that you will not tolerate mistreatment, mislabelling or negligent medical care and that you'll be consulting your attorney,

You do not have to agree to any tapering of your opioid medication unless you wish to. Forced tapering of pain patients is medical malpractice. It can make you very sick, worsen your health, and in some cases, lead to an early death due to physical deterioration. Point out to any medical professional who is intent on robbing you of your prescription opioid that you intend to sue them for your suffering. Then get busy getting similarly-affected patients to mount a class action. The trick will be to find a sympathetic attorney, maybe one with a pain-sufferer family member, who will take on this challenge. If you are too sick and disabled to do the necessaries yourself, try to locate family, friends, allies in the pain community who are not in pain, to help you succeed in getting an attorney and your case heard and compensated. The more of these negligent practices that can be punished, the sooner the public will stop putting up with the murdering of American pain care promulgated by the DOJ, the DEA and the VA.

You do not have to put up with cold-turkeying of your opioid medication. This is flat out medical malpractice, will lead to rapidly declining health, unbearable pain, thoughts of suicide and too often to suicide itself. Apply the same instructions as with nonconsentual tapering. Don't tolerate government medical directives. Don't tolerate fourth world health care. Because, without normal opioid medications when warranted, as they have been for over a century, the United States falls well below even Third World nations. Which amounts to human rights violations.

Make sure your local journalists and the national media are updated on all you are doing to hold various individuals, institutions and government agencies liable for harming you and millions of others, to publicize what you won and how you got your prescription opioids restored to you and millions of other Americans in pain.

Build alliances with individuals and organizations and philanthropists who are not suffering a painful condition and, thus, are able to take the time, do the necessary travel, find the necessary funds to fight for your rights and for the rights of all patients in all kinds of pain everywhere. Mount class action lawsuits (see below for specifics). Come at all the malfeasors in your painful existence from as many angles as you and your allies can identify. Millions of pain patients are all counting on the critical mass of such actions coalescing to effect a sea change in the pain, deteriorations and suicides millions are now victims of.

Families of Pain Patients who've Suicided should sue for wrongful death, medical malpractice, personal injury, negligence, for whatever applies to your loved one's pain circumstances. Veterans' family members should litigate against VA doctors and the VA itself. (See below for Class Actions and suing government agencies.)

THE AMERICAN MEDICAL ASSOCIATION (AMA) and the large numbers of other medical, surgical, pediatric, neurologic and psychiatric associations throughout our country need to stand up, en masse, countering this American holocaust against suffering patients in pain, and against the mounting suicides that are still being ignored by the powers that caused these to occur. (Various sections in this book discuss the patient-positive role the AMA and its leaders have taken to counter the misguided 2016 *CDC Guideline* and to dispute government overreach which is tampering with normal medical prescribing of opioids for pain.)

Memini: Vince malum bono. Remember, good triumphs over evil. *Maybe the ACLU can help.*

Action Essentials: Freedom for All Physicians in America
What American physicians must do – both those imprisoned by DOJ overreach and those who must now practice "defensive" medicine due to DOJ/DEA operatives-gone-amok against opioid prescribing MDs and other clinicians:

***AMNESTY* FOR ALL WRONGFULLY CONVICTED PHYSICIANS (Over 1200 in U.S. Prisons).** (Please read Chapter 16, "Plight of the Pain Physician") for these shame-on-America imprisonments of fine clinicians...and some have died.)

***IMMUNITY* FOR ALL PHYSICIANS TO PRESCRIBE OPIOIDS AS THEY NORMALLY WOULD FOR PATIENTS IN PAIN**

What Opioid-Prescribing Clinicians Worried about DOJ/DEA Scrutiny and Prosecutions Should Do It's a shame that, in effect, based on the ramped-up government intrusions into doctors' and patients' healthcare activities, you'll now have to be practicing "Defensive Medicine" to protect yourself from allusions and prosecution. To help you with this ever-looming problem, I sought some solid answers from a friend of a colleague. As a result, I can pinpoint key elements of what this retired DOJ prosecutor (for anonymity, I'll call him Mr. Price) told me about how you should deal with these stringent DOJ constrictions still being imposed on physicians and other clinicians prescribing opioid medications.

Here's the rundown of cautions you – as an opioid prescriber not yet DEA scrutinized or raided, nor DOJ prosecuted, yet – should be instituting in your medical practice to avoid being the focus of these agencies' punitive misinterpretations of the normal care of patients in pain.

With the DOJ's hardline goal of prosecuting doctors and other clinicians who prescribe narcotic analgesics, it's prudent, Mr. Price says, to institute certain medical practice protections that can divert government suspicions from your normal care of your pain patients.

Bearing in mind that the DOJ has recently further tightened its prosecutory noose by inaugurating its Opioid Fraud and Abuse Detection Unit – aimed at scrutinizing the amounts of opioids you prescribe, whether you've some arrangement with opioid dispensers, and whether any of your patients died of overdoses – here are some anticipatory actions Mr. Price suggests you take to kind of "vaccinate" you and your medical practice from being targeted by ill-informed but overzealous DEA operatives seeking to ingratiate themselves with their DOJ counterparts and superiors:

1. *To, hopefully, immunize yourself against suspicion and prosecution, you must keep keenly accurate, up-to-date records of all your opioid prescribing for each individual pain patient.* Remembering that prosecutors are *en garde* to closely scrutinize physicians who provide opioid paincare for a high patient census. Medical auditors can comprehensively review your chartings to be sure you've documented, in detail,

your rationale for each patient's opioid prescription, as well as accounting for the dosages and timings of these medications for each such patient. Clarity to the DOJ/DEA about each patient's pain diagnosis and opioid-prescription-justification can go a long way to mitigate government suspicions, motivating exclusion of your practice from further federal scrutiny.

2. *To further mitigate government suspicions, periodic examinations of your pain patients' medical records, with an eye to assure watchdogs that every patient you are treating is not a cookie-cutter copy of each other's paincare plan,* Mr. Price warns, will go a long way to demonstrate to the non-medical government eye that you're one of "the good doctors". Because, such a practice, every three months for example, could prevent civil or criminal actions against you.
3. The following is a tough instruction because – though it may seem to have some bearing on the government's prosecutory focus – it usually wouldn't make sense in a normal medical practice. Why? Because, when a patient appears in a doctor's office suffering pain, that patient wants and deserves pain relief right away. Too, empathic, moral, and standard-of-care excellence requires immediate addressing of pain. It's inappropriate to do otherwise.

   Nevertheless, DOJ stringency requires their focus on the length of time between your pain patient's first visit and your first narcotic prescription for that patient. Unfortunately, reports Mr. Price, government-think assumes the sooner you prescribe an opioid relative to a patient's first appointment, the more likely this leads to addiction. Where the DEA police and DOJ lawyers got that idea is a mystery because it has zero to do with medical treatment realities. Still, Mr. Price warns against opioid prescribing for a patient upon first meeting that patient. Of course, such an exclusionary action hinders all kinds of normal medical care. For example, pain care for root canal work by a dentist-prescriber as well as TMJ pain care. For another example, Emergency Department patients, just injured or with other urgent medical conditions evidencing pain where stat opioids are justified. Similary, such one-time pain, or ongoing pain, can present itself in your office, as you know, which justifies immediate narcotic analgesia. I don't know how you can get around this crazy government platitude.

The DOJ sees opioid prescribing before you get the drug urinalysis results back as a bull sees a red flag. Never in years of nursing practice did my patients in pain get their urines analyzed before we'd provide narcotic pain relief!

In these first visit cases, though, Mr. Price advises that you definitively chart everything essential about your patients' disorder and your justification for prescribing an opioid on their first visits.

4. *Similar detailed documentation, Mr. Price advises, is essential when it comes to monitoring urine for any drugs the patient may be taking.* This is because the DOJ will scrutinize whether you are adapting your prescribing for each patient based on such urinalysis results. Apparently, the DOJ wants doctors to adapt drug test panels individually, as different patients' conditions reflect different drug class requirements. Such DOJ stringencies, of course, hogtie clinicians into a bind – stripped of time for actual pain patient care – while they're having to spend time in a paranoid state of worry about infinitesimal record-keeping, unnecessary urine testing of normal pain patients (wasting these patients' time and privacy), unable to have enough time to attend to the medical care of their non-pain patients.
5. *Be observant and cautious if you treat, with opioids, some family members or others who live at the same address.* The government will fault you if you've neglected to notice that you've more than one or two family members or people living in the same house for whom you're prescribing narcotic analgesics. In such instances, Mr. Price advises that you be in touch with such patient's other doctors and prior health records to protect yourself from prescribing for addicts.

6. *Mr. Price also warns that the DOJ is suspicious of clinicians who see patients who live in other states.* The DEA notices, short-sightedly, car licenses in doctors' parking areas and jumps to its ridiculous conclusions. However, due to the opiohysteria, whipped up by public relations releases from the DOJ to the broadcast and print media, here's the catch-22 the government has created: Pain patients, whose doctors' practices have been shut down or whose doctors are imprisoned, can't find any other physician to treat their pain in their home state, so they drive to where some pain doctors have not yet been arrested. These are not "drug-seeking addicts", as short-sighted DEA watchdogs have mislabeled them. These are patients in pain looking for pain relief.

My advice in such cases: When out-of-state pain patients call your office for an appointment, instruct them not to come to your office in their own cars. Instead, tell them to park them at the hotel and take a taxi to your office. Sadly, such gross inconvenience and expense, for already severely suffering and maligned pain patients is essential to protect these patients from being labeled "drug-seekers". And to protect you from prosecution because narrow-focused DEA police can't see the pain patient forest for the trees of opiohysteria they themselves have whipped up. It appears that government operatives are complacently clueless that they themselves caused the pain patient exodus from home state to elsewhere state.

More In-Depth Lawsuit Information to Help You Restore Normal Prescription Opioid Pain Relief

Despite the fact that:

1. Physicians, other clinicians and pharmacists are also victims of our government's stirred up opiohysteria, particularly by ***carte blanche overreach of the Veterans Administration, the Department of Justice and its Drug Enforcement Administration***...

2. And that I've also provided, here, actions they too must take to extricate themselves and their careers from VA, DOJ, and DEA government oppression, prescription intrusions, prosecutions and imprisonments...

   ...we must all attack totalitarian, mortally-wounding government entities, and their frightened functionaries (the latter, particularly professionals working in the VA hospital system) from every angle possible!

   Because, if enough doctors, other prescribing clinicians, pharmacists, clinics, and hospitals are sued (even if they don't lose, they have to pay high legal fees to combat such litigations) this may motivate them to grow some testicular strength against illegal, unconscionably substandard medical behaviors thrust upon them by DOJ, DEA, and VA administrators clueless about quality patient care. Your determination to not let them get away with denying you your rightful analgesic medications could motivate them to return to their Hippocratic obligations to "First do no harm". To return to the normal prescribing, for specific levels and durations of pain, the opioid medications that have always optimally ameliorated such suffering. That is, before this government insanity against treating pain appropriately, and with opioids as decided by a patient's physician only!

BRING LAW SUITS AGAINST THOSE DENYING OPIOID PAIN CARE

You should consider these individuals, institutions, hospitals, emergency facilities, dental clinics, dentists, general clinics, doctors, surgeons, pain clinics and whoever and whatever facility is keeping you from getting your opioid pain reliever, and whoever is insulting you, labeling you a "drug seeker," forcing you to have your urine and blood tested (which no doctor or nurse has ever had to do for patients in pain, that's ridiculous, intrusive and embarrassing) as your targets as potential defendants in your own individual case(s) against such malfeasors. However, if, as in the case of a large institution, like a hospital, you are able to gather together enough complainants who've suffered similarly by the defendant's actions, or inactions, you ought to consider a Class Action Lawsuit against that hospital, pain clinic, or other at-fault institution or facility. Remember, such entities often have directives, policies that coerce staff into denying you appropriate opioid paincare.

In such cases, you, of course, will have yours and other pain patients' records of your diagnoses, treatment histories showing positive pain-relief results from your opioids before being tapered without your consent, suddenly *cold-turkeyed*, summarily discharged from your pain clinic. Those records noting you were able to remain employed and have reasonable mobility. Subsequent records showing that you could no longer keep your job, that you are now homebound, bedridden, on Disability payments, ironically from this same government whose actions have sidelined you, whose hardline is causing you to suffer, even though there's opioid medication available in the world to soothe at least some of it away.

Here, I can't resist wishing that the American Civil Liberties Union (ACLU) would step in and help American patients in pain fight for your civil rights, human rights, and rights against the daily torture of untreated pain.

BRING CLASS ACTIONS TO RESTORE OPIOID PAIN CARE

You may sue a corporation in a class action if you are injured physically (or financially) and others are similarly injured because of the corporation's wrongful actions. Hospitals, clinics, medical practices, freestanding emergency clinics, and such are often incorporated. In the case of pain patients suing as a class action, you have a decided advantage: there are millions and millions of you, 50,000,000 in pain, now disabled by denial of their usual and effective opioid medications. And you can point to, in your tort case, the many pain patients who've died prematurely due to heart attacks and neurologic deficits from the drastic effects of *cold-turkeying*. And also to those who could no longer bear the torture of unremitting pain and committed suicide.

A Class Action permits such large numbers of people to bring litigation against an individual, a business, or other group when each filing separately would be financially prohibitive.

You may start a class action alone, if you can afford legal fees. Or a small group may start a class action. Either would then be on behalf of the huge numbers of pain patients who are similarly suffering due to the defendant's actions or lack of action. Once filed, a judge determines whether enough people in pain are similarly injured by the defendant to propel your class action suit forward:

1. Find an attorney or law practice which specializes in bringing class action suits
2. Usually, there are no legal fees unless you win your class action. In which case, your legal team receives a percentage of your court-awarded monies, or of the agreed settlement.
3. As the initiator of, and active participator in your class action, you and your co-plaintiffs may be financially compensated for representing the many similarly-injured people in the class.

When you approach a malpractice attorney, she or he will ask for records, photos, anything to prove the worthiness of your contentions. Not to worry. In addition to your own medical records and those of others who've joined you as plaintiffs, add these:

1. The Tweets of many veterans in pain, many other pain patients, pain-treating physicians and pain-studying scientists who are daily on Twitter...
2. Photos of injuries, hospitalizations, surgeries, proof of job termination and Disability payments
3. Photos of gravestones of untreated pain patients who've suicided
4. Consider giving your lawyer this book because it's filled will evidence of the medical wrongdoing you are fighting.

Once satisfied with the validity of your Class Action case, your attorney will file a Class Action Complaint which presents the details of your case. You, the filer, will be called "the Lead Plaintiff".

In order for your class action to be allowed to proceed, the judge reviewing it will need to know:

1. The numbers of people affected. Huge numbers of pain patients are convincing.
2. All in the class must similarly be suffering, or have suffered.
3. All must have similar legal issues.
4. The lead plaintiffs (you and the others who've started your Class Action) must suffer similar issues
5. The lead plaintiff and the case attorney must be totally committed to the case issues and the lawyer should have complex litigation and class action expertise.

Once the judge certifies that your class action may proceed, your defendant is now threatened with a legally-justified litigation. For more in-depth information about class actions, visit these sites.

https://www.classaction.org

https://www.sheppardmullin.com/healthcare-industry

CONSIDER SUING THE GOVERNMENT

Even government entities can cause injury and suffering, physical and/or financial to citizens. Government workers (doctors, other hospital staff, clinics, etc.) can be targeted by neglected pain patients. There's such a thing as "a standard-of-care," especially in medical practice. Not being prescribed your usual, very effective medication, an opioid, is "below standard-of-care". Government hospitals – municipal, county, state, federal, VA – and their physicians, pharmacists and other professional staff members can and should be sued for negligence, suffering, loss of income...whatever services and care your attorney says you have a right to and do not receive by neglect, omission, by accusation of "you're a drug seeker," you should consider pursuing. So, if a government employee or entity has been negligent or harmed you in any way, especially related to their deprivation of your usual opioid medication, you can and should sue.

Needed are Funds to Mount these Law Suits

Imagine what a turnaround is possible, with opioids returned to every hospital and neighborhood drug store pharmacopeia. With doctors no longer fearing to write opioid prescriptions for patients in pain. With pain patients no longer eyed like they were drug addicts.

Naturally, many people in pain don't have enough discretionary funds to pay for an attorney willing to take on such a challenging litigation. Somehow, though, of those *50 million Americans in under-treated or untreated pain*, most of whom have benefited from opioid pain relief, there have to be some with money willing to invest in this cause, which will benefit many as well as them. And, of the many grass roots pain advocacy organizations, it would be great if somehow they were funded enough to hire attorneys specializing in medical cases, highly skilled, and empathic with your cause.

Powerful Government Agencies Use Our Tax Billions in their Defense Even When Harming the Public

Despite things so heavily weighted in their favor, despite egregious behaviors on their part, you still have civil rights, human rights and your right to medically-ethical pain care.

1. **File a Notice of Claim** with the agency that wronged you, for example, the Department of Justice. Consider that its DEA has easy access to your confidential medical records via your state's Prescription Monitoring Drug Program (PDMP), via your Electronic Medical Records, via your doctors' office records.
2. **If you're a DEA-targeted physician, or other prescribing clinician, consider suing** for wrongful seizure of your assets, for wrongful intrusion on your patient care, for curtailing the normal

supply of opioids for sick-in-pain patients...., for intimidating telephone "warnings" and intimidating "warning" letters instructing you how to practice medicine, what lowered opioid doses to prescribe, who not to prescribe opioids for...

3. **Pain patients should acquire Form 95, known as SF95**. It must show a monetary claim which is called "a sum certain claim".

Timely Filing of Your Claim against a Government Entity

Note the statute of limitations, the period during which your claim is actionable. In the case of SP95, this would be two years from the date you knew of the negligence you are claiming.

Once filed, your defendant government agency has six months to act on your claim. They can settle after looking into your situation or, if they don't, your suit can move forward. Your suit is then brought against the United States in the United States District Court. Often, you won't get a jury trial; thus a federal judge will decide whether you win and how much money you are awarded.

Nota bene: Where there are legal constraints against you directly suing a government agency, you have recourse to sue individuals in that agency who've directly harmed you. Please discuss this possibility with the attorneys you engage.

FEDERAL TORT CLAIMS ACT (FTCA)

Consider suing the government for negligence. If you're a veteran in pain, for instance, did a nurse make you worse at a VA hospital? (One case against the VA arose in September of 2019 when a veteran patient at a VA hospital was found covered with ants.)

The FTCA is the law under which you can most likely have your claim against a federal agency adjudicated. You can sue the VA in a medical malpractice case against a VA doctor, for example. You can sue for careless actions and tortious (wrongful) actions against any federal agency or federal employee.

To determine whether you have a viable case to sue the government or a government employee under the FTCA, access this wise article at Nolo! **https://www.nolo.com/legal-encyclopedia/negligence-the-duty-care-fault-accident.html**

SUITS AGAINST STATE GOVERNMENTS

Like the federal government, state governments are also protected by "sovereign immunity" from law suits. Fortunately, however, each state has created tort legislation to enable citizens to be protected against tortious actions by state entities and state employees. Most states call these the "Tort Claims Act" so that a state government agency or its employee(s) can be sued for personal injury and property damage. Find out about your state's tort laws here! **https://www.nolo.com/legal-encyclopedia/injury-claim-against-state**

About the Professionalism of Pharmaceutical Manufacturers

It is baffling how such medically-essential corporations, doing so much good in the healthcare arena, are continually victimized by many state Attorneys-General to the tune of millions upon millions of dollars which would do much more good in those companies' Research and Development coffers.

Importantly, manufacturers of prescription medicine's have zero to do with who prescribes what and how much to whom and how many of those whoms are patients in a pain specialist's practice. Also, bearing in mind that less than 1% of patients prescribed opioids ever become addicted to them, how'd legitimate opioid manufacturers become targets of prosecutors nationwide? What's going on here? It's time for these A-Gs to cease indicting fine drug companies. These A-Gs are wasting the time and money of fine companies. What would the world do without the medicines they make for all of us? Do these A-Gs wish to have no more pharmaceutical companies manufacture opioid analgesics? Okay. Back to the Dark Ages...snakes and newts in broths, leeches, amputations without anesthesia. Go. Go back there.

Countering Baseless Lawsuits against Pharmaceutical Manufacturers of Opioids

The American public needs to learn these simple facts:

1. All prescription medications, and the science that supports their applications for various conditions, are scrutinized by the Food and Drug Administration (FDA).
2. Then the FDA approves each drug for marketing.
3. And the FDA monitors all medical journal advertising of drug products.
4. Finally, if there's something dangerous or ineffective about a drug, the FDA takes it off the market.
5. Each drug is accompanied by a thorough disclosure sheet in both medical and lay terminology describing the intricacies of the medication: its indications, contraindications, side effects, warnings, allergenic potential, etc., etc.
6. Physicians' prescriptions for medications are also very explicit giving the name of the drug, its dosage, how many times a day and how many hours between doses a patient must wait. Also, the doctors may or may not prescribe a refill. And physicians discuss with patients the reason for and how to use this medication.
7. The pharmacist fills each script according to the doctors orders and provides the Pharm manufacturer's insert.
8. Medical advertising agencies create advertising campaigns for broadcast and print media. And they create other promotional materials, as well as sales brochures for highly skilled medical sales forces to personally visit physicians to introduce any new, often life-saving products pharmaceutical companies have just researched and developed, like a new era antibiotic or a new generation antidepressant or antipsychotic which can save more lives from infection and suicide. Such medical

> educational materials and on-the-spot doctor discussions are essential if physicians are to keep up with the burgeoning world of therapeutic solutions to many severe, life-shortening and painful conditions suffered by patients everywhere.

A Few Ideas from a Healthcare Professional and Medical Writer (Me):

1. Pharmaceutical Manufacturers, particularly those now under heavy fire for having the good conscience to provide prescription opioids for pain relief, should fight back. Purdue Pharma recently won against an Attorney General when the judge pointed out some of the facts, mentioned here, about how the FDA oversees each drug's efficacy and safety, as well as its marketing. Unfortunately, other entrenched A-Gs so attacked Purdue Pharma that Purdue was forced to declare bankruptcy in September 2019.
2. Pharmaceutical Manufacturers should consider convening a consortium of some kind to develop a center for the education of the public of what exactly a pharm corporation does, how it operates, its science arm, its medical educational activities, its sales teams, its advertising aims.
3. Tours could be arranged where groups, maybe of college students, maybe premeds, maybe of interested citizens, to view close-up how a drug is manufactured physically.
4. Out of such activities might come some future scientists, doctors, marketing experts, pharmacists, and science teachers. Also, such in-person experiences could generate more allies to ally with pharm corporations when our government and sometimes clueless press and broadcast media malign your patient-centered products.

Part II THE VICTMIZERS: The VA, DOJ, DEA, CDC, State Medical Boards, State Attorneys-General, and Federal Legislators Must Act Now

ALL STATES MUST ENACT WASHINGTON STATE'S ENLIGHTENED OPIOIDS-FOR-PAIN POLICIES:

It's Medical Board has a Heart!

Unlike all the other American states' Medical Boards, one stands out as unique, the Washington Medical Commission (WMC). On May 24, 2019, the WMC, through Deputy Director Micah Matthews, released the following medically ethical approach of the state of Washington toward prescription opioids for patients in pain. It points out that **doctors are not mandated to taper chronic pain patients**. That pain over 12 weeks is chronic and that **there are no restrictions on the number of pills a patient can be prescribed.**

Furthermore, Washington physicians and other prescribing clinicians are warned that tapering and cutting off opioid medications to such patients is not accurate nor acceptable. And, going along with this state's pioneering pro-patient and pro-physician stance, the WMC has addressed these misrepresentations of the 2016 *CDC Guideline* by actively doing outreach to the medical community "to ensure confusion and concern is addressed." These pro-patient activities included over 30 presentations to hospitals around the state, and licensees received a booklet of information. There were also several Twitter Town Halls, a Live Webinar, and a myriad of inter-agency events all in the name of assuring that patients in pain continue to receive their opioid analgesics as they always have.

The WMC also instructed prescribers on "Opioid Prescribing and Monitoring" addressing the problems of tapering and discontinuing opioid treatment for pain patients like so: "A practitioner who refuses to treat the condition (chronic pain) properly, including the appropriate utilization of opioids when opioids are clearly indicated, would be practicing below the standard of care." Then the WMC warns: "Practicing below the standard of care falls under the WMC regulative authority and the Uniform Disciplinary Act"; and that "tapering without the patient's consent or without consideration of the patient's function or quality of life is "a violation of WMC prescribing rules."

Finally, the Washington Medical Commission declares: "It was never our goal, nor is it permissible, to keep appropriate pain medications from people who need them. Our interpretive statements should offer comfort and education to anyone who believes otherwise." Thus, as should the remaining forty-nine states, the WMC has bravely lived up to its motto: "Listening Accountability Leadership". **Medical.commission@doh.wa.gov**

Bravo Washington State. You are the leading Medical Board in the nation to ease the pain of millions, to save the lives of many pain patients who, in other states, have been driven to choose suicide.

DOJ Mandatories Relative to Patients in Pain and Opioid Prescribers

Hands off! You're not doctors! You've already ruined millions of pain patients' lives by your nooses around the necks of opioid medication prescribers. You've imprisoned hundreds of innocent doctors on bogus "conspiracy" charges for the rest of their lives because they did the medically-correct thing, they prescribed opioids appropriately for pain – but they wouldn't plead to yet other bogus lesser charges, so were trapped in the legal maze of "conspiracy" carrying sentences of 25 years each. (See Chapter 16, " Plight of the Paincare Physicians".)

Not only, DOJ, do pain patients need their rights to their pain-relieving opioids restored, these physicians in prison due to questionable DOJ prosecutorial tactics, demand immediate **AMNESTY** and immediate release from unjust confinement. It's on you prosecutors at the DOJ that some of those physicians and other clinicians have either become ill and died shortly after these questionable cases and incarcerations, or several have committed suicide. Their blood is on your hands.

(Need I mention the many fine American medical practitioners who've exiled themselves to Canada, Greece and elsewhere, to escape these totalitarian DOJ/DEA entrapments and life and career ruinations. Not to mention all the patients who've relied on these good doctors for care over decades, who now are abandoned due to DOJ/DEA invasions and threats.)

Why doesn't the DOJ investigate where all the money, State Attorneys-General get from Big Pharma, goes. To whom? And that DOJ bonanza of $1.4 billion from Reckitt Benckiser and Suboxone "lapses"; who gets that? What about us taxpayers? What about the destruction of Pharm manufacturers who provide us all with health-preserving, life-saving, mental-health improving, and pain-relieving drugs? What hath you wrought, DOJ? An America without prescription medications altogether? A world turned back to medieval doctors with leeches and potions and "double-double, toil and trouble" witches' brews? Medi-EVIL is what the DOJ has created.

Now some brave *juris doctor* at the DOJ needs to halt this torture of pain patients and their doctors; halt the DOJ and state A-G assaults on Pharm companies doing nothing wrong but providing us all with the medicines we need to live better and longer lives.

You need to butt out of medical practice and concentrate on real criminal matters. And, immediately, you need to reform or dissolve your DEA altogether because they've gone so far as to be analogous to the infamous Gestapo.

Rid the DOJ and its DEA of their dangerous *carte blanche* behaviors Rescind the DOJ's and its DEA's carte blanche to victimize physicians, patients and pharmaceutical companies by hounding them without evidential justification. Throwing everything at their innocent targets that might stick like adhesive tape, then prosecuting them, ruining health, lives, careers, corporations, and access by all Americans to the prescription medications that save our lives and modulate our pain.

Dissolve the Drug Enforcement Administration! This DEA subdivision of the Department of Justice should never have had anything to do with normal medical practice and prescription medications which physicians utilize for varied and complex clinical disorders. It was, supposedly, set up to deal with criminals who import and sell adulterated, counterfeit, and stolen opioid narcotics and other street drugs like questionably-concocted anxiolytics such as Xanax® (alprazolam) and tainted ethanol. Worse, tainted, high-powered fentanyl being swallowed which causes fatalities – since medically-pure fentanyl products, manufactured by reputable pharmaceutical companies, are available only in skin-patch and lollipop formulations to assure very slow absorption because rapid absorption oral formulations (as in fentanyl illicits) the DEA was supposed to intercept, are killing people because these are swallowed.

(One also wonders how these dealers make profits from such tainted and fast-acting fentanyl products, and its far more powerful analog carfentanil, when due to oral administration their customers are dying off.)

Ergo, there's plenty of work there for the DEA to focus on and effect widespread deterrence of illicits dealings and deaths. Therefore, the DEA needn't be bothering normal pain patients' legal prescription opioid supply. Pain patients are not addicts and DEA operatives know this. Yet they persist in the diversion of their mandated role from criminal activities related to chemical illicits to tricking the public into blaming doctors who prescribe opioids for pain and their patients who require opioids to manage their pain so they can work and participate in life.

Nonetheless, escalating out-of-control DEA police have been dogging American doctors, raiding their practices, sending them "warning letters" about numbers of pain patients, numbers of opioid medications prescribed, and (like these clowns have a medical degree) instructing physicians how many fewer MMEs (morphine milligram equivalents) to order for their patients. Even phoning doctors, in the middle of their care of all their office patients and "warning" them about such normally confidential medical matters, thereby spying and criminalizing the normal medical treatment of patients in pain.

Right now, the DEA is functionally kaput! It's not doing the job it supposedly exists to do. Drug addicts are dying in droves, these deaths escalating exponentially, even as the DOJ/DEA clamp-down with greater and greater ferocity on normal medical opioid analgesia which has been almost brought to a halt.

Add to that, the gut-level fear these DEA spyings, oppressions, and physician-arrests have injected into all the other innocent physicians doing their normal jobs treating patients in pain with appropriate opioids. Cringing in fear of license forfeiture, lengthy court cases, asset seizures, there's been a mass exodus of excellent, empathic physicians and other clinicians from taking care of patients in pain at all. Patients abandoned. Dying from effects of sudden withdrawal. Dying from suicides due to unbearable pain. This is what the DEA inaction against illicits has wrought; and what its effect on pain patients has caused and is still causing.

No more Drug Enforcement Administration! Dissolve it! Prosecutory divisions of government should have nothing to do with the manufacture, distribution, dispensing, or prescribing of normal medicines used for everyone's health. Those include opiate and opioid analgesics used to combat pain in acute ER, Postsurgical, Dental conditions; as well as in Cancer, Hospice, and End-of-Life circumstances; plus in long-term, even lifelong pain, as in IPPs (Intractable Pain Patients).

Inaugurate a New Entity:

ILLICITS DRUG ENFORCEMENT AGENCY (IDEA)

The **IDEA** would focus on the appropriate roles of dealer arrests, illicits interdictions, and helping addicts. Period! Those are enough challenges to keep one agency busy. Thus, the **IDEA** will have four major functions, none of which relate to legally-prescribed opioid medications:

1. **Interdiction of Illicits** – from China, Mexico, the Internet, Wheresoever
2. **Arrests and Jailing** – of drug importers, sellers, dealers

3. **Murder Charges** – against dealers identified as having sold a substance to an addict who died of it. That's murder by poisoning, right? There's a murder-by-poisoning epidemic which the IDEA must confront directly!
4. **Transportation of drug addicts to detox facilities.** In this regard, the IDEA could, alternatively as is done successfully in other countries, set up safe places for self-administration of addictive substances where there are medical and other healthcare professionals available to assure sterile syringes, infection prevention, naloxone availability and counseling, where addicts might then become motivated to take advantage of in-depth services toward recovery from addiction.

The **IDEA** will have no interaction with normal pain patients' medical care, nor will it disrupt paincare physicians' and other opioid-prescribing clinicians from their appropriate medical duties.

Finally, the DOJ and the IDEA Must be Honest!

No more fancy footwork when it comes to Suboxone® (buprenorphine/naloxone). You guys have been sleight-of-hand magicians in this regard: You've been demonizing all the opiates and semi-synthetic and synthetic opioid analogs in the American pharmacopeia, labeling them bad, erroneously targeting them for extermination, while blithely helping the addictions industry fall into the lap of Suboxone largesse. That because you government magicians have managed to force Prescription Drug Monitoring Programs (PDMPs) to exclude Suboxone, "THE LEGAL MORPHINE," from oversight during your spying-on-pain-patients'-records forays. Either list Suboxone with its morphine component or don't list any opioids for oversight. (See Chapter 20, "The Suboxone Hoax".)

CONGRESS MUST REIN IN THE DOJ and its Rogue DEA

No more PDMP access, nor access to patients' EMRs (electronic medical records).

HIPAA (Health Insurance Portability and Accountability Act) rules of privacy and confidentiality apply. **Congress must:**

1. **Publicly interrogate, sanction and imprison wrongfully-acting DOJ prosecutors and their DEA subordinates.** Up to now, they've been exempting themselves from professional integrity, increasingly upping the antes of bogus charges against innocent physicians, other clinicians, pharmacists and pain clinic principals. With that, they've severely negatively impacted the increasingly unlivable lives of 50,000,000 Americans in pain, causing daily suicides due to doctors' increasingly mortal fear of DOJ/DEA tactics, because of which, many physicians have stopped prescribing opioid pain relief at all.
2. Congress must assure all of America that neither the DOJ, nor any of its subordinate agencies will ever again interfere in the practice of medicine, nor in the doctor-patient relationship.

DUTIES OF THE VETERANS ADMINISTRATION TO PROTECT AND TREAT SICK VETERANS, NOT TO DENY THEM PAINCARE

Our valiant veterans in pain DEMAND restoration of their rights to opioid paincare and also to adequate dosage levels of these analgesics. Change your damaging VA rules against opioid therapy that are causing mounting veteran suicides. No! Do not broadcast the lie any longer that these, sometimes daily, veteran suicides around the country are due to posttraumatic stress disorder (PTSD). That's a crock of spent bullets. There are many treatments for PTSD including cognitive processing therapy, certain psychotropic medications, EMDR (Eye Movement Desensitization and Reprocessing), and others. And these can greatly help real veterans with PTSD.

But, for unrelenting, unbearable pain there is a class of pharmaceuticals that are irreplaceable: Opiates (Morphine, Codeine) and their opioid analogs, the semi-synthetics and the synthetics. To deprive pain-suffering veterans of these essential opioid analgesics is criminal torture. And the perpetrators of these denials should be on trial for their crimes against patients in pain. Like the Nuremberg trials, these would act as ominous warnings to current and future government functionaries who believe it's acceptable to torture people already disabled, especially our veterans.

With Its Huge Taxpayer-Funded Budget, the VA Owes Veterans Empathic Opioid Paincare

With over 1700 hospitals, clinics and living facilities, the Veterans Administration runs the largest healthcare system in America. It's medical component is known as the Veterans Health Administration but is commonly referred to as the VA, as in "VA hospitals". In 2015, its yearly budget was $65 billion and its workforce consisted of 298,546 professional and ancillary employees. The VA system, thus, is amply equipped to provide the best medical care to its more than 9 million veteran patients.

Military Medicine and Common Sense Should Not Be Mutually Exclusive

Strict VA policies denying opioid treatment to veterans with conditions where they are clearly medically-indicated are based on lack of scientific knowledge, myth and also upon the rising tide of misinformation about medical use of opioids. The latter fed copiously to, and swallowed whole by, VA functionaries such as managers, administrators, business-minded types far removed educationally and emotionally from the healing and empathic goals of quality physicians and nurses.

Having decided, erroneously, that prescription opioid use automatically creates addicts (despite scientific truth that less than 1% of patients so prescribed ever go on to addict), these nonmedical overseers have decided that elimination or abatement of pain is not the goal. As a result, elimination of common sense about what's essential in paincare medicine, to treat the pain, is rampant in VA medical settings.

VA managers, administrators, whosoever, lacking medical education and lacking intimate knowledge of individual veteran-patients' paincare history and analgesic needs, are making medical decisions about opioid therapy. Who are these empty-headed, feelingless, *dumbchucks* battling our valiant vulnerable veterans by denying them pain relief? Who gave them this power? Where is Congress to rein in their heartless stupidity, to order them "hands off the medical care of veteran patients"?

VA nonmedical department heads: Get out of the practice of medicine. You are killing our veterans by forcing them to choose suicide because of your insensitivities which result in cruelties most foul.

VA physicians are frightened to buck the system that demands: "Abandon all dope ye who enter here"! But, if a veteran suffers pain and is not an addict, too bad. No opioid prescription for you, soldier! This is VA madness on stilts. Because opioids, throughout modern, and pre-modern, medical history have proven their dependable effectiveness against all kinds of acute, intermediate, chronic, and lifelong pain. The quandary that the VA has found itself drowned in is its baffling conflation of drug addicts with pain patients.

Once again, just like other government agencies severely mistreating patients in pain, learn this: **Drug addict patients and paincare patients are two entirely different diagnostic categories of illness**. And the treatments for addictions – detoxing from illicit drugs – are entirely different than the most appropriate medical treatment for pain, prescription opioids. So stop torturing our American heroes. Stop sending them to early graves by suicides because you stubbornly refuse to allow VA physicians to prescribe the opioids known to help them. And when you do restore normal opioid prescribing to our veterans, remember this:

Don't demand the dosages be in such low MMEs (morphine milligram equivalents) that they wouldn't ease the pain of a flea.

It's very important that Congress also interrogate these guilty VA non-medical supervisors who have instituted cruel, inhuman policies against our valiant veterans who are suffering war injuries and/or illnesses occurring since their military careers ended. It's very important that medical staff at VA hospitals and other VA healthcare facilities rebel against anti-patient policies. Medical care is based on this fundamental instruction, Hippocrates' *Primum non nocere*. First do no harm. VA head honchos have been harming sick and injured veterans for years, even before the CDC's misguided 2016 *CDC Guideline* burst upon the general healthcare world and destroyed the normal, empathic medical treatment of pain.

STATE ATTORNEYS-GENERAL MUST STOP VICTIMIZING THE PHARMACEUTICAL INDUSTRY

Americans know you *juris doctors* have moved from your baccalaureate degree to your J.D. in 3 years beyond that undergraduate work. Americans are puzzled, though, by the many attorneys like yourselves (including many DOJ prosecutors) who appear to have taken upon yourselves the aura of having graduated medical school. Like you lawyers have morphed into medical doctors. This idea is not arrived at lightly. It's because, along with the horrendous misapplication of DOJ and DEA policing and prosecutions against the normal medical prescribing of opioid analgesics for pain patients – such as the asset seizures from, and imprisonments of, innocent physicians – there is the destruction of millions of pain patients' lives. Those are due to iatrogenic incapacitation of patients denied their opioid relief, and of those in desperation choosing suicide over unbearable pain.

Such sufferings having been generated by this new legion of juris doctors who are practicing medicine – the DEA by its spying on, raiding of, targeting of real doctors, and telling real doctors how low their opioid dosages must go "or else". And by the DOJ who, as plaintiffs, drum up everything short of surgical glue to see what sticks against prosecuted physicians. Further worsening this war on pain patients and their physicians, the whole bunch of government juris doctors are colluding to further shrink the legal supply of opioid analgesics for their legitimate medical use.

Given that the aforementioned mindset so blatantly afflicts federal police (DEA operatives) and federal prosecutors (DOJ juris doctors), it's not surprising that many of the top attorneys in each state government have been contaminated by the same erroneous thinking and questionable judgement under the delusion that they too know how to practice medicine without having attended medical school. That they understand the intricacies of encephalic behavior, of neurochemistry, of pharmacology, of nociception, of all the varied diseases, heritable conditions, and injuries that inflict varied kinds and levels of pain. But you guys don't.

Instead, state Attorneys-General must protect the Pharmaceutical Industry from ceaseless litigations. Because you lawyers are not physicians, or pharmacologic scientists, you can't possibly understand the research and development processes that pharmaceutical manufacturers invest in long before a medicine is FDA-approved for marketing. Finances, years, and valuable scientific talent during which no earnings are accruing to that company for that prescription medication.

Therefore, it's imperative, Madam or Sir Attorney General of your state, that you carefully consider the effects incessant litigations against legitimate makers of our medicines have on all Americans with all kinds of ailments.

What are you doing to the one industry that accounts for infection-curing, life-saving, de-hospitalization of the mentally ill, seizure-preventing, and pain-relieving medications? Please! Stop the bogus suits against legitimate pharmaceutical manufacturers whose ongoing research and development activities continue to bring us better and safer curative and pain-relieving medicines.

Pharm companies have sales forces with salespeople educated about their products, the conditions they treat, their drugs' benefits, side effects, cautions, allergenic potential, and so forth. Such are the facts the medical salesperson discusses with the physicians in the sales territory he/she covers. There's no attempt to mislead physicians to put patients at risk by giving doctors misinformation. Such would be marketing stupidity. For, if your drug harms your demographic of patients, you won't be making any profit on that medication.

State Attorneys-General Must Stop anti-Pharm Company Litigations

- **Pharm companies obey all Food and Drug Administration (FDA) regulations**
- **Pharm companies might someday consolidate an action against such suits**
- **Don't go after pharm corporations because of hidden "perks" at winning**
- **Companies you sue are FDA-approved to market their medications**
- **All businesses hold internal and external conferences, meetings and seminars discussing sales strategies**
- **Advertising their products is not illegal**
- **Discussing their products is legal**
- **Ads in medical journals and promotional materials to physicians are all FDA-monitored**
- **If anything about a drug is concerning, the Pharm manufacturer will hear from the FDA**

Egregiously, some officials are so enmeshed in such nonsensical thinking about medical care and pain care, that they are totally overlooking how ceaseless litigations interfere with pharmaceutical manufacturers' need to focus on research and development of new and better medications and the ongoing safe manufacture of vital pain-relieving opioids to be prescribed by physicians to prevent the pain-overwhelmed from dying by suicide!

How any "settlement' monies are spent should be publicized in detail. Who gets what? And what are the perks for various staff members of each A-G's office, such as promotions, raises, bonuses – for working on these too-often questionable litigations? Where, exactly, do these millions and billions go?

Speaking of "diversion," any monies so acquired are diverted from Big Pharma's research and development of new and better life-saving and pain-relieving drugs. This is tragic. Lawsuits like these should be rare. Instead, they're ever-accruing, a legal feeding frenzy by short-sighted emboldened prosecutors all poised to execute this gaggle of Pharma golden geese.

State Attorneys-General should investigate the addiction treatment industry's Suboxone bonanza. (See Chapter 20, "The Suboxone Hoax".) Refocus, instead of on the makers of medicines that help all of us, on the harm to patients – both drug addicts and those in pain – of clinics and other facilities' questionable use of Suboxone® (buprenorphine/naloxone). Because nobody can yet prove that it's actually effective for addicts. (Let alone for pain patients now being wrongly labeled "drug seekers" so they too can be forced onto Suboxone). Many addicts have to stay on it for life. Just another morphine, "The Legal Morphine", replacing the illicit one.

Prevent the infliction of the scurrilous diagnosis "addict" on patients in pain who are then, without medical justification, referred to Suboxone prescribers. A morphine tamed with its naloxone component is unlikely to provide analgesia for pain patients.

State Attorneys-General should investigate Brandeis University and Stanford University. Both of these esteemed institutions have research arms which receive grants (from private donors and taxpayer dollars from government) focused on opioid-related research. That'd be fine if there weren't principals associated with such institutions who are decidedly against opioid therapy for pain patients but pro-buprenorphine, "The Legal Morphine" for drug addicts and sometimes forced on pain patients.

CDC DUTIES TO PATIENTS NEEDING OPIOIDS FOR PAIN

What about the Epidemic of American suicides due to untreated pain? The Centers for Disease Control and Prevention (CDC) is famous for its marvelous work against epidemics of bacterial and viral infections, of its work against many other epidemics, even worldwide, and of toxic dangers. Unfortunately, the CDC seems oblivious to the epidemic of suicides of patients in pain who have been tapered to such low doses of their usual opioids or who've been cold-turkeyed altogether that they are committing suicide in droves. These same tragedies are afflicting, daily, our valiant military veterans who've long been cut off their opioid analgesics. Why this epidemic of suicides of pain patients has not galvanized the CDC to bring it to a halt, STAT, is a mystery. And it's unconscionable. Immediately, the CDC must:

1. Announce this epidemic of pain patient suicides to the public.
2. Investigate and remedy this suicide epidemic of pain patients STAT!
3. Tear up the misguided *2016 Guideline for Prescribing Opioids for Chronic Pain* (See Chapter 7, "Critique of the *CDC Guideline for Prescribing Opioids for Chronic Pain*".)
4. If the CDC ever again attempts to create a set of principles for pain management, be sure you have a large number of pain specialists as expert contributors, not like the pitifully disingenuous handful of anti-opioid zealots who are addictions specialists, unconcerned about pain sufferers.
5. Cease promoting the falsehood that conflates two entirely different patient groups – drug addicts seeking "highs" and pain patients depending on an opioid medication to alleviate enough of their pain so they can hold a job and have some modicum of a life.

THIS IS A NATIONAL EMERGENCY: CONGRESS MUST ACT IMMEDIATLELY TO SAVE PATIENTS' LIVES, TO PREVENT PHYSICIAN IMPRISONMENTS

It's your congressional duty to help quell an epidemic. I'm speaking of the epidemic of horrible suffering and illness befalling millions upon millions of Americans in pain who've, suddenly, had their dependable legal opioid pain relievers ripped from them due to the misguided direction of zealots unschooled in the intricacies of nuanced opioid paincare.

1. A commission must be formed to interrogate both DOJ leadership and its prosecutors about their questionable *carte blanche* targetings and prosecutions of responsible, ethical physicians and other clinicians who legally prescribe opioids for patients in pain.
2. Such government employees ought to be made liable for their actions that harm pain patients and their doctors.
3. Uncovered criminal behaviors of such government functionaries ought to be prosecuted.
4. Vital interrogations are essential to uncover motivations, that have zero medical validity, for shrinking the supply of legally manufactured opioid analgesics. Because such DOJ/DEA behaviors that harm all patients in pain, that kill others who die from failing health and suicides due to deprivation of pain relief are escalating, even as users of illicits are dying in droves because the DOJ/DEA officials can't figure out that, while practicing medicine (not their strong suit) they've shirked their responsibilities to get illicits off the street.
5. Interrogate these agency leaders about their scare-tactics publicity campaigns, pulling the wool over journalists' eyes, creating a national hysteria worthy of dark era witch hunts about two

innocent groups – patients in pain and their physicians. Ask these government persons, "Why the diversion from your duties to focus on illicits, dealers, and the care of addicts?"

6. Legislate the DOJ and the DEA out of patients' confidential records, including Electronic Medical Records (EMRs) and state PDMPs (Prescription Drug Monitoring Programs).
7. Remove the DOJ's and its DEA's *carte blanche* to harm patients by shrinking the opioid analgesic drug supply, by incriminating innocent doctors. They've been making up their own rules as they go along and getting more and more autocratic as more and more Americans patients and physicians fall victim to their out-of-control actions.
8. Create legislation that prevents government interference in pain-care medicine.
9. Mandate that all government agencies must have Congressional oversight to protect American citizens from totalitarian behaviors of government operatives.
10. The DOJ shall no longer be able to menace and threaten physicians, other prescribing clinicians, or anyone else for that matter, with the nebulous, catch-22 charge of "conspiracy". A charge that, when adjudicated guilty, remands your physician to prison for a quarter century. A charge that, to avoid, forces doctors to plead to a lesser charge, that though also bogus, incarceration for it is somewhat shorter. You see, "conspiracy" doesn't have to be explicated to the judge. Your physician gets convicted on the meaning of the word, not on any facts. What kind of America is this? I call those prisons "The American Gulag"!
11. Congress shall see to it that the DEA no longer gives its renegades free rein to send "Warning Letters" to doctors about their opioid prescribing, nor to make ominous, "threatening phone calls" informing doctors about what these police incorrectly decide is overprescribing. Nor shall they bother doctors' pain patients via

any form of communication about the doctors opioid analgesic prescribing as has been happening, too.

12. Congress: You need to do your job and get these federal police and prosecutors OUT OF THE PRACTICE OF MEDICINE!
13. **ENACT AMNESTY for imprisoned physicians, other prescribing clinicians, pharmacists and pain clinic staff and owners whose only "crime" had been providing pain relief for pain sufferers.**
14. **ENACT IMMUNITY FROM PROSECUTION for all MDs and related healthcare professionals and personnel**, absent absolute proof (no bogus "conspiracy" or "lesser charges" prosecutorial trap) absent absolutely solid proof of wrongdoing. This is imperative so that more physicians and other prescribing clinicians don't also abandon patients in pain due to intimidation, insinuation, raids, asset-confiscations, and baseless imprisonments due to confiscatory, venal motives of out-of-control federal forces. American physicians and other healthcare professionals should not have to feel the sword of Damocles hanging over the beneficent head of Hippocrates, the Healer. American medical professionals need to be free to do the very best for their patients. Which includes the removal, or at least the lessening, of their patients' experiences of pain.
15. **OVERSEE AND CURTAIL THE WANTON MUNICIPAL, COUNTY AND STATE LITIGATIONS AGAINST THE PHARMACEUTICAL COMPANIES WE RELY ON FOR MEDICINES TO SAVE OUR LIVES**

    The FDA monitors everything scientific, clinical, marketing, and advertising that relates to prescription medications. Enough. No one needs the DOJ or the DEA practicing medicine. Nor deciding what wordings a drug manufacturer should use in print or broadcast media, nor how drug salespeople should introduce new medications to physicians in their sales territories.

Apparently neither the DEA police, nor the DOJ lawyers have ever seen the lengthy, somnolence-inducing detailed package inserts that come with all prescription medications, nor the very long ones in plainer language for nonprofessionals. These are filled to the brim with the good, the worrisome, the possibilities, the warnings...everything a person needs to know about his/her medications; everything a doctor will find in the current PDR (Physicians' Desk Reference).

Therefore, in the advertising of prescription medications, not only does this full PDR information accompany every medical journal ad, it's information can't be deviated from by advertising copywriters. Thus, its incomprehensible that these lawyers-playing-doctor find some words they worry about, or a conference where sales matters are discussed (Anyone know of a business where you don't discuss sales, earnings projections, in addition to product improvements and new research?)

16. **ENACT LEGISLATION PROVIDING COMPENSATION FOR ABANDONED PAIN PATIENTS (LIKE THE HORRORS OF 911) WITHOUT PAIN RELIEF due to DEA and DOJ Overreach**
17. **ENACT LEGISLATION PROVIDING COMPENSATION TO THE FAMILIES OF THOSE LOST TO SUICIDE FROM DESPAIR OF EVER AGAIN BEING FREE OF PAIN**
18. **Enact legislation preventing anyone untrained in medicine from dictating medical practices, categories of analgesics, and drug dosages to physicians**
19. **Enact legislation preventing the DOJ's DEA from curtailing our prescription opioid supplies.** If you don't, they're coming for your insulin, for your anti-epileptic, for your antihypertensive, for your anxiolytic, for your antidepressant, for your life-saving epinephrine, maybe soon for an addicts' essential naloxone. That's

how far afield DEA overreach has extended itself. If you don't rein them in, next the DEA will be rationing our water.

Behind-the-Scenes Manipulators against Opioid Therapy for Pain

It's not necessary for me to mention who these individuals are who've managed to time-warp our entire country back into the medical dark ages. Nor do I have to name the organizations, or universities complicit in the promotion of their "never prescribe opioids for pain" agenda. Millions upon millions of pain-suffering Americans know exactly who these individuals are and what anti-opioid groups and universities they heavily influence. Suffice that these anti-opioid zealots' actions and interferences in quality paincare medical practice must be continually scrutinized and monitored, and must continue to be:

1. **challenged** by pain patients and by scientific evidence.
2. **exposed** by honest journalists who take the time to do in-depth research.
3. **investigated** for misuse of grant funds for biased "research results" based on an anti-opioid agenda which amounts to this rigid stance before any experiment begins: "These are the conclusions upon which my facts are based."

Part III SUMMARY OF ESSENTIAL ACTIONS TO END THE OPIOID WAR AGAINST PAIN PATIENTS

All victims (see Part I, above) of the government's anti-opioid crusade against patients in pain, against opioid-prescribing doctors, and against opioid manufacturers must be proactive. The more you muster your strength and resolve to do this, the sooner you'll achieve your goals of (1) life with opioid pain relief restored, (2) amnesty for imprisoned opioid-prescribing physicians, (3) Immunity for all American physicians, other prescribing clinicians, and pharmacists against DEA spying and gestapo tactics, against DOJ prosecutions for providing normal opioid prescriptions, and (4) surcease from endless, frivolous litigations against opioid manufacturers who can be relied upon to provide prescription medications in consistent FDA-approved forms, in accordance with all FDA regulations.

No more forced taperings, sudden *cold-turkeyings*, useless urinalyses, pointless pill counts. No more being labeled a "drug seeker". No more useless Suboxone "treatments". (See Chapter 20, "The Suboxone Hoax".) No more premature deaths due to patient-abandonment by DOJ/DOE-intimidated physicians, due to fear of a state medical board rescinding one's MD license. No more having to move to another state, or even to exile oneself out of America, in order to find quality pain care including one's reliable opioid analgesic. And, no more pain-desperation suicides.

Of the five categories in this segment, families, Big Pharma and Physicians are in better positions to be proactive. For patients in pain, including pain-racked veterans, lacking their usual opioids, they're often wheelchair-bound, home-bound, even bed-bound. Such incapacities make it nearly impossible to participate in proactive activities which require easy ambulation and focus, abilities slashed from pain patients' lives without their opioid medications.

Whichever category you fall into, do your utmost to fight for your rights. Remember, if you're bringing a lawsuit, your lawyer can come to your home if you can't ambulate to an office.

Consider lawsuits based on your specific perspectives. For instance, patients can sue doctors, hospitals, clinics, pharmacies, etc. Also, review Part I, above, on mounting Class Actions as well as on suing both Federal and State government agencies and government employees. Veterans can sue the Veterans Administration.

If enough victims of government opioihysteria – pain patients, opioid prescribers, and other paincare advocates – sue, the mainstream press will notice, legislators will notice, the tide will turn, the pendulum of sane opioid prescribing will swing back to normal from its current, government-induced, oxymoronic position of "helping addicts while killing off pain patients". That, even though neither the DOJ nor the DEA is helping addicts since deaths from the opioid fentanyl, in its illicit oral formulation, are rising exponentially. That too, even though the prescribing of opioids for pain has plummeted.

ACTIONS FOR PAIN VICTIMS AND ADVOCATES

Don't let government *OxyMORONS* spoil your life. Instead:

1. **Demand that politicians and legislators prevent DEA police and DOJ prosecutors from practicing medicine.** Too long have they been ordering physicians around, threatening them with asset-seizure and imprisonment, while demanding that doctors prescribe such low MMEs (morphine milligram equivalents) of an opioid, that these would provide the patient no pain relief at all.
2. **Vote out of office** all representatives, senators, state legislators, governors, and other clueless officials who won't uphold yours and your loved ones' rights to medically-selected opioids at individually-determined dosages by qualified physicians and other prescribing clinicians.

3. **Tell your pain story to Human Rights Watch. https://www.hrw.org**
4. **Tell your pain story to the Print and Broadcast Media.**
5. **Refuse any elective surgery unless your surgeon signs a contract that you'll be prescribed an appropriate opioid**, at an appropriate dosage, for as long as is necessary to control the pain you'll be experiencing.
6. **Pursue individual legal actions against Emergency Rooms, Intensive Care Units, Clinics, Hospital Administrators, and Hospitals in instances where you were refused opioid medication for pain** where you know it should have been ordered by the physician on your case. (Remember, for example, when suing a physician for not prescribing "standard of care" narcotic analgesia, you also should sue the hospital and its administrator(s) because they are responsible for the actions and inactions of their employees. In legalese, that is known as *Respondeat Superior*.)
7. **If you know of other pain patients similarly mistreated by the same facility and its staff, get yourselves together to an attorney.** If you have mobility issues and ambulation is a problem, or if bedridden, many attorneys will come to your home. Your co-litigants (complainants) can gather there. In a group like this, your case will be even stronger. And your charts, medical records, and radiologic exhibits will show that your valid pain was not treated. Or that, if you were given an ineffective substance like acetaminophen (Tylenol®), you were still left in enormous pain. That would be if the nurse on your case charted your suffering accurately.

Sadly, none of us yet know the entirety of all the damage the DOJ/DEA cabal has inflicted on quality medical and nursing practice relative to empathic care of patients in pain and what all health professionals are mandated to do for all patients. If neither the doctor who treated you nor the nurse who carried out his or her instructions, such as they were, didn't chart your lack of pain relief from the ineffective thing they gave you, I don't know how you overcome this in court. But I believe a smart lawyer, skilled in medical cases, can find an expert to say what the standard of care should have been in your case(s) as to the type of analgesic and dosage strength that would have and should have been given to you. So don't let bad charting, or absence of an accurate description of your ill-treated pain deter you from suing such bad healthcare practitioners.

8. **Get together with a number of pain patients using the same doctor, hospital or pain clinic who are refusing you all appropriate pain care they've up to now provided.** Are they now, instead, trying to foist implants and other invasive procedures on you instead of the ease of opioids to protect the quality of your life by relieving enough of your pain so you can live and breathe and keep your job? Tell your story to local and national journalists. Mount a class action lawsuit against these medical practices.
9. **Sue government agencies in class actions.** Where lawsuits against government agencies are disallowed, you can sue individual government employees whose actions or negligence have harmed you.
10. **Get petitions out warning of Class Actions to every public figure you can locate.** Be demanding of their cooperation!
11. **Perhaps Class Action suits are possible for Families of Pain Patients who've Suicided.** Speak to a lawyer about "wrongful death" lawsuits. Sue also for compensation for negligence, medical malpractice, lack of treatment of opioid-level pain. Refer to the new Washington Medical Commission (WMC of Washington state) which urges opioid therapy for patients in pain and will punish physicians who don't so prescribe, referring to that as "below the standard of care". (See Part II, above, describing Washington state's leadership in protecting pain patients from being deprived of their opioid analgesics.)

12. **Consider Personal Injury, Medical Malpractice, and Negligence lawsuits** against any prescriber or facility for nonconsensual tapering, *cold-turkeying* and dismissing you from their practice without a lifeline of care to another pain management facility, without referral to another physician.
13. **Our Valiant Veterans in Pain should take Legal Actions against the Veterans Administration (VA)**. Here is one pain physician and patient-advocate who is also an attorney. He can refer you to specific laws enacted to help veterans. He is the very empathic Daniel Laird, MD, JD with a new law practice in Las Vegas, who also treats patients in pain. (Read more about Dr. Laird and how to contact him in Chapter 23, "Heroines and Heroes....).

Robert Rose is one veteran in pain seeking a groundswell of other veterans, suffering under-treated or untreated pain, in order to mount a class action lawsuit against the Veterans Administration for its callous mistreatment of veterans in pain and to compensate families of veterans who've suicided due to the VA's intransigent below-medical-standards pain care.

In a September 15, 2019 **nationalpainreport.com** article about Veteran Robert Rose, the author Ed Coghlan said that Rose urged him to "...publish his phone number if an attorney wants to reach him [about a class action law suit on behalf of Veterans in Pain vs. the Veterans Administration]." It is 423-794-8241. Veteran Rose is on Twitter @ RobertDroseJr1.

Again, the VA is yet another government agency literally "getting away with murder" as administrators without medical degrees are making opiophobic decisions for, and intimidating, VA staff physicians, leaving the latter in tears (as reported to me by VA nurses) because they know what their veteran patients really need to quell their painful conditions – an opioid.

ACTIONS FOR HEALTHCARE PROFESSIONALS AND THEIR ORGANIZATIONS

1. **AMNESTY** *for hundreds of wrongfully imprisoned opioid-prescribing physicians, and other clinicians and pharmacists caught up in the DOJ/DEA witch-hunt.* Demand immediate amnesty and immediate release from prison for these scapegoats of government Oxy-Morons. Consider appealing to the governor of your state to pardon these wrongfully convicted innocents. Demand immediate release of these innocents and prompt return of their assets "confiscated" by that league of OxyMorons.

   A brave lawyer or courageous law firm must do this work pro bono – at least at first until you begin to receive some legal winnings – because the DOJ has been having its DEA seize all these clinicians' professional and personal assets leaving them with no funds with which to defend themselves to pay for a talented attorney.

   Where the American Civil Liberties Union (ACLU) is in these cases is baffling. So far, the ACLU doesn't seem to be interested in helping these wrongfully prosecuted and wrongfully imprisoned clinicians.

2. **IMMUNITY** *for all American Physicians, now in trepidation of ever again treating any patient in pain with an opioid due to the OxyMoronic behaviors of the DOJ and its DEA.* **Demand that all American physicians, other prescribing clinicians, pharmacists and nonmedical staff of pain clinics** be protected from spying-scrutiny, raids, paranoid suspicions, seizures, arrests, prosecutions, and imprisonments by overreaching out-of-control DOJ/DEA autocrats. Complete immunity from such government tyranny is essential if medical care in America is ever again to be considered the world's best. Right now, because of unprecedented government intrusions into paincare medicine, the resulting 24-hour suffering of millions upon millions of pain patients, and the ever-mounting

suicides of patients in unbearable untreated pain, I consider this country's medical care sinking so low that it falls below the depths of Third World health. Thus, the opiophobes and the OxyMorons have rendered America, Fourth World in healthcare.

In the meantime, follow the advice of my anonymous informant, retired DOJ prosecutor "Mr. Price" in Part I of this chapter.

3. **What the American Medical Association and All Other Medical, Surgical, and Psychiatric Organizations Must Do to Protect Your Patients and Your Colleagues Careers:** *You must all band together, becoming a mighty voice and a mighty force against government intrusion* including spying into confidential medical matters. Particularly related to pain care and opioid prescribing. You must raise funds for the legal protection of your co-professionals. Each of your organizations, or consider banding together to create a mightier force, can mount class actions against whatever government agencies or individuals – that may be legally culpable – which are interfering in the doctor-patient relationship and normal opioid prescribing for pain.

Also, physician-leaders in these organizations, please take note of the intricate advice from the identity-protected Mr. Price, retired DOJ prosecutor, whose advice I elaborated in Part I of this Chapter. Isn't it an outrageous shame that doctors should be forced to practice "defensive medicine" – not against a disease, injury, or genetic condition – but against our spying government of interlopers who've deputized themselves to criminalize normal, Hippocratically-empathic opioid prescribing for pain?

In the case of Pharmaceutical Manufacturers of pure and dependably consistent opioid medications, that have been carefully researched and are reliably available for prescribing paincare physicians – before the current DOJ/DEA blitz against medicinal opioids – there are some suggestions I hope you'll counter the blitzkrieg of State Attorneys-General and other juris doctors with, who have been getting away with outrageously unfounded litigations that eat into your companies' earnings earmarked for Research and Development to bring into existence new and better life-saving, emotion-easing, and pain-relieving drugs.

In Your Defenses: Prescriptions to Fight Frivolous Lawsuits Against Pharmaceutical Manufacturers

- Drugs are all approved, after much science is carefully reviewed, by the FDA
- Marketing and Advertising is overseen by the FDA
- Quantities of ethical drugs – whether insulin, antibiotics or opioids – in any given community, are reflective of that specific community's population needs. For example, the needs of elderly and disabled, or a large community will likely have more pain patients than a sparsely populated neighborhood.
- Pharm manufacturers shouldn't be wasting time worrying about "quantities" of any medications shipped to distributors, then from distributors to pharmacies.
- Neither should distributors be forced by government to be concerned with this nonsense. Because these are opioid medications, along with many other classes of ethical drugs, that are legally prescribed and end up solely in the hands of the patients they are prescribed for. Thus, these "quantities" have zero to do with the loads of illicits our clueless DEA is letting into our country from China, Mexico, the Internet and via the U.S. Postal Service.
- Marketing and targeting medication information to specialists and other physicians is appropriate – and so are conversations, conferences and meetings about company earnings and sales goals among sales executives and salespersons – the same as for any business on the planet. And, in the case of the ethical pharmaceuticals industry, a huge chunk of those earnings is plowed right back into the research and development of advanced medicines for a healthier nation.

- Conversations about marketing, profits and company growth occur in all businesses. Since when are marketing discussions a crime?

Pain patients, their physicians, and all Americans need principled public servants. Not self-serving oligarchic tyrants – DOJ prosecuting juris doctors and DEA invading rogue police – counting pills, prescribing opioid doses, practicing medicine.

You've read, herein, about the unconscionable human toll the misguided policies of the HHS, its CDC and the DOJ with its DEA have been forcing upon anyone in pain. Now you have some suggested actions you can take against them and their medically-nihilistic tactics.

Massive class actions against indivduals and institutions can tilt the opioid treatment pendulum in your favor. Similarly, challenging government agencies and government employees in court as a class of millions upon millions in pain will get the real American public's attention (a groundswell up to now ignored by the press) and could turn the tide in pain patients' favor.

Now read on about what the government perpetrators, of your non-stop pain-suffering, must be mandated to do. Because of their naked interference in opioid paincare, I enjoy calling these Cold Turkeys "OxyMorons".

Defective Detectives DEA police must be stopped from targeting physicians, from spying on their patients' records (Electronic Medical Records and Prescription Drug Monitoring Programs), from seizing doctors' assets, from making threatening phone calls and sending warning letters to clinicians demanding they lower patients' opioid doses and abandon the care of pain patients above a government-decided census.

Instead, the DEA must be commanded to focus solely on the problem of illicit drugs in America and drop it's unwarranted fixation on legally-prescribed opioids. Additionally, the DEA should have zero control over normally-prescribed legal medications, not even over their manufacture or their distribution. Right now, in its "defective detective" mode, DEA operatives are preparing to cut even further (they've already reduced the medicinal opioid supply) much-needed opioid narcotic quantities so that shortages exist. Tragic since, not only does this lack of availability of opioid pain relief affect long-suffering Intractable Pain Patients (IPPs), it also causes great suffering to cancer patients in the last months, weeks, and days of their lives, and those in hospice and end-of-life care.

Imprudent Jurisprudence DOJ prosecutors are, these days, killing American medical practice. They're disrupting quality healthcare by their stranglehold on things medical they have no clue about. Their autocratic actions against innocent physicians and other clinicians who dare to provide normal opioid medications for pain are off the charts irresponsible. Right now, they proceed apace to prosecute innocent physicians and other opioid prescribers across the nation. Their modus operandi? Throw everything, including surgical collodium, at doctors they've targeted for imprisonment, to see if anything sticks. But, when a physician won't agree to bogus charges that will require some jail time, fines, house arrest, and so forth, fancy footwork DOJ prosecutors belch forth with the charge of "conspiracy". And, since a "conspiracy" conviction exposes the doctor to a 25-year prison sentence – even though the DOJ plaintiff need not disclose to the judge what "conspiracy" entails in each case – good doctors are forced by this catch-22 legal maneuver to plead to the lesser untrue charges. This underhanded "legal" trick against doctors must stop.

Empty of Empathy The misguided 2016 *CDC Guideline* had been doomed from its government "task forces" inception. It was just plain wrong for the Centers for Disease Control and Prevention (CDC) to convene many and varied experts to contribute to a "guide" for physicians prescribing pain medications, particularly opioids, which didn't include highly skilled and intensely specialized pain management medical professionals. Instead, the CDC had the nerve to include anti-opioid zealots from an organization rabidly opposed to any opioid pain medications whatsoever. (Read in depth about this misguideline and my contretemps to it in Chapter 7.)

Vacuous VA Shame on the Veterans Administration for its "...and to the republic for **Rigid Stands....**" heartless mistreatment of our valiant veterans in pain. The VA knows those nearly daily suicides of American veterans are not due to posttraumatic stress disorder. (Known physiologic and psychologic treatments for PTSD abound.) These suicides are caused by an insane administrative VA policy, that has nothing to do with quality medical practice, that has cruelly cold-turkeyed double-amputees, elder vets in deteriorating health, brain-injured former soldiers, and many more. These are the causes of the many veteran suicides we all read about in our local papers. So far, the VA is doing zero for our military heroes. The VA must immediately rescue its veteran pain patients, all side-lined, by freeing VA staff doctors to prescribe opioids when these physicians' in-depth training tells them opioids are indicated in various veteran pain cases.

Litigious Lawyers Revamp all state attorneys-general thinking about their actions that are killing the golden geese of research and availability of life-saving, sanity-restoring, and pain-relieving pharmaceuticals. State A-Gs are disrupting and bankrupting ethical pharmaceutical manufacturers' higher duties to the public. These are our reservoir of breakthrough, life-preserving and opioid analgesic medications. Imagine a world, an America, without these health-preserving products and the daring companies whose caring scientists created them for us.

Congressional Oversight Here "oversight" has a double meaning. Thus far, Congress has given certain government agencies free reign (sic) to get away with anything they please. This problem of dying patients in pain, patients suiciding, patients whose pain is going untreated due to nonsensical opiophobia has got to end now. STAT! That's medical-speak for IMMEDIATELY! RIGHT NOW!

DEA police have no medical knowledge to justify their interference in any medication prescriptions, so it is unsafe for pain patients, to allow these know-nothings to continue prescribing opioid MMEs (morphine milligram equivalents) so low they wouldn't ease the pain of a flea.

Due to DEA sneaky actions, it's pitiful that highly-educated, caring and ethical MDs need to worry about being spied upon. The DOJ/ DEA conglomerate treats MDs like they're criminals. In advance of anything criminal having happened, without cause targeted because of simply treating pain patients with the opioids that have eased pain from time immemorial, and certainly over a century of paincare in American hospitals. And they've been getting away with this for years because of Congressional laxness which, by default, has granted this government cabal carte blanche to raid and invade the lives and careers of physicians everywhere.

Congress you've missed all the signs and symptoms of an autocracy, the DOJ/DEA cabal, operating with impunity, right under your noses and you've done zero about this injustice. You must take oversight command of these entities STAT! You must rein them in. Their carte blanche must be rescinded STAT!

Congress must declare or legislate that "There shall be no CDC, DOJ, DEA, or VA intrusions in the normal medical care of patients in pain when a physician, or other prescribing clinician, determines an opioid is indicated."

Congress, you have to monitor – and interrogate in public when necessary – what the DOJ and its sub-agencies are doing, how their actions affect all Americans. Otherwise, Congress's inaction in this regard amounts to a gross American oversight that leads to pain torture and suicides for millions.

It is sad that I felt forced to write this book and, upon researching it, shocking to have found a bilious undertow of festering, fulminating rot within the inner sanctum (underbellies) of key federal and state agencies, purportedly existing to help Americans maintain good health and secure longevity.

However, what has been building in recent years, by way of *carte blanche* fiat, has been, not merely government impotence, but deliberate programs against public health on a scale reminiscent of 1933 Germany.

Yes, I mean that. It's not just a few patients here or there with some rare disease which has no life-saving treatment yet. Everyone is affected when the best analgesics in the galaxy, opioids, the class of pharmaceuticals for chronic moderate to severe pain, and for several other levels of pain (e.g., acute conditions such as nephrolithiasis, postsurgery, and dental pain) are demonized and virtually expunged from the American pharmacopeia.

And the public has been deliberately misled by DOJ inventors of federal and state publicity campaigns shamelessly linking deaths from illicit drugs to the prescription of medicinal opioids for patients in pain. Widely acknowledged as scientifically false, this specious juxtaposition of two vastly different patient categories has nevertheless infected press releases and television announcements all over our country, obviously meant to brainwash all Americans against legal prescription narcotics, causing a crusade of tirades against prescription opioid medications everywhere you turn.

Glue together a medically-naive public and vacuous, irresponsible government leadership – the DOJ's and the DEA's severe demonizing of normal medicinal opioid use, a diversionary tactic to remove the spotlight from their failure to control illicits importation, sales, and deaths – and you've got:

~ **50,000,000 million Americans in severe pain** (acute, chronic, or lifelong) who are being mistreated, labeled drug addicts, and denied their usual beneficial opioid medications.

~ **Scores of patients weekly, including military veterans, suiciding due to denial of opioid pain relief.**

~ **Over 1200 physicians and other clinicians**, who dared prescribe analgesic narcotics, criminalized and **imprisoned.**

~ **Ethical pharmaceutical manufacturers of FDA-approved opioids** for pain therapy litigated against in a feeding frenzy by clueless state prosecutors.

This diversion of the public mind from government's mindless goal – kill the prescription opioid supply so patients can't get any for pain relief – somehow has loosed upon the public a tidal wave of DOJ-generated, DEA-executed searches, seizures and suicides. Disastrously, these federal microcephalics have also decided to practice the profound profession of medicine. Seems, hidden from the public, DOJ and DEA juris doctors and police actually majored in medical subjects at the police academy and in law school.

What I wish would be made clear to the public is this: How did two agencies, the DOJ and its DEA – empowered to interdict illicit chemicals, to prosecute dealers and drug lords, and who should also "escort" all street addicts directly to mandated detox to save their lives – how did these agencies turn these legitimate and urgent responsibilities of theirs into a mass extermination of patients in pain all over our America? Including the annihilation of our revered veterans? By premature deaths due to severe debilities caused by untreated pain? By suicides due to despair of ever again being free of unbearable pain?

And how did this anti-opioid mindset also morph into a killing game against our nation's empathic, ethical physicians, and other clinicians, who've dedicated their lives to treating pain? Because doctors are, not only losing their cherished medical careers and their livelihoods, but some are dying from duress and suicide brought on by these malicious life-invasions by DOJ and DEA operatives.

This question is addressed directly to our Congress and other publically-accountable legislators and officials: How in the world did anyone allow this rogue band of DOJ lawyers and their DEA enforcers to supercede and circumvent citizen-protective laws and healthcare rights? To break into noncriminal medical practices? To fatally impact millions of innocent humans' lives, wreaking havoc, inducing greater suffering, causing suicides? Who do these truth-twisters answer to?

From the perspectives of millions of suffering and dying patients in pain – and from those of physicians and pharmaceutical company executives – it appears these miscreants have morphed into gods to divert public attention from their impotence in achieving their assignment: interdicting illicit drugs and dealing with related criminal issues.

Victims of Federal and State Lawless Lawyers

SCAPEGOATS: MORPHINE and its synthetic and semi-synthetic analogs, OPIOIDS demonized by government ignorance

SCAPEGOATS: PAIN PATIENTS did well on prescribed opioids, now suffering and dying without their reliable pain relief

SCAPEGOATS: MILITARY VETERANS who are victims of inhumane VA denial of prescription opioids for pain

SCAPEGOATS: CLINICIANS very brave in this gestapo climate to prescribe opioids for patients benefiting medically from them

SCAPEGOATS: ETHICAL PHARMACEUTICAL COMPANIES which research, develop and manufacture legal opioids

Ominously, as this book goes to press, I've learned of yet two other innocent but major targets of the DOJ/DEA war against patients in pain: **Your Children** and **Your Pets. Veterinarians** are being cowed by this cabal to deny opioid scripts for postop, injured, and ailing pets. The cuckoo DOJ/DEA rationale:"Owners will ingest their pets' opioids." Patients of **Pediatricians** – from infancy to late teens – no matter how severe their injuries, post-surgical pain, or pain from an inherited or other incurable illness, are being left to suffer needlessly due to the ever-looming ominous threat to pediatric clinicians by the DOJ/DEA horde.

Until Americans empower Congress to get rid of the whole bunch of government functionaries and agencies that have so botched the goal of stemming the mortality rate from illegal drugs – by diversion of public focus to the unrelated opioid treatment of pain – the torture of pain patients will continue and the suicides of retired soldiers and civilians in pain will soar.

America, HELP! S.O.S.! Mayday! Reverse this ghost-of-1933 holocaust against patients in pain. And in this 21st Century, restore American physicians' rights to prescribe pain-relieving opioids for their patients in pain. Remove all nonphysicians from overseeing the prescribing of any medications. Stop, already, with the endless, mindless litigations against our quality opioid medication manufacturers. Finally, shut down all government activities that impinge on quality medical care, the doctor-patient relationship, and the normal prescribing of opioid analgesics.

A Petition and a Resource section follow. I wish you the best. If a pain patient, may you have your trusty opioid medicine restored immediately. If a physician, other clinician or pharmacist in prison, I wish you amnesty and release from prison immediately. If a physician or other prescribing clinician not yet targeted by DOJ/DEA forces, I wish you immunity from government interference. If an ethical pharmaceuticals corporation, Americans appreciate your diligent research and development of medicines that save lives, keep us healthy, and free us from pain. The time has come for the victims of American Agony to be victors. To multi-quote Puccini, "VINCEREMO"! VINCEREMO! VINCEREMO!

About the Petition

The following ***American AGONY* Petition** is intended to help you enlighten all governors, state attorneys-general, state legislators, community leaders, state medical boards, congressional representatives, and senators; plus federal agencies, especially HHS, its CDC; the DOJ, its DEA; and the VA about the urgency of:

1. **Restoring Normal Opioid Medications to Patients in Pain**
2. **Protecting the Legal Opiate and Opioid Supply from Shortages**
3. **Protecting Opioid-Prescribing Physicians and Other Clinicians from baseless DEA raids,** asset-seizures, invasions of patients' medical records via PDMPs, eroding HIPAA privacy laws. And from wrongful targeting, threatening, arresting, prosecuting and imprisoning opioid-prescribing professionals.
4. **Stopping DOJ Lawyers and DEA Police from Practicing Medicine** \Stop them from sending ominous "warning letters" and from making "warning phone calls" telling clinicians how much they must lower Morphine Milligram Equivalent (MME) doses of opioids per day, or else!

This petition is one way to help you and/or your organization – whether you're a pain patient, an opioid prescriber, or other advocate for the restoration of common sense in the practice of paincare medicine, currently wrested from physicians' hands by clueless government functionaries – impress upon those in powerful government positions the urgency of making essential policy changes to restore medical opioid prescribing to normal. In the professional hands of physicians. For a return to quality pain patient care.

A key to reversing the ominous trend of unmedicated severe sufferings and suicides of patients in pain is to rein in the activities of the DEA or dissolve it altogether. Because it is chiefly the DEA's irresponsible actions that are causing such human misery, subjecting millions to unrelieved pain and ongoing suicides. See (in Chapter 24, Part II The Victimizers) how its dissolution and, potential, restructuring as IDEA, Illicits Drug Enforcement Agency, will strictly limit it to interdicting illicits, arresting dealers, arresting for murder those whose illicits caused deaths, and transporting known addicts to detox facilities.

Use your***American AGONY*** **Petition** to ensure that the DEA no longer has anything whatever to do with legal, medically-prescribed opioids – is no longer ruining the lives of pain patients and their doctors, no longer causing suicides, no longer decimating supplies of legal narcotics, no longer intimidating physicians nationwide, no longer emboldening State Attorneys-General to flood the courts with questionable litigations against the makers of medicines we all need for a healthy nation.

You have my permission to quote from this page, or from this whole book. anything you wish in order to communicate your urgent message. A message you may also wish to send to your local print journalists and broadcast media.

You may use the***American AGONY*** **Petition** as is. Or, you have my permission to adapt it – to your pro-prescription-opioids-for-pain position – in ways specific to your particular objectives. I cheer you on to **S.O.S. SAVE OPIOID SCRIPTS** success!

American AGONY Petition
TO RESTORE, FOR ALL CATEGORIES OF PAIN, PATIENTS' RIGHTS TO OPIOIDS PRESCRIBED BY MEDICAL CLINICIANS

To: ______________________________ Date: / /

Address: ________________________ Phone: ( )

________________________________ Email: ____________________

________________________________ Website: ____________________

Dear ____

Because of years of government intrusions into the medical profession's legal opioid prescribing for patients suffering pain, these are the dire consequences I/we implore you to bring to an end:

- **Millions of Americans Forcibly Tapered:** Intractable Pain Patients (IPPs), in unceasing pain, are suffering on ineffective low doses of their years-long, even decades-long well-working opioids. Many **die prematurely** from cardiac and neurologic effects of forced taperings. **These tortures must cease Stat!**
- **Millions of Americans Suddenly Cold-Turkeyed:** Pain Patients, long-stabilized on prescribed opioids, abandoned to neverending pain, are suffering severely, many suiciding.
- **Millions More Sick and Dying Americans Denied Opioids Prescribed Safely for Over a Century in:**
  - Cancer Care . Palliative Care . Hospice Care
  - End-of-Life Care . Acute Injuries and Illnesses . Postop Pain
  - Acute ER Diagnoses . Dental Pain and Surgeries
  - Children in Serious Pain . Even Pets, Postop Cats and Dogs
- **Countless American Veterans Forcibly Cold-Turkeyed:** Veterans Administration anti-opioid dictates prevent pain relief in amputees, and other battle-injured and retired soldiers leading to almost **daily suicides the VA falsely attributes to PTSD**.

- **Hundreds of Innocent Clinicians Imprisoned for high-quality care of patients in pain**: Clueless DEA police and DOJ prosecutors presume to prescribe, either blanket denial of essential opioids or one-size-fits-all MMEs (Morphine Millegram Equivalents) so low they wouldn't relieve the pain of a flea. And they scare, raid, imprison physicians. **I/we demand AMNESTY for those in prison, IMMUNITY for all other opioid prescribers Stat!**
- **49 State Medical Boards Collude with the DEA and DOJ by Intimidating Opioid-Prescribers:**

Except for brave Washington State's Washington Medical Commission supporting its pain patients and physician opioid prescribers, shame on all other state medical boards for colluding with DOJ and DEA renegades, non-MDs practicing medicine unlicensed, deciding MMEs, forcing abandonment of pain patients to zero analgesic help, forcing good doctors to retire. **State Boards Must Support Physicians Stat!**

Anything you can do to reverse the severe damage the CDC, VA, DOJ and DEA have been inflicting on pain patients (propelling many to suicide), on their families, on innocent doctors, on our valiant veterans, while assuring normal supplies of essential opioids from Pharm manufacturers to patients in pain will be most appreciated.

I and my growing Group______________________ will be watching for your positive actions toward restoring legal opioid treatments to pain patients nationwide without CDC, VA, DOJ, or DEA interferences. We are 50 million American patients deprived of the opioids medically known to best treat our pain. Others of us are paincare physicians. We are watching your legislative and related actions on these pain-related prescription opioid issues. We intend to vote out of office anyone who won't help restore ours and our doctors' rights to utilize legal opioids according to medical exigencies.

Name (print): ____

Organization: ____

Address: _____________________ Phone: ______________

___________________________ Email: ______________

Signature of Petitioner __________________________________

RESOURCES

PROFESSIONAL PAIN ORGANIZATIONS, PATIENT ADVOCACY GROUPS AND OTHER SERVICES

Demonstrating how far and wide PAIN affects Americans are the numbers and diversities of organizations, Medical, Varied Other Professional, and Lay Advocates which exist to tackle this multifactorial sensate symptom. A symptom that interrupts the lives of 50,000,000 Americans who, with appropriate medical care, often using opiates or opioids, can live some kind of a quality of life, albeit never as free completely of some level of pain. However, the bedridden may then get around in a wheelchair, the wheelchair-bound with a cane, the cane dispensed with in pain well-controlled by an opioid, so such patients can even go to work.

A number of painful conditions are enumerated in Section I. These do not include other than chronic, intractable pain, those conditions in which pain never fully relents. Because of unconscionable actions by American governmental agencies–HHS, CDC, DOJ, DEA,VA, particularly–and specious individuals looking out for their own self-aggrandizement and financial enrichment, American millions are cruelly suffering, against all medical Hippocratic goals, against all common sense. These are patients dying from medical conditions such as myocardial infarctions, brain disorders and related ailments brought on by cruel rapid-tapering or sudden cold-turkeying of such patients' normal narcotic analgesic medications. Others, whose pain is so neverendingly unbearable, choose SUICIDE. These are avoidable tragedies. These should really be labelled HOMICIDES BY GOVERNMENT FIAT. Instigated by the infamous, callous 2016 *CDC Guideline* and stampeded into tragedy after tragedy by the Drug Enforcement Administration gestapo-style raids of innocent physicians' practices, physicians then imprisoned, pain clinics closed, pain patients abandoned. All while the Department of Justice, overseeing this catastrophe, proceeds to charge innocent physicians, and other clinicians of "conspiracy," a charge to which "there is no defense". Such catch-22 government fools fooling around with patients' and physicians' lives. Who will have the courage to make a clean sweep of these microcephalics murdering our citizens?

In the meantime, here is a list, by no means covering every existing organization trying to help patients in pain, but it's a start. We probably wouldn't need so many of them if federal, state and municipal governments kept their noses out of confidential patient care and out of the physician-patient relationship. To pain patients everywhere, best of luck in your search for quality pain care in this era of evil engendered by wrong-headed government operatives and by certain individuals and groups intent on depriving patients in pain of surcease.

The following list of resources for pain patients, pain management physicians and other prescribing clinicians is by no means all-encompassing. That's because there are far too many professional organizations in America, and around the world, that deal with varied aspects of pain research, and its diagnosis and treatment to encompass herein.

Also, especially here in the States, there are ever-increasing grass roots organizations of patients in dire need of their well-working opioid medications which have been ripped from them by the clouded thinking of government bureaucrats overreaching, way beyond their education – the DEA closing down physicians' medical practices, leaving abandoned patients in their wake, the DOJ prosecuting doctors on bogus "conspiracy" charges, leaving all American medical practitioners quaking in their offices if they dare prescribe an opioid that has always worked well for specific patients.

Patients in pain are no longer going to put up with this government annihilation by pain-torture and suicides reminiscent of the homicides of 1939 Nazi Germany.

The following are a small example of some professional and grass roots pain-concerned organizations and other resources. Pain patients with specific conditions can Google these and organizations will appear which you may contact for help. (Note that the **Practical Pain Management** listing, below, highlights many painful conditions that are explicated at that website.)

I sincerely wish the reader the best in finding useful help with your condition and in allying with medical professional and grass roots communities that exist to help you.

Also, please bear in mind you have human rights against torture, you have legal rights to medical privacy (see HIPAA regulations), you have patients' rights against unethical medical care and inadequate or zero pain relief. To these ends, your other resources are legal and legislative. You have to teach government a lesson at the voting booth. You have to demand legislators reverse all laws that interfere with physician autonomy in medical practice and patient autonomy in choosing the appropriate pain care. And physicians have to be rendered immune to government discussion of pharmaceuticals and dosages of any and all pharmaceuticals. Reason: Lawyers and Police didn't go to medical school.

What follows are several professional and grass roots organizations, as well as other helpful groups and websites that offer valuable general information and some low-cost and even free services and products.

American Academy of Pain Medicine Professional organization of pain medicine clinician specialists. https://painmed.org/

American Board of Pain Medicine This medical board is "committed to the certification of qualified physicians in the field of Pain Medicine." http://www.abpm.org/

American Chronic Pain Association Located in California, reach them at https://the acpa.org ACPA@acpa.org

American Headache Society Located in New Jersey, reach them at http://americanheadachesociety.org/

American Society of Anesthesiologists Specialists in anesthesiology are often the medical professionals who are also specialists in pain management.https://www.asahq.org/

American Society of Pain Management Nursing Promotes "best nursing practices for people in pain". http://www.aspmn.org/Pages/default.aspx

Arthritis Foundation Located in New York City. https://www.arthritis.org help@arthritis.org

The Centers for Medicare and Medicaid Services From this site, you can ascertain whether your physician has any financial relationship with any pharmaceutical or medical device manufacturer such as payment for speeches, research or consulting. https://openpaymentsdata.cms.gov/search/physicians/by-name-and-location/

Chronic Pain Research Alliance This organization is the "voice for the millions suffering with multiple pain conditions". The latter, known as Chronic Overlapping Pain Conditions (COPCs) "come at a high cost – to the individuals affected, their loved ones, our health care system and society at large." Misdiagnosis, lack of coordinated medical care, and the absence of safe, effective treatments must be exposed and must change for the better. Research dedicated to this huge group of pain sufferers ailments is the goal here. http://www.chronicpainresearch.org/site/index

Dental Lifeline Network Offers donated dental services. https://dentallifeline.org/

The Foundation for Peripheral Neuropathy This is "...a public charity foundation committed to fostering collaboration among today's most gifted and dedicated neuroscientists and physicians." That, in their effort to ease the lives of people suffering this painful condition. https://www.foundationforpn.org/

Free Lifeline Cell Phones Here's your access to free cell phones. https://www.tagmobile.com/

Give Pain a Voice This is a grassroots Canadian organization that Americans may wish to ally with to conquer similar lack-of-access-to-opioids issues within our U.S. borders. "We are the INVISIBLE PAIN PATIENTS....not readily recognized [because] we may not use a wheelchair or cane, and we may look just fine on the outside". However, lab tests may reveal nothing definitive but these patients' pain is just as real as those easily diagnosed. Though tests do not deliver a definitive diagnoses, pain-suffering persists, just like that of pain patients definitively diagnosed. http://www.givepainavoice.org/

Healthcare Bluebook This vast data base can help reduce your healthcare costs for tests, operations and medications. https://www.healthcarebluebook.com

Healthfinder You can access patient assistance programs at this federal site. https://healthfinder.gov/rxdrug/

Migraine Research Foundation Located in New York City, you can find important information about this unusual kind of brain pain at http://www.migraineresearchfoundation.org

Hospital Compare For patients and healthcare professionals, this site rates the quality of care of over 4,000 hospitals. https://www.medicare.gov/hospitalcompare/search.html#

Human Rights Watch has a 99-page report on the negative social and health consequences of DEA and DOJ intrusions into the medical treatment of pain. It reports, too, on the trepidation–instilled by these government intruders–in physicians who dare to prescribe opioids for patients in pain. https://www.hrw.org

The International Association for the Study of Pain This professional organizaton brings together scientists, clinicians, health-care providers, and policymakers to stimulate and support the study of pain and translate that knowledge into improved pain relief worldwide. https://www.iasp-pain.org/

Lilly Cares Foundation This is Eli Lilly company's nonprofit which helps patients, who qualify, receive their prescription drugs for heart disease, diabetes, cancer, osteoporosis and psoriasis. http://www.lillycares.com/

The National Association of Free & Charitable Clinics These various clinics, available to low-income citizens, cover the gamut of health-care services – psychiatric, general medical, pharmacy, opththalmology, and dental. You'll also find, at their site, access to charities that offer to help, with companionship, safety checks, and meals, mobility-challenged elders and others needing similar help. https://www.nafcclinics.org/

National Headache Foundation Located in Chicago, Illinois, you can find information on all kinds of headaches at https://headaches.org/

National Institutes of Health - Chronic Pain site https://www.ninds.nih.gov/Disorders/All-Disorders/Chronic-Pain-Information-Page/2872/organizations/962

National Pain Report Visit this very informative site which provides up-to-date information on various imperative topics related to patients struggling to get treated appropriately for their pain. http://nationalpainreport.com

1-800-Charity Cars This charity helps a variety of people, with donated vehicles, including the medically needy. http://www.1-877-Charity.org

Pain Advocacy Coalition The Pain Advocacy Coalition is a grass-roots, patient-centric movement empowering patients and caregivers to successfully advocate through the use of collaborative tools, social media platforms and social media strategy....advocating to bring about social and healthcare policy reform impacting patients diagnosed with acute, chronic or intractable pain." This organization is determined to educate the public about pain issues being trampled on by government bureaucrats. And its members are hell-bent on changing the current malignant policies fostered by the ignorance of government functionaries and the reprehensible intrusions on the medical care of pain patients by DEA and DOJ police and prosecutors preventing normal opioid prescribing for patients in pain. https://painadvocacycoalition.com/

Pain and Pain Management This is **Pain Management Expert Forest Tennant, MD's website**. (See Chapter Twelve about Dr. Tennant's work and its disruption by the DOJ's DEA interference with his professional work.) If you're a patient with any level of pain, chronic, intractable or acute, this site is dedicated to you. It is sponsored by the Tennant Foundation, 334 S. Glendora Avenue, West Covina, California 91790-3043 http://foresttennant.com

Also, Dr. Tennant's work extends to the diagnosis arachnoiditis. Get help here http://www.arachnoiditishope.com Tennant Foundation, Dr. Forest Tennant's site, here, provides you with a FREE download of his Handbook for patients with intractable pain and those with adhesive arachnoiditis. It includes research studies and treatment information.

Pain Management This is a program at the Stanford Medicine Department of Anesthesiology, Perioperative and Pain Medicine. https://med.stanford.edu/anesthesia/education/fellowships/clinical-fellows/pain_management.html

Pain News Network Another very valuable site to catch up with all the latest in the, sorry to say, world of neverending pain. This will continue to be one of the many valuable resources for pain patients, their physicians and empathic legislators...until the DEA and DOJ can be ousted from practicing medicine, prescribing opioid dosages, and jailing innocent clinicians. https://painnewsnetwork.org

Partnership for Prescription Assistance Here you'll have access to free or low-cost prescription medications via 475 sources.. https://medicineassistancetool.org/

Practical Pain Management Their motto: Conquer Chronic Pain, Reclaim Your Life. Here is this site's shortlist of conditions they help you navigate and help you fight for your rights to effective pain care.

Cancer Carpal Tunnel Syndrome CRPS/RSD Diabetic Neuropathy Ehlers-Danlos Syndrome (EDS) Fibromyalgia Gout Amyloidosis Low Back Pain Lupus Lyme Disease Migraine and Headaches Neck Pain Osteoarthritis Osteoporosis Plantar Fasciitis Postherpetic Neuralgia Pelvic Pain Psoriatic Arthritis Rheumatoid Arthritis Sickle Cell Disease Thigh Pain Traumatic Brain Injuries TMJ Disorders https://www.practicalpainmanagement.com/

PubMed Scientific medical research studies and medical reports on vast and varied conditions and treatments. https://www.ncbi.nlm.nih.gov/pubmed

RateMDs Information about more than one million doctors and medical facilities are accessible here. https://www.ratemds.com/ny/forest-hills/

Surgeons Scorecard This site rates surgeons who perform common operations like hip and knee replacements and spinal fusions. https://projects.propublica.org/surgeons/

U.S. Pain Foundation This organization is "dedicated to serving the 50 million Americans who live with chronic pain through its free programs and services." It sponsors a wide variety of activities – that even many pain patients volunteer to help with – assuring public exposure of this EPIDEMIC OF UNTREATED PAIN, education of communities about this dire issue, and concerted efforts to get politicians and legislators involved in ousting the DEA and the DOJ from the medical care and prescribing for patients in pain. https://uspainfoundation.org/

Vitals This is a site to find physicians in various specialties. https://www.vitals.com/

WellRx With this discount program, you can get up to 45% discounts on brand and generic medications. https://www.wellrx.com/family-prescription-savings?gclid=EAIaIQobChMIyNiNz7ut1QIVTW1-Ch19uwx4EAAYASAAEgIQVvD_BwE

Additional Suggested Subjects to Google

American Cancer Society

Global Healthy Living Foundation

International Pain Foundation

Interstitial Cystitis Association

Mayday Pain Project

National Fibromyalgia Chronic Pain Association

National Patient Advocate Foundation

Pain Connection

PAINS

Reflex Sympathetic Dystrophy Syndrome Association

State Pain Policy Advocacy Network

The Foundation for Peripheral Neuropathy

The Pain Community

TMJ Association

Worldwide Headache Information Center

References

Ahn JS, Lin J, Ogawa S, et al. Transdermal buprenorphine and fentanyl patches in cancer pain: a network systematic review. J Pain Res. 2017;10:1963-1972.

American Academy of Pain Medicine. Minimum Insurance Benefits for Patients with Chronic Pain. Chicago, IL. Author; 2014

American Academy of Pain Medicine. Use of opioids for the treatment of chronic pain. February 2013. http://www.painmed.org/files/use-of-opioids-for-the-treatment-of-cronicpain.pdf

American Academy of Pain Medicine. Comments to the Centers for Disease Control and Prevention on the 2016 proposed guideline for prescribing opioids for chronic pain. January 2016. http://www.painmed.org/

American Board of Pain Medicine. American Board of Pain Medicine FAQs. Published 2018. http://www.abpm.org/faq

American Medical Association. AMA suggests changes to CDC policies on opioids. 2016. http://www.ama-assn.org/

American Medical Association. Combating the Opioid Abuse Epidemic: Professional and Academic Perspectives. Chicago, IL.: American Medical Association; 2015.

American Society of Regional Anesthesia and Pain. The specialty of chronic pain management. Published 2018. https://www.asra.com/page/44/the-specialty-of-chronic-pain-management/

Anie KA, Grocott H, White L, et al. Patient self-assessment of hospital pain, mood and health-related quality of life in adults with sickle cell disease. BMJ Open. 2012;(4):e001274.

Anson P. AMA: 'Inappropriate Use" of CDC Guideline. Pain News Network editor reports on American Medical Association's warning on the misuse of the guideline. Published November 14, 2018. https://www.painnewsnetwork.org/stories/2018/11/14/ama-calls-for-misapplication-of-cdc-opioid-guideline-to-end/

Anson P. Pain patients forced to go 'cold turkey' from hydrocodone. National Pain Report. November 2014. http://nationalpainreport.com/

Anson P. PROP [Physicians for Responsible Opioid Prescribing] helped draft the CDC opioid guidelines. Pain News Network. September 2015. http://painnewsnetwork.org/

Anson P. Should the CDC opioid guidelines be revised? Pain News Network. February 2019. http://painnewsnetwork.org/

Anthony M. Headache and the greater occipital nerve. Clin Neurol Neurosurg. 1992;94(4):297-301.

Armstrong D. OxyContin maker explored expansion into 'attractive' anti-addiction market. Medscape. January 31, 2019. http://medscape.com/

Aronoff GM. How did we get here? A past society president on the opioid crisis. Pain Med News. March 2014. http://www.painmedicinenews.com/

Artemiadis AK, Zis P. Neuropathic pain in acute and subacute neuropathies: a systematic review. Pain Physician. 2018;21(2):111-120.

Ataga KI, Kutlar A, Kanter J, et al. Crizanlizumab for the prevention of pain crises in sickle cell disease. N Engl J Med. 2017;376(5):429-439.

Atkinson TJ, Schatman ME, Fudin J. The damage done by the war on opioids: The pendulum has swung too far. J Pain Res 2014;7:265-8.

Bandewar SV. Access to controlled medicines for palliative care in India: pains and challenges. Indian J Med Ethics. 2015;12:77-82.

Bazazi AR, Zelenev A, Fu JJ, Yee I, Kamarulzaman A, Altice FL. High prevalence of non-fatal overdose among people who inject drugs in Malaysia: Correlates of overdose and implications for overdose prevention from a cross-sectional study. Int J Drug Policy. 2015;26:675-81.

Beal BR, Wallace MS. An Overview of Pharmacologic Management of Chronic Pain. Med Clin North Am. 2016;100(1):65-79.

Beck JG, Clapp JD. A different kind of co-morbidity: Understanding posttraumatic stress disorder and chronic pain. Psychol Trauma theory Res Pract Policy. 2011;3(2):101-108.

Bicket MC, Chakravarthy K, chang D, Cohen SP. Epidural steroid injections: an updated review on recent trends in safety and complications. Pain Mang. 2015;5(2):129-146.

Bicket MC, Mao J. Chronic Pain in Older Adults. Geriatr Anesth. 2015;33(3):577-590.

Bonnet CS, Walsh, DA. Osteoarthritis, angiogenesis and inflammation. Rheumatol Oxf Engl. 2005;44(1):7-16.

Bosco MA, Murphy JL, Clark ME. Chronic pain and traumatic brain injury in OEF/OIF service members and veterans. Headache. 2013;53(9):1518-1522.

Brandow AM, DeBaun MR. Key components of pain management for children and adults with sickle cell disease. Hematol Oncol Clin North Am. 2018;32(3):535-550.

Brandow AM, Zappia KJ, Stucky CL. Sickle cell disease: a natural model of acute and chronic pain. Pain. 2017;158 Suppl 1:S79-S84.

Broida RI, Gronowski T, Kalnow Af, Little AG, Lloyd CM. State emergency department opioid guidelines: current status. West J Emerg Med. 2017;18(3):340-344.

Brousseau DC, Owens PL, Mosso AL, Panepinto JA, Steiner CA. Acute care utilization and rehospitalization for sickle cell disease. JAMA. 2010;303(13):1288-1294.

Brousseau DC, Panepinto JA, Nimmer M, Hoffmann RG. The number of people with sickle-cell disease in the Unites States: national and state estimates. Am J Hematol. 2010;85(1):77-78.

Bruehl S. Complex regional pain syndrome. BMJ. 2015;351:h2730.

Bruera E. Parenteral opioid shortage - treating pain during the opioid-overdose epidemic. N Engl J Med. 2018;379(7)c601-603.

Burkill S, Montgomery S, Kockum I, Piehl F, Strid P, Hillert J, Alfredsson L, Olsson T, Shahram B. The Association Between Multiple Sclerosis and Pain Medications. Pain. 2019;160(2):424-432.

Busse JW, Juurlink D, Guyatt GH. Addressing the limitations of the CDC guideline for prescribing opioids for chronic noncancer pain. CMAJ Can Med Assoc J J Assoc medicale Can. 2016;188(17-18):1210-1211.

Carlson CL. Effectiveness of the World Health Organization cancer pain relief guidelines: an integrative review. J Pain Res. 2016;9:515-534.

Centers for Disease Control and Prevention. Fentanyl. Opioid Overdose. 2017. http://www.cdc.gov/drugoverdose/opioids/fentanyl.html

Centers for Disease Control and Prevention. Guideline for prescribing opioids for chronic pain. Washington DC:US Department of Health and Human Services; 2016.

Centers for Disease Control and Prevention. Injury Prevention and Control: Prescription Drug Overdose. Opioid Data Analysis. Atlanta, GA: Center for Disease Control and Prevention; 2016. http://www.cdc.gov/drugoverdose/data/analysis.html

Centers for Disease Control and Prevention. Rising numbers of deaths involving fentanyl and fentanyl analogs, including carfentanil, and increased usage and mixing with non-opioids. Published 2018. https://emergency.cdc.gov/han/HAN00413.asp

Chambers J, gleason RM, Kirsh KL, et al. An online survey of patients' experiences since the rescheduling of hydrocodone: The first 100 days. Pain Med 2016;17(9):1686-93.

C.heng J. Cryoanalgesia for refractory neuralgia. J Perioper Sci. 2015;2(2):1-7.

Chew M. Researchers, like politicians, use "spin" in presenting their results, conference hears. BMJ 2009;339:b3779.

Chou R, Clark E, Helfand M. Comparative efficacy and safety of long-acting oral opioids for chronic non-cancer pain: A systematic review. J Pain Symptom Manage. 2003;261026-1048.

Chou R, Deyo R, Devine B. The Effectiveness and Risks of Long-Term Opioid Treatment of Chronic Pain. Evidence Report/Technology assessment No. 218. AHRQ Publication No.14-E005-EF. Rockville, MD: Agency for Healthcare Research and Quality; 2014.

Chou R, Fanciullo GJ, Fine PG, et al. Clinical guidelines for the use of chronic opioid therapy in chronic noncancer pain. J Pain Off J Am Pain Soc. 2009;10(2):113-130.

Chou R, Gordon DB, deLeon-Casasola OA, et al. Management of Postoperative Pain: A Clinical Practice Guideline from the American Pain Society, the American Society of Regional Anesthesia and Pain Medicine, and the American Society of Anesthesiologists' Committee on Regional Anesthesia, Executive Committee, and Administrative Council. J Pain. 2016;17(2):131-157.

Chua NHL, Vissers KC, Sluijter ME. Pulsed radiofrequency treatment in itnerventional pain management: mechanisms and potential indications–a review. Acta Neurochir (Wien) 2011;153(4):753-771.

Ciccone TG, Kean N. Responses and criticisms over new CDC opioid prescribing guidelines. Pract Pain Manag 2016;16. http://www.practicalpainmanagement.com/resources/news-and-research/responses-criticisms-over-new-cdc-opioid-prescribing-guidelines/

Cole C, Jones I, McVeigh J, Kicman A, Syed Q, Bellis M. Adulterants in illicit drugs: a review of empirical evidence. Drug Testing Analysis. 2011;3:89-96.

Cooney MF. Postoperative Pain Management: Clinical Practice Guidelines. J Perianesth Nurs. 2016;31(5):445-451.

Cornelius R, Herr KA, Gordon DB, Kretzer K, Butcher HK. Evidence-Based Practice Guidelines: Acute Pain Management in Older Adults. J Gerontol Nurs. 2017;43(2):18-27.

Curatolo M. Regional anesthesia in pain management. Curr Opin Anaesthesiol. 2016;29(5):614-619.

CVS pharmacy expands naloxone access in 12 more states. Pharmacist. Sep 24, 2015. http://www.pharmacist.com/

Dahlhamer J, Lucas J, Zelaya C, et al. Prevalence of chronic pain and high-impact chronic pain among adults - United States, 2016. MMWR Morb Mortal Wkly Rep. 2018;67(36):1001-1006.

Dampier C, Palermo TM, Darbari DS, Hassell K, Smith W, Zempsky W. AAPT diagnostic criteria for chronic sickle cell disease pain. J Pain Off J Am Pain Soc. 2017;18(5):490-498.

Darbari DS, Ballas SK, Clauw DJ. Thinking beyond sickling to better understand pain in sickle cell disease. Eur J Haematol. 2014;93(2):89-95.

Davis CS, Carr D, Southwell JK, Beletsky L. Engaging law enforcement in overdose reversal initiatives: authorization and liability for naloxone administration. Am J Public Health 2015; 105:1530-7.

De la Rosa MB, Kozik EM, Sakaguchi DS. Adult Stem Cell-Based Strategies for Peripheral Nerve Regeneration. Adv Exp Med biol. August 2018.

Demidenko MI, Dobscha SK, Morasco BJ, et al. Suicidal ideation and suicidal self-directed violence following clinician-initiated prescription opioid discontinuation among long-term opioid users. Gen Hosp Psychiatry 2017;47:29-35.

Dong Y, Luo L, Hu Y, Fang K, Liu J. Clincial practice guidelines for the management of neuropathic pain: a systematic review. BMC Anesthesiol. 2016;16:12.

Dowell D, Haegerich TM, Chou R. CDC guideline for prescribing opioids for chronic pain–United States, 2016. MMWR Morb Mortal Wkly Rep 2016;65(1):1-52.

Doyon S, Benton C, Anderson BA, et al. Incorporation of poison center services in a state-wide overdose education and naloxone distribution program. Am J Addict. 2016;25(4):301-306.

Drug Enforcement Administration. 2015 National drug threat assessment summary. DEA-DCT-DIR-008-16; October 2015.

Drug Enforcement Administration. The DEA reduces amount of opioid controlled substances to be manufactured in 2017. 2016. https://www.dea.gov/

Dunn K, Saunders K, Rutter C, Banta-Green C, Merrill J, Sullivan M, et al. Opioid prescriptions for chronic pain and overdose: A cohort study. Ann Intern Med. 2010;152:85-92.

Elman I, Borsook D, Volkow ND. Pain and suicidality: Insights from reward and addiction neuroscience. Prog Neurobiol 2013;109:1-27.

Elmofty DH, Anitescu M, Buvanendran A. Best practices in the treatment of neuropathic pain. Pain Manag. 2013;3(6):475-483.

Erie County Opiate Epidemic Task Force. Erie County Community-Wide Guidelines: Acute Pain Management. Buffalo, NY: Erie County Department of Health; 2016. http://www2.erie.gov/health/sites/www2.erie.gov.health/files/uploads/pdfs/ECAcutePain MgmtGuidelines12062016.pdf

European Monitoring Centre on Drugs and Drug Addiction (EMCDDA). European drug report 2015: trends and development. Lisbon: 2015.

Fairbairn N, Coffin PO, Walley AY. Naloxone for heroin, prescription opioid, and illicitly made fentanyl overdoses: challenges and innovations responding to a dynamic epidemic. Int J Drug Policy. 2017;46:172-179.

Fishman MA, Kim PS. Buprenorphine for Chronic Pain: A Systematic Review. Curr Pain Headache Rep. 2018;22(12):83.

Fishman SM, Young HM, Lucas Arwood E, et al. Core competencies for pain management: results of an interprofessional consensus summit. Pain Med Malden Mass. 2013;14(7):971-981.

Fishman SM, Carr DB, Hogans B, et al. Scope and nature of pain- and analgesia-related content of the United States Medical Licensing Examination (USMLE). Pain Med Malden Mass. 2018;19(3):449-459.

Food and Drug Administration. Abuse-Deterrant Opioids - Evaluation and Labeling Guidance for Industry. Silver Spring MD: US Department of Health and Human Services; 2015.

Food and Drug Administration. Identifying the Root Causes of Drug Shortages and Finding Enduring Solutions; Public Meeting; Request for Comments. Fed Regist. 2018;83(175):45640-45642.

Food and Drug Administration. Key Facts about "Abuse-Deterrent" Opioids. Published 2016. https://blogs.fda.gov/fdavoice/index.php/2016/10/key-facts-about-abuse-deterrent-opioids/

Fredheim OM, Kaasa S, Fayers P, et al. Chronic non-malignant pain patients report as poor health-related quality of life as palliative cancer patients. Acta Anesthesiol Scand 2008;52(1):143-8.

Frieden TR, Houry D. Reducing the risks of relief–the CDC opioid-prescribing guideline. N Engl J Med 2016;374(16):1501-4.

Fudin J. Walgreens shirks pain patients. PainDr. August 2013. http://paindr.com/walgreens-shirks-pain-patients/ *

Fudin J, Atkinson TJ. Opioid prescribing levels off, but is less really more? Pain Med 2014; 15(2):184-7.

Fudin J, Cleary JP, Schatman MD. The MEDD myth: The impact of pseudoscience on pain research and prescribing-guideline development. J Pain Res 2016;9:153-6.*

Gallagher RM. Advancing the pain agenda in the veteran population. Anesthesiol Clin. 2016;34:357-378.

Gardner K, Douiri A, Drasar E. Survival in adults with sickle cell disease in a high-income setting. Blood. 2016;128(10):1436-1438.

Gatchel RJ, Okifuji A. Evidence-based scientific data documenting the treatment and cost-effectiveness of comprehensive pain programs for chronic nonmalignant pain. J Pain Off Am Pain Soc. 2006;7(11):779-793.

Genev IK, Tobin MK, Zaidi SP, Khan SR, Amirouche FML, Mehta AI. Spinal Compression Fracture Management: A Review of Current Treatment Strategies and Possible future Avenues. Glob Spine J. 2017;7(1):71-82.

G**ereau RW, Sluka KA, Maixner W, et al.** A pain research agenda for the 21st century. J Pain Off J Am Pain Soc. 2014;15(12):1203-1214.

Gladden RM, Martinez P, Seth P. Fentanyl law enforcement submissions and increases in synthetic opioid-involved overdose deaths–27 states, 2013-2014.MMWR Morb Mortal Wkly Rep 2016;65(33):837-43.

Global Commission on Drug Policy. The negative impact of drug control on public health: the global crisis of avoidable pain. Rio de Janeiro: 2015.

Goadsby PJ, Holland PR, Martins-Oliveira M, Hoffmann J, Schankin C, Akerman S. Pathophysiology of migraine: a disorder of sensory processing. Physiol Rev. 2017;97(2):553-622.

Gordon AL, Connolly SL. Treating pain in an established patient: sifting through the guidelines. RI Med J. 2017;100(10):41-44.

Gotbaum R. Pain patients say they can't get meds after illegal Rx drug crackdown. MedPage Today. August 2015. http://www.medpagetoday.com/search/? *

Grant M. Terminally ill cancer patients denied prescription drugs at pharmacy. February 2015. http://www.wesh.com/news/terminally-ill-cancer-patients-denied-prescription-drugs-the-pharmacy/

Green TC, Mann MR, BowmanSE, et al. How does use of a prescription monitoring program change medical practice? Pain Med Malden Mass. 2012;13(10):1314-1323.

Grover A. Report of the Special Rapporteur on the right of everyone to the enjoyment of the highest attainable standard of physical and mental health. 2010 Human Rights UN General Assembly, 65th Session. UN doc. A/65/255

Haddox JD. Opioids with abuse-deterrent properties: A regulatory and technological overview. J Opioid Manag. 2017;13(6):397-413.

Hall W, Carter A, Forlini C. The brain disease model of addiction: challenging or reinforcing stigma? Author's reply. Lancet Psychiatry. 2015;2:292.

Hassett AL, Aquino JK, Ilgen MA. The risk of suicide mortality in chronic pain patients. Curr Pain Headache Rep 2014;18(8):436-43.

Hayek SM, Deer TR, Pope JE, Panchal SJ, Patel VB. Intrathecal therapy for cancer and non-cancer pain. Pain Physician. 2011;14(3):219-248.

Health and Human Services (U.S. Dept. of) Interagency Pain Research Coordinating Committee. National pain strategy. 2016. http://iprac.nih.gov/National_Pain_Strategy/NPS_Main.htm

Hollingsworth H, Herndon C. The parenteral opioid shortage: causes and solutions. J Opioid Manag. 2018;14(2):81-82.

Hooten W, Timming R, Belgrade M, et al. Assessment and Management of Chronic Pain. Inst Clin syst Improv. November 2013:106.

Horgas AL. Pain Management in Older Adults. Nurs Clin North Am. 2017;52(4):e1-e7.

Hudson S, Wimsatt LA. How to monitor opioid use for your patients with chronic pain. Fam Pract Manag. 2014;21(6):6-11.

Huntoon L. The disaster of electronic health records. J Am Physicians surg. 2016;21(2):35-37. Institute of Medicine (U.S.) Committee on Advancing Pain Research Care and Education. Relieving Pain in America: A Blueprint for Transforming Prevention, Care, Education, and Research. Washington, DC: National Academies Press; 2011.

Institute for Safe Medication Practices. A shortage of everything except errors: harm associated with drug shortages. ISMP Medical Saf Alert. 2012;17:1-3.

Institute for Safe Medication Practices. Weathering the storm: managing the drug shortage crisis. ISMP Medical Saf Alert. 2010;15(20):1-4.

Inturrisi CE. Clinical pharmacology of opioids for pain. Clin J Pain. 2002;18:S3-S13.

Irvine JM, Hallvik SE, Hildebran C, Marino M, Beran T, Deyo RA. Who uses a prescription drug monitoring program and how? Insights from a statewide survey of Oregon clinicians. J Pain Off J Am Pain Soc. 2014;15(7):747-755.

Jackman RP, Purvis JM, Mallett BS. Chronic nonmalignant pain in primary care. Am Fam Physician 2008;78(10):1155-62. 1164.

Jamison RN, Scanlan E, Matthews ML, Jurck DC, Ross EL. Attitudes of primary care practitioners in managing chronic pain patients prescribed opioids for pain: A prospective longitudinal controlled trial. Pain Med 2016;17:99-113.

Jann M, Kennedy WK, Lopez G. Benzodiazepines and Opioids: a major component in unintentional prescription drug overdoses with opioid analgesics. J Pharm Pract. 2014;27(1):5-16.

Jawahar R, Oh U, Yang S, Lapane KL. A systematic review of pharmacological pain management in multiple sclerosis. Drugs. 2013;73(15):1711-1722.

Ji R-R, Xu Z-Z, Gao Y-J. Emerging targets in neuroinflammation-driven chronic pain. Nat Rev Drug discov 2014;13(7):13533-48.

Jones CM, Lurie PG, Throckmorton DC. Effect of US Drug Enforcement Administration's rescheduling of hydrocodone combination analgesic products on opioid analgesic prescribing. JAMA Intern Med 2016;176(3):399-402.

Joshi G, Gandhi K, Shah N, Gadsden J, Corman SL. Peripheral nerve blocks in the management of postoperative pain: challenges and opportunities. J Clin Anesth. 2016;35:524-529.

Kapur BM, Lala PK, Shaw JLV. Pharmacogenetics of chronic pain management. Clin Biochem. 2014;47(13-14):1159-1187.

Kato GJ, Piel FB, Reid CD, et al. Sickle cell disease. Nat Rev Dis Primer. 2018;4:18010.

Kerensky T, Walley AY. Opioid overdose prevention and naloxone rescue kits: what we know and what we don't know. Addict Sci Clin Pract. 2017;12(1):4.

Kishk NA, Gabr H, Hamdy S, et al. Case control series of intrathecal autologous bone marrow mesenchymal stem cell therapy for chronic spinal cord injury. Neurorehabil Neural Repair. 2010;24(8):702-708.

Kolodny A. Opioid Policy Research Collaborative (OPRC). Heller School. Brandeis University. (Accessed March 1, 2019) https://heller.brandeis.edu/opioid-policy-research-collaborative/

Kolodny A. Responding to the prescription opioid and heroin crisis: an epidemic of addiction. Opioid Policy Research Collaboration (OPRC). Slide Show. (Accessed March 2, 2019) https://heller.brandeis.edu/opioid-policy-research-collaborative/

Kozlov N, Benzon HT, Malik K. Epidural steroid injections: update on efficacy, safety, and newer medications for injection. Minerva Anestesiol. 2015;81(8):901-909.

Krebs EE, Becker WC, Zerzan J, Bair MJ, McCoy K, Hui S. Comparative mortality among Department of Veterans Affairs patients prescribed methadone or long-acting morphine for chronic pain. Pain. 2011;152:1789-1795.

Krebs EE, Gravely A, Nugent S, et al. Effect of Opioid vs Nonopioid Medications on Pain-Related Function in Patients with chronic Back Pain or Hip or Knee Osteoarthritis Pain: The SPACE Randomized Clinical Trial. JAMA. 2018;319(9):872-882.

Kuczynska K, Grzonkowski P, Kacprzak L, Zawilska JB. Abuse of fentanyl: An emerging problem to face. Forensic Sci Int. 2018;289:207-214.

Lanzkron S. Carroll CP, Haywood CJ. The burden of emergency department use for sickle-cell disease: an analysis of the national emergency department sample database. Am J Hematol. 2010;85(10):797-799.

Lanza FL, Chan FKL, Quigley EMM; The Practice Parameters Committee of the American College of Gastroenterology.

Guidelines for prevention of NSAID-related ulcer complications. Am Coll Gastroenterol 2009;104(3):728-38.

Larance B, Campbell G, Moore T, et al. Concerns and Help-Seeking Among Patients Using Opioids for Management of Chronic Noncancer Pain. Pain Med Malden Mass. 2018.

Law L, Derian A. Cryoanalgesia. In: StatPearls. Treasure Island (FL): StatPearls Publishing;2018. http://www.ncbi.nlm.nih.gov/books/NBK482123/

Lee JH, Kim DH, et al. Comparison of Clinical Efficacy of Epidural Injection with or without Steroid in Lumbosacral disc Herniation: A Systematic Review and Meta-abaktsus, Pain Physician. 2018;21(5):449-468.

Lewis CR, Vo HT, Fishman M. Intranasal naloxone and related strategies for opioid overdose intervention by nonmedical personnel: a review. Subst Abuse Rehabil. 2017;8:79-95.

Lin D, Jones C, ComptonW. Prescription drug coverage for treatment of low back pain among US Medicaid, Medicare Advantage, and commercial insurers. JAMA Netw Open. 2018;1(2).

Lintzeris N, Nielsen S. Benzodiazepines, methadone and buprenorphine; Interactions and clinical management. Am J Addictions. 2009;19:59-72.

Lynch ME. A review of the use of methadone for the treatment of chronic noncancer pain. Pain Res Manag. 2005;10:133-144.

Lundberg GD. The Sacklers meet El Chapo. Medscape. February 4, 2019. http://medscape.com/

Major JM, Zhou EH, Wong H-L, et al. Trends in rates of acetaminophen-related events in the United States. Pharmacoepidemiol Drug Saf. 2016;25(5):590-598.

Manchikanti L, Kaye AM, Knezevic NN, et al. Responsible, safe, and effective prescription of opioids for chronic non-cancer pain: American

Society of Interventional Pain Physicians (ASIPP)guidelines. Pain Physician 2017;20(2S):S3-S92.

Martin J, Cunliffe J, Decary-Hetu D, Aldridge J. Effect of restricting the legal supply of prescription opioids on buying through online illicit marketplaces: interrupted time series analysis. BMJ. 2018;361:k2270.

Matthie N, Ross D, Sinha C, Khemani K, Bakshi N, Krishnamurti L. A qualitative study of chronic pain and self-management in adults with sickle cell disease. J Natl Med Assoc. September 2018.

McAllister MW, Aaronson P, Spillane J, et al. Impact of prescription drug monitoring program on controlled substance prescribing in the ED. Am J emerg Med. 2015;33(6):781-785.

McCance-Katz E, Sullivan LS, Nallani S. Drug interactions of clinical importance among the opioids, methadone and buprenorphine, and other frequently prescribed medications: A review. Am J Addictions. 2009;19:4-16.

McIntosh G, Hall H. Low back pain (acute). BMJ Clin Evid. 2011, https://www.ncbi.nlm.nih.gov/pmc/articles/PMC3217769/

Metzack R. The tragedy of needless pain. Sci am 1990;262(2):27-33.

Moore PQ, Weber J, Cina S, Aks S. Syndrome surveillance of fentanyl-laced heroin outbreaks: Utilization of EMS, Medical Examiner and Poison Center databases. Am J Emerg Med. 2017;35(11):1705-1708.

Mounteney J, Giraudon I, Denissov G, Griffiths P. Fentanyl: Are we missing the signs? Highly potent and on the rise in Europe. Int J Drug Policy. 2015;26:626 -31.

Nadeau SE. Opioids for chronic noncancer pain. To prescribe or not to prescribe–what is the question? Neurology 2015;85(7):646-51.

National Academies. Pain management and the opioid epidemic: balancing societal and individual benefits and risks of prescription opioid use. Washington DC: National Academies of Sciences, Engineering, and Medicine; 2017.

National Alliance for Model State Drug Laws. Prescription Drug Monitoring Programs. 2018. http://www.namsdI.org/prescription-monitoring-programs.cfm

National Institute on Drug Abuse. Benzodiazepines and Opioids. Drugs of Abuse. March 2018. https://www.drugabuse.gov/drugs-abuse/opioids/benzodiazepines-opioids/

National Institutes of Health. Division of Blood Diseases and Resources. The management of sickle cell disease. NIH publication no. 02-2117, 4th ed. June 2002.

National Spine & Pain Centers. Joint Injection Facts & Information. Published 2018. https://treatingpain.com/treatment/joint-injections

Ngo SCA, Bartolucci P, Lobo D, et al. Causes of death in sickle cell disease adult patients: old and new trends. Blood. 2014;124:2715.

Nelson LS, Juurlink DN, Perrone J. Addressing the Opioid Epidemic. JAMA. 2015;314(14):1453-1454.

Network for Public Health Law. Legal interventions to reduce overdose mortality: naloxone access and overdose Good Samaritan laws. St Paul, MN (USA): 2015.

Nicholson B. Benefits of extended-release opioid analgesic formulations in the treatment of chronic pain. Pain Pract 2009;9(1):71-81.

North RB, Kidd DH, Farrokhi F, Piantadose SA. Spinal cord stimulation versus repeated lumbosacral spine surgery for chronic pain: a randomized, controlled trial. Neurosurgery. 2005;56(1):98-106.

O'Brien T, Christrup LL, Drewes AM, et al. European Pain Federation position paper on appropriate opioid use in chronic pain management. Eur J Pain 2017; 21:3-19.

O'Connor AB. Neuropathic pain: Quality-of-life impact, costs and cost effectiveness therapy. Pharmacoeconomics 2009;27(2):95-112.

Ohio Academy of Family Physicians. Opioid Prescribing Guidelines - Ohio Academy of Family Physicians. 2017. https://www.ohioafp.org/public-policy/state-legislative-regulatory-issues/opioid-prescribing-guidelines/

Okomo U, Meremikwu MM. Fluid replacement therapy for acute episodes of pain in people with sickle cell disease. Cochrane Database Syst Rev. 2017;(7):CD005406.

Open Society Foundatioon. Stopping overdose: peer-based distribution of naloxone. New York:2013.

Paice JA, Portenoy R, Lacchetti C, et al. Management of Chronic Pain in Survivors of Adult Cancers: American Society of Clinical Oncology clinical Practice Guideline. J clin Oncol Off J Am Soc Clin Oncol. 2016;34(27):3325-3345.

Pain and Policy Studies Group. Achieving balance in state pain policy: A progress report card (CY 2013). University of Wisconsin Carbone Cancer Center; Madison, Wisconsin: 2014.

Park CJ, Shin YD, Lim SW, Bae YM. The effect of facet joint injection on lumbar spinal stenosis with radiculopathy. Pak J med Sci. 2018;34(4):968-973.

Passik SD. Issues in long-term opioid therapy: Unmet needs, risks, and solutions. Mayo Clin Proc 2009;84(7):593-601.

Payne FL. An integrated approach to undertreatment of pain; In: Worley SL. New directions in the treatment of chronic pain. National Pain Strategy will guide prevention, management and research. P T 2016;41:107-15.

Pearlstein M. Taking aim at America's opioid crisis. Heller magazine. Brandeis University. May 26,2017. [relative to Dr. Kolodny's assertions]

Peh W. Image-guided facet joint injection. Biomed Imaging Interv J. 2011;7(1).

Peng PWH, Narouze S. Ultrasound-guided interventional procedures in pain medicine: a review of anatomy, sonoanatomy, and procedures: part I: nonaxial structures. Reg Anesth Pain Med. 2009;34(5):458-474.

Peng PWH, Tumber PS. Ultrasound-guided interventional procedures for patients with chronic pelvic pain - a description of techniques and review of literature. Pain Physician. 2008;1192):215-224.

Pergolizzi J, Pappagallo M, Stauffer J, et al. The role of urine drug testing for patients on opioid therapy. Pain Pract Off J World Inst Pain. 2010;10(6):497-507.

Petrosky E, Harpaz R, Fowler KA, et al. Chronic pain among suicide decedents, 2003 to 2014: findings from the National Violent Death Reporting System. Ann Int Med. September 2018.

Pincher MH, Von Korff M, Bushnell MC, Porter L. Prevalence and Profile of High-Impact Chronic Pain in the United States. J Pain Off J Am Pain Soc. August 2018.

Platt OS, Thorington BD, Brambilla DJ, et al. Pain in sickle cell disease. Rates and risk factors. N Engl J Med. 1991;325(1):11-16.

Pollack AB, Tegeler ML, Morgan V, Baumrucker SJ. Morphine to methadone conversion: An interpretation of published data. Am J Hosp Palliat Care. 2011;28:135-140.

Polomeni P, Schwan R. Management of opioid addiction with buprenorphine: French history and current management. Int J Gen Med. 2014;7:143-8.

Practical Pain Management. Suicide and suffering in the elderly: We must do better. Pract Pain Manag 2012;12:6. http://www.practicalpain-management.com/pain/

President's Commission on Combating Drug Addiction and the Opioid Crisis. Draft of the Final Report. Washington, DC: 2017. https://www.whitehouse.gov/ondep/presidents-commission/

President's Commission on Combating Drug Addiction and the Opioid Crisis. Interim Report. Published July 31, 2017. https://www.whitehouse.gov/sites/whitehouse.gov/files/ondep/commission-interim-report.pdf

Qaseem A, Wilt TJ, McLean RM, Forciea MA. Clinical Guidelines Committee of the American College of Physicians. Noninvasive Treatments for Acute, Subacute, and Chronic Low Back Pain: A clinical Practice Guideline from the American College of Physicians. Ann Intern Med. 2017;166(7):514-530.

Radnovich R, Scott D, Patel AT, et al. Cryoneurolysis to treat the pain and symptoms of knee osteoarthritis: a multicenter, randomized, double-blind, sham-controlled trial. Osteoarthritis Cartilage. 2017;25(8):1247-1256.

Radomski TR, Bixler FR, Zickmund SL, et al. Physicians Perspectives Regarding Prescription Drug Monitoring Program Use within the Department of Veterans Affairs: a Multi-State Qualitative Study. J Gen Inter Med. 2018;33(8):1253-1259.

Reddy S, Patt RB. The benzodiazepines as adjuvant analgesics. J Pain Symptom Manage. 1994;9(8):510-514.

Rees DC, Olujohungbe AD, Parker NE, et al. Guidelines for the management of the acute painful crisis in sickle cell disease. Br J Haematol. 2003;120(5:744-752.

Renton T. Dental (Odontogenic) Pain. Rev Pain. 2011;5(1):2-7.

Reuben DB, Alvanzo AAH, Ashikaga, R, et al. National Institutes of Health Pathways to Prevention Workshop: the role of opioids in the treatment of chronic pain. Ann Int Med. 2015;162(4):295-300.

Rigaud J, Delavierre D, Sibert L, Labat J-J. Sympathetic nerve block in the management of chronic pelvic and perineal pain. Progres En Urol J Assoc Francaise Urol Soc Francaise Urol. 2010;20(12):1124-1131.

Rosenberg JM, Bilka bM, Wilson SM, Spevak C. Opioid Therapy for chronic Pain: Overview of the 2017 U.S. Department of Veterans Affairs and U.S. Department of Defense Clinical Practice Guideline. Pain Med Malden Mass. 2018;19(5):928-941.

Rowbotham MC, Twilling L, Davies PS, et al. Oral opioid therapy for chronic peripheral and central neuropathic pain. N Eng J Med 2003;348(13):1223-32.

Rudd RA, Aleshire N, Zibbell JE, Gladden RM. Increases in drug and opioid overdose deaths–United States, 2000-2014. Am J Transplant 2016;16(4):1323-7.

Salwan AJ, Hagemeier NE, Harirforoosh S. Abuse-Deterrent Opioid Formulations: A Key Ingredient in the Recipe to Prevent Opioid Disasters? Clin Drug Investig. 2018;38(7):573-577.

Samp RA, Chenoweth MS. Letter to Tom Frieden and Debra Houry re: Guideline for prescribing opioids for chronic pain. Washington Legal Foundation. November 2015. http://www.wlf.org/

Schatman ME. The American chronic pain crisis and the media: About time to get it right? J Pain Res 2015;8:885-7.

Seers T, Derry S, Seers K, Moore RA. Professionals underestimate patients' pain: a comprehensive review. Pain. 2018;159(5):811-818.

Serafini M. The Physicians' Quandary with Opioids: Chronic Pain vs. Addiction. NEJM Catalyst. Published April 26, 2018. https://catalyst.nejm.org/quandary-opioids-chronic-pain-addiction/

Shaiova L, Berger A, Blinderman CD, Bruera E, et al. Consensus guideline on parenteral methadone use in pain and palliative care. Palliat Support Care. 2008;6:165-176.

Shim E, Lee JW, Lee E, et al. Facet joint injection versus epidural steroid injection for lumbar spinal stenosis: intra-individual study. Clin Radiol. 2017;72(1):96.e7-96.e14.

Sinatra R. Causes and consequences of inadequate management of acute pain. Pain Med Malden Mass. 2010;11(12):1859-1871.

Smith TJ, Staats PS, Deer T, et al. Randomized clinical trial of an implantable drug delivery system compared with comprehensive medical management for refractory cancer pain: impact on pain, drug-related toxicty, and survival. J Clin Oncol Off J Am Soc Clin Oncol. 2002;20(19):4040-4049.

Smith WR, Penberthy LT, Bovbjerg VE, et al. Daily assessment of pain in adults with sickle cell disease. Ann Intern Med. 2008;148(2):94-101.

Soin A, Cheng J, Brown L, Moufawad S, Mekhail N. Functional outcomes in patients with chronic nonmalignant pain on long-term opioid therapy. Pain Pract Off J World Inst Pain. 2008;8(5):379-384.

Staats P, Wallace M. Just the Facts. Pain Medicine. 2nd ed. New York, NY: McGraw-Hill;2015

Starrels JL, Wu B, Peyser D, et al. It made my life a little easier: primary care providers' beliefs and attitudes about using opioid treatment agreements. J Opioid Manag. 2014;10(2):95-102.

Substance Abuse and Mental Health Services Administration, Office of the Surgeon General. Facing Addiction in America: The Surgeon General's Report on Alcohol, Drugs, and Health. Washington, DC: US Department of Health and Human Services; 2016. http://www.ncbi.nlm.nih.gov/books/NBK424857/

Sun E, Dixit A, Humphreys K, Darnall B, Baker L, Mackey S. Association between concurrent use of prescription opioids and benzodiazepines and overdose: retrospective analysis. BMJ. 2017;356:j760.

Suri P, Saunders KW, von Korff M. Prevalence and characteristics of flare-ups of chronic non-specific back pain in primary care: a telephone survey. Clin J Pain. 2012;28(7):573-580.

Szalavitz M. Why are patients shut out of the debate over prescription pain medicine? The Washington Post. March 2014. http://www.washingtonpost.com/news/the-watch/wp2014/06 *

Tait RC, Chibnall JT, House K, Biehl J. Medical judgments across the range of reported pain severity: Clinician and lay perspectives. Pain Med 2016;17(7):1269-81.

Tighe P, Buckenmaier CC, Boezaart AP, et al. Acute Pain Medicine in the United States: A Status Report. Pain Med Malden Mass. 2015;16(9):1806-1826

Tobin DG, Andrews R, Becker WC. Prescribing opioids in primary care: Safely starting, monitoring, and stopping. Cleve Clin J Med. 2015;83(3):207-215.

Todd KH. A Review of Current and Emerging Approaches to Pain Management in the Emergency Department. Pain Ther. 2017;6(2):193-202.

Torrance N, Elliott AM, Lee AJ, Smith BH. Severe chronic pain is associated with increased 10 year mortality. A cohort record linkage study. Eur J Pain 2010;14(4):380-6.

Trescot AM, Datta S, Lee M, Hansen H. Opioid pharmacology. Pain Physician. 2008;11(2 Suppl):S133–153.

Turk DC, Wilson HD, Cahana A. Treatment of chronic non-cancer pain. Lancet Lond Engl. 2011;377(9784):2226-2235.

U.S. Department of Health and Human Services. 5-point strategy to combat the opioid crisis. HHS.gov/opioids. https://www.hhs.gov/opioids/about-the-epidemic/hhs-response/index.html Published August 7, 2018.

U.S. Department of Health and Human Services. National Pain Strategy. Washington, DC; 2016. https://iprcc.nih.gov/sites/default/files/HHSNational_Pain_Strategy_508C.pdf

U.S. Department of Veterans Affairs, U.S. Department of Defense. Management of opioid therapy (OT) for chronic pain (2017) - VA/DoD Clinical Practice Guidelines; 2017.

Vallerand AH, Cosler P, Henningfield JE, Galassini P. Pain management strategies and lessons from the military: a narrative review. Pain Res Manag. 2015;20(5):261-268.

Vallerand A, Nowak L. Chronic opioid therapy for nonmalignant pain: the patient's perspective. Part II-Barriers to chronic opioid therapy. Pain Manag Nurs Off J Am Soc Pain Manag Nurses. 2010;11(2):126-131.

Vanderhave KL, Perkins CA, Scannell B, Brighton BK. Orthopedic manifestations of sickle cell disease. J Am Acad Orthop Surg. 2018;26(3):94-101.

VOCAL-NY Users Union. Beyond methadone: improving health and empowering patients in opioid treatment programs. New York: 2015.

Walker FO, Cartwright MS, Wiesler ER, Caress J. Ultrasound of nerve and muscle. Clin Neurophysiol Off J Int Fed Clin Neurophysiol. 2004;115(3):495-507.

Wallwork RS, Cipidza FE, Stern TA. Obstacles to the prescription and use of opioids. Prim Care Companion CNS Disord 2016;18(1):10.4088/PCC.15f01900.

Warner M, Trinidad JP, Bastian BA, Minino AM, Hedegaard H. Drugs Most Frequently Involved in Drug Overdose Deaths: United States, 2010-2014. Nat Vital Stat Rep Cent Dis Control Prev Natl Cent Health Stat Natl Vital Stat Syst. 2016;65(10):1-15.

Watson CPN. Opioids in chronic noncancer pain: More faces from the crowd. Pain Res Manag 2012;17(4):263-75.

Webster L. The pain epidemic versus the opioid crisis; in Worley SL. New directions in the treatment of chronic pain. National pain strategy will guide prevention, management, and research. PT 2016;41:107-15.

Webster LR. Risk factors for opioid-use disorder and overdose. Anesth Analg. 2017;125(5):1741-1748.

Webster LR. Pain and suicide: The other side of the opioid story. Pain Med 2014;15(3):345-6.*

Weiner SS, Nordin M. Prevention and management of chronic back pain. Best Pract Res Clin Rheumatol. 2010;24(2):267-279.

Wong CSM, Wong SHS. A New Look at Trigger Point Injections. Anesthesiol Res Pract. 2012;2012.

Woolf SH, Grol R, Hutchinson A, Eccles M, Grimshaw J. Potential benefits, limitations and harms of clinical guidelines. BMJ 1999;318(7182):527-30.

World Health Organization. Ensuring Balance in National Policies on Controlled Substances: Guidance for Availability and Accessibilty of Controlled Medicines. Geneva: World Health Organization, Dept. Of Essential Medicines and Pharmaceutical Policies, 2011.

World Health Organization. Community management of opioid overdose. Geneva:2014.

Ziegler SJ. Patient abandonment in the name of opioid safety. Pain Med 2013;14(3):323-4.*

About Dr. Helen Borel

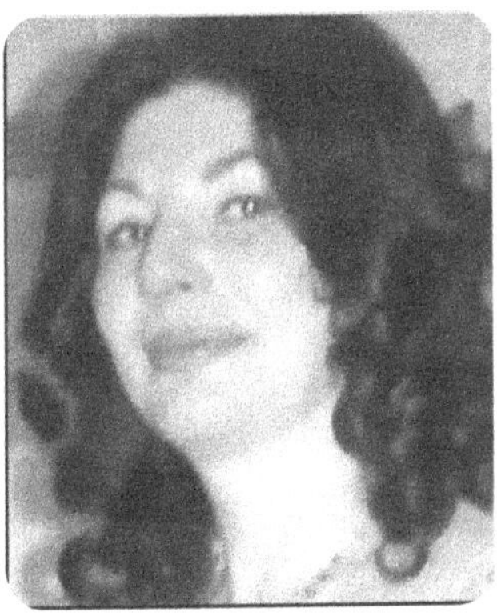

Dr. Helen Borel spent her childhood until age 17 writing poetry and playing piano as she grew up in two orphanages. She became a registered nurse, then earned a master's degree in creative writing. And, after 18 years as a medical, psychiatric and pharmaceutical copywriter on "Medicine Avenue," she published books, literary criticism, satire and short fiction. Later, she became a doctor in psychoanalytic studies with her own website, PsychDocNYC.com. From a creative heritage, third cousin of playwright Arthur Miller, she's proud of her talented son Jonathan, his wife Andrea, and her grandboy, Sean James – all having been actors.

Recently, after publishing *The Hippo Campus*, her playful pictorial-tutorial for children about the brain, she was heartbroken to learn of millions suffering and hundreds suiciding because their opioids were no longer prescribed due to federal interference in physicians' paincare. Always outspoken for the underdog, her intense research is the basis for her passionate exposê of government wrongs and the legal rights pain victims must assert.

Fresh Ink Group

Publishing
Free Memberships
Share & Read Free Stories, Essays, Articles
Free-Story Newsletter
Writing Contests

Books
E-books
Amazon Bookstore

Authors
Editors
Artists
Professionals
Publishing Services
Publisher Resources

Members' Websites
Members' Blogs
Social Media

Twitter: @FreshInkGroup
Google+: Fresh Ink Group
Facebook.com/FreshInkGroup
LinkedIn: Fresh Ink Group
About.me/FreshInkGroup
FreshInkGroup.com

Fresh Ink Group

www.ingramcontent.com/pod-product-compliance
Lightning Source LLC
Chambersburg PA
CBHW060959280326
41935CB00009B/758
9781947867680